Supporting the Caregiver in Dementia

Supporting the Caregiver in Dementia

A Guide for Health Care Professionals

Edited by

SHEILA M. LOBOPRABHU, M.D.

VICTOR A. MOLINARI, PH.D.

JAMES W. LOMAX, M.D.

The Johns Hopkins University Press

Baltimore

2 4 6 8 9 7 5 3 1

The Johns Hopkins University Press
2715 North Charles Street
Baltimore, Maryland 21218-4363
www.press.jhu.edu

Library of Congress Cataloging-in-Publication Data
Supporting the caregiver in dementia : a guide for health care professionals / edited by
Sheila M. LoboPrabhu, Victor A. Molinari, and James W. Lomax.
p. ; cm.
Includes bibliographical references and index.
ISBN 0-8018-8343-1 (hardcover : alk. paper)
1. Dementia—Patients—Care. 2. Caregivers—Mental health. I. LoboPrabhu,
Sheila M., 1969– . II. Molinari, Victor, 1952– . III. Lomax, James W., 1944– .
[DNLM: 1. Dementia—nursing. 2. Caregivers—psychology.
3. Patient Care. WM 220 S959 2006]
RC521.S87 2006
362.196'83—dc22   2005027389

A catalog record for this book is available from the British Library.

Contents

Preface

Read, sweet how others strove,

Till we are stouter;

What they renounced,

Till we are less afraid;

How many times they bore

The faithful witness,

Till we are helped,

As if a kingdom cared!

—*Emily Dickinson*

Dementia is one of the greatest challenges facing seniors all over the world. Hopes for a leisurely retirement and fulfilling old age are wrecked by the devastation of this disorder. Alzheimer disease and other dementias cost the health care system billions of dollars, while severely undermining the quality of life for whole families. Because of the loss of skills and resulting disability experienced by the person with dementia, families sacrifice to maintain the person in the community; at later stages they maintain their strong ties even as more formal caregiving shifts to institutional settings. Emily Dickinson, the famous poet, uses the words "faithful witness"—words that may represent the family members of the patient, who experience the pains, losses, and joys of caregiving. As with bereavement and mourning, it is only in sharing the experience with others that we derive the ability to bear suffering with a sense of meaning.

There was little systematic research into caregiving until the late 1970s and early 1980s, when Steven Zarit, Robert Kahn, Marjorie Lowenthal, and others pioneered the field by defining the concept, identifying it as a topic worthy of scientific interest, and promoting it as an important area for federal research funding. When the idea of a volume on caregiving was first suggested to us by the editors at the Johns Hopkins University Press, we saw an opportunity to better explore the experience of caregiving in dementia. We wanted to write a text for health care professionals, summarizing the current research in the field and demonstrating how this research could be translated into state-of-the-art clinical practice. Our approach has been that of a multidisciplinary team in a geriatric setting examining the situation from varying clinical perspectives and thereby providing a multidimensional framework of care for both the patient and the caregiver. Pluralism requires an integration of ideas from a diversity of sources. We propose such an approach to the caregiver–care recipient dyad in the health care setting and, by extension, to the training of mental health professionals from varied disciplinary backgrounds. We should pay attention to a wide variety of medical, social, environmental, and psychological factors affecting their health and well-being and integrate these findings into a coherent multidisciplinary treatment plan.

The chapter topics were determined by the editors as ones that have immediate practical salience for mental health professionals "in the trenches." The chapters are grouped from more "micro" to more "macro" levels of analysis. They transition from topics that are relevant to the caregiver as an individual, proceeding to the interpersonal aspects of caregiving, then turning attention to how the mental health professional team collaborates with the caregiver and care recipient to address common caregiving problems, and ending with aspects of overarching societal issues that the United States will continue to struggle with for years to come. The guiding principle for this volume has been to cover issues of relevance to the mental health clinician, so that reading of this material will have immediate pragmatic translatability into optimal professional practice. Although the focus is on older adults with dementia, the research findings are also readily applicable to a significant number of family members managing the care of individuals with early-onset dementia.

Addressing the needs of mental health professionals from multiple disciplines for guidance on this far-ranging subject requires a special ensemble of authors. Schultz and Patterson note in their introduction to a special issue of the *American Journal of Geriatric Psychiatry* devoted entirely to caregiving (12:234–37, 2004) that there are more than 150,000 references to caregiving on the worldwide web, and that nearly 2,000 articles have been published on this topic. The selection of authors stemmed from our belief that the time was ripe to gather a cadre of experienced scientist-practitioners who could draw on clinical wisdom informed by this voluminous research to help guide the practice of generalist mental health professionals. Therefore, literature reviews for the chapters are written as broad overviews and forums intended to make possible a translation of this knowledge into practical treatment guidelines with obvious training implications.

We needed a blend of scholar and practitioner: scientists well trained in the methodology of geriatric research to condense clinical pearls from the published literature; clinicians with years of experience working in the "front lines" with older adults to ensure relevance; and educators with a keen interest in geriatric mental health training to provide easy translation from written word to practice. We also wanted to showcase a variety of disciplinary perspectives across diverse health care settings. Clinical psychology, counseling psychology, developmental psychology, psychiatry, psychoanalysis, nursing, social work, and public health are represented. Chapter authors have provided clinical services in medical center, veterans hospital, outpatient, inpatient, primary care, long-term care, and community settings. In the course of their careers, contributors have been challenged to assimilate the latest research to direct "best practices" training for both students and nongeriatrician mental health professionals, who with increasing frequency in the normal course of their work will be confronted with caregiving issues.

There are five parts to this book. Part I explores the history of caregiving, defines formal and informal caregiving, discusses early assessment and intervention studies, and discusses current research directions in the field.

Part II focuses on individual caregivers of persons with dementia: who they are, what their problems are, and how they become caregivers. In this part, we describe the demographics of caregivers and care recipients, the tasks caregivers perform, and the economic outcomes of caregiving. We provide an overview of the literature on caregiver burden and caregiver resiliency. An overarching transtheoretical model is used as a framework to understand decisions leading to placement in various settings.

Part III examines caregiving from an interpersonal context. The affective bond between individuals and its role in caregiving is discussed. We review the literature on attachment with respect to the disruption and repair of the interpersonal bond between patient and family members in family caregiving. We proffer a spiritual perspective within a psychodynamic framework to explain joy in caregiving as resulting from creative illusion formation, analogous to the comfort and peace derived from religion. Caregiving is also considered from a sexual perspective, with a discussion of how intimacy and sexuality are affected in dementia. Grief and loss are discussed with respect to the "living death" in dementia.

Part IV draws clinical implications from the research on the individual and interpersonal aspects of caregiving. A biopsychosocial model is outlined addressing the mental health needs of the patient with dementia and the caregiver across formal and informal settings. Pharmacological options are explored for the care of the patient with behavioral disturbance. Psychotherapy, family therapy, and social supports are discussed as they apply to the care of a person with dementia in clinical and home settings.

Part V addresses overarching social concerns. Diversity issues, the legal and health care environment, and current delivery system for dementia care are investigated. Various health policies and their impact on caregiving in the United States today are explored, followed by a discussion of the ethical dilemmas often faced by caregivers and of strategies to guide ethical decision making.

We recognize some limitations to the organization of this volume. A multidisciplinary team approach may have imperfect applicability in some practice contexts (e.g., private practice or consultation psychiatry). In such settings, we recommend that the health care professional primarily in charge of care consider using this volume as an educational tool for appropriately identifying, reaching out, and making referrals to staff of other disciplines in the care of persons with dementia. Activities such as music therapy, occupational therapy, art therapy, and spiritual counseling can be of value to the patient's emotional well-being and quality of life, but these have not been discussed in detail. Such therapies may also have beneficial effects for the caregiver by supplying an emotional outlet and release, as well as providing an opportunity for the caregiver to participate in the patient's efforts to remain productive and creative. In the absence of the availability of these modalities, the individual clinician should at least be aware of a variety of biological, social, psychological, and spiritual frameworks in order to gain a multifaceted picture of the patient and caregiver. Paying attention to all such aspects helps in the appreciation of the patient and caregiver as unique individuals. All patient visits can therefore be used therapeutically to address the changing spectrum of needs in a flexible manner, allowing the clinician to remain alert to changes along each particular dimension as dementia progresses. We could not cover every issue in caregiving, and we devote limited attention to some new developing areas, such as caregiving for those with mild cognitive impairment, for which there remains a restricted knowledge base. But we do attempt to summarize key scientific findings in the most important and practitioner-relevant areas and to use case examples to illustrate how research can be used to plan care in various clinical settings. Before the conclusion, each chapter contains a section summarizing clinical implications of the presented material.

Acknowledgment is due to our wonderful chapter authors, who have been unstinting in giving of their time and expertise to make this volume a success. We were greatly helped by the support staff of the Mental Health Care Line at the Michael E. DeBakey Department of Veterans Affairs Medical Center, the Department of Aging and Mental Health of the Florida Mental Health Institute at the University of South Florida, and the Baylor College of Medicine. This material is the result of work supported with resources and the use of facilities at the Michael E. DeBakey Department of Veterans Affairs Medical Center and the University of South Florida. We are indebted to Wendy Harris and Sarah Shepke, editors at the Johns Hopkins University Press, for their sage editorial advice. All these contributions have been tremendously valuable, as have the experiences with the courage and resilience of the family members of our patients with dementia, to whom we dedicate this book.

Contributors

F. M. Baker, M.D., M.P.H., professor, Department of Psychiatry, University of Maryland School of Medicine, and medical director, Lower Shore Clinic, Salisbury, Maryland

David A. Chiriboga, Ph.D., professor, Department of Aging and Mental Health, Florida Mental Health Institute, University of South Florida, Tampa, Florida

Irving Hellman, Ph.D., assistant clinical professor, Department of Psychiatry, University of California, Davis

Michele J. Karel, Ph.D., staff psychologist, Veterans Affairs Boston Healthcare System, and assistant professor, Department of Psychiatry, Harvard Medical School, Boston, Massachusetts

Deborah King, Ph.D., associate professor and director of training in clinical psychology, director of Geriatric Psychiatry Services, and clinical director of psychology, Department of Psychiatry, University of Rochester Medical Center, Rochester, New York

Mark E. Kunik, M.D., M.P.H., associate director, Houston Center for Quality of Care and Utilization Studies of the Health Services Research and Development Service, Michael E. DeBakey Department of Veterans Affairs Medical Center; core investigator at the Veterans Affairs South Central Mental Illness Research, Education, and Clinical Center; and assistant professor, Menninger Department of Psychiatry and Behavioral Sciences, Baylor College of Medicine, Houston, Texas

Sheila M. LoboPrabhu, M.D., staff psychiatrist, Michael E. DeBakey Department of Veterans Affairs Medical Center; affiliate investigator at the Veterans Affairs South Central Mental Illness Research, Education, and Clinical Center; and assistant professor, Menninger Department of Psychiatry and Behavioral Sciences, Baylor College of Medicine, Houston, Texas

James W. Lomax, M.D., professor and Karl Menninger Chair for Psychiatric Education, and associate chairman and director of educational programs,

Menninger Department of Psychiatry and Behavioral Sciences, Baylor College of Medicine, Houston, Texas

Melissa Martinez, M.D., psychiatry resident, Menninger Department of Psychiatry and Behavioral Sciences, Baylor College of Medicine, Houston, Texas

Victor A. Molinari, Ph.D., professor, Department of Aging and Mental Health, Louis de la Parte Florida Mental Health Institute, University of South Florida, Tampa

Jennifer Moye, Ph.D., director, Geriatric Mental Health, Brockton VA Medical Center, and assistant professor, Department of Psychiatry, Harvard Medical School, Boston, Massachusetts

Naomi D. Nelson, Ph.D., co-associate director of education, Parkinson's Disease Research, Education and Clinical Center, Michael E. DeBakey Department of Veterans Affairs Medical Center, and assistant professor and psychologist, Baylor College of Medicine, Houston, Texas

Margaret P. Norris, Ph.D., private practice, College Station, Texas

Hana Osman, Ph.D., M.S.S.W., assistant professor, Department of Community and Family Health, College of Public Health, University of South Florida, Tampa

Sharon K. Ostwald, Ph.D., R.N., professor and Isla Carroll Turner Chair in Gerontological Nursing and director, Center on Aging, University of Texas Health Science Center, Houston

Martin Pinquart, Dr.Phil.Habil., associate professor, Department of Developmental Psychology, University of Jena, Germany

Silvia Sörensen, Ph.D., senior instructor, Program in Geriatrics and Neuropsychiatry, Department of Psychiatry, University of Rochester Medical School, Rochester, New York

Steven H. Zarit, Ph.D., professor and head, Department of Human Development and Family Studies, Pennsylvania State University, University Park, Pennsylvania

Supporting the Caregiver in Dementia

PART I

Introduction

This section explores the background of caregiving research. In chapter 1, Steven H. Zarit, one of the pioneers of research in caregiving, offers his perspective on the history and development of the field in the last half-century. In the past, families came together to care for their loved ones in the final stages of life. With the changing social trends and the lengthened life expectancy in recent times, there has been a shift in the nature and locus of care provided to elderly persons. This is especially noted in the care of persons with dementia. Dr. Zarit describes the work of leaders in the interrelated fields of stress research, community mental health, and the deinstitutionalization movement, and how the principles generated from these efforts may guide a multidimensional approach to caregiver burden. In doing so, he explores the tremendous stresses entailed in caregiving at the familial, institutional, and societal levels. He discusses such important concepts as the effects of caregiving on the health of caregivers and interventions for the relief of caregiver burden within the framework of the stress process model. He ends with guidelines directing future research, including the need for a more family-centered methodological focus accompanied by longitudinal data collection, family intervention studies, and investigations of the social and policy implications of caregiving.

CHAPTER ONE

The History of Caregiving in Dementia

STEVEN H. ZARIT, PH.D.

In 1979, two of my graduate students, Karen Reever and Julie Bach, and I presented the results of a small study of caregiver burden at the Gerontological Society of America meetings in San Diego, and subsequently we published that paper in *The Gerontologist* (Zarit, Reever, and Bach-Peterson, 1980). Before that time, there had been only a limited amount of research on family care of older adults and little interest in the topic among researchers or clinicians. Indeed, our presentation was one of only a small number of papers on caregiving at that conference. Within a few years, however, caregiving had become a major focus for research and practice with older people. This interest reflects the confluence of social trends that have made caregiving, as Elaine Brody (1985) once characterized it, a normative and stressful event in people's lives. In this chapter, I look at the social trends that led to the emergence of caregiving as a focus of research and practice, the intellectual traditions that contributed to the development of the field, and the concepts and issues that have emerged in research in the past twenty-five years.

THE EMERGENCE OF FAMILY CARE

Families have always cared for their older relatives, but in the past it was a rare and usually short-lived event. Most people did not survive to old age, and death at any age was likely to be relatively sudden, due to infectious disease or other acute medical problems. During the first half of the twentieth century, the development of antibiotics and other treatments for infectious diseases, as well as improvements in immunization, water, sanitation, and other public health measures made it likely that most children born in a particular birth cohort would survive to adulthood, and beyond to old age. In the second half of the twentieth century, further improvements in life expectancy resulted from better treatment for chronic conditions, as well as health behaviors that have delayed or lowered the risk of particular diseases, such as cardiovascular disease. As a result, life expectancy increased from 47 in the year 1900 to 77 by the year 2000, and most people born in the United States now can expect to live to old age (U.S. Census Bureau, 2000).

An overwhelming majority of older people function independently, but the increase in life expectancy means that more people are reaching ages at which the probability of developing one or more chronic conditions and accompanying disabilities is high. Moreover, since there is now better control of acute and infectious diseases, people tend to live longer after the onset of a disability (Cassel, Rudberg, and Olshansky, 1992). Much of the care for the elderly with disabilities is provided in community settings, usually by family and sometimes with support from formal helpers. Rates of institutionalization have held steady or dropped a little over the past forty years (Hetzel and Smith, 2001).

Coinciding with the increasing need for care, the family's resources for providing care have been diminishing. Several factors have contributed to this change. One consequence of the monumental movement of women into the work force is that there is less likely to be someone at home available to provide care. Lower rates of fertility mean that there are fewer children from whom a caregiver for a parent might emerge. The increase in divorce may weaken ties between some parents and children, resulting in conflicted commitments to providing help, or no assistance at all. The low rate of economic growth for the working class during the past twenty-five years also means that many families have only limited finances for providing help. There has also been little help from the formal sector. Despite the huge increases in Medicare expenditures in recent decades, it remains primarily a program for acute medical care and pays only a little toward the cost of community-based services. Services such as adult day care, which may enable many caregivers to provide care to an aged relative, are not reimbursed through Medicare. Thus, although more older people need help than ever before, the family's resources for providing assistance are more limited.

By the 1970s, the increase in the number of people providing help to an elderly relative was sufficient to get attention in the media. The term "sandwich generation" was applied to the dilemma of a middle-aged woman who simultaneously rears adolescent children while assisting a disabled parent (Schwartz, 1979). Caregiving, however, had not yet become the focus of research or practice. Neugarten (1979) observed that she was more likely to hear about the difficulties in caring for an older relative from women at the beauty parlor than from her professional colleagues.

In the mid- to late 1970s, people who were providing care to severely disabled individuals began finding one another, forming support groups and advocacy organizations. One of the earliest of these organizations, Family Survival Project (now called Family Caregiver Alliance), was founded in San Francisco in 1976 as a coalition of family members of adults with brain disease and injury, including dementia and stroke. While Family Survival Project remained committed to serving a diverse population of brain-injured adults, four other grassroots organizations that focused on care of people with dementia came together in 1979 to form the Alzheimer's Association (see Fox, 1989). Chapters of the Alzheimer's Association soon developed throughout the country.

My own work with caregivers began during this period, in response to the growing public awareness about caregiving and the initiative taken by families to get information and assistance that would help them with their daily efforts. In the late 1970s, my students and I were operating a counseling program in a community setting for older adults that was funded by an Administration on Aging grant. The most common problem for which people sought help was caring for a relative with dementia or another disability. We were one of the few agencies in a large metropolitan area willing to work with families of people with dementia. Indeed, one caller to our program said she had telephoned 44 other agencies before reaching us and finding someone who would talk with her about her mother's condition. Word must have gotten around that we could be helpful, because we were quite busy, despite a limited budget and a staff made up only of graduate students and volunteers. In response to the problems families presented, we developed clinical strategies for managing people at home with dementia (Zarit, 1979; Zarit and Zarit, 1982; Zarit, Orr, and Zarit, 1985) and became interested in understanding better the stresses and adaptation made by families (Zarit, Reever, and Bach-Peterson, 1980). One of my students, Karen Reever, and several family members from our program also helped establish the local Alzheimer's Association chapter. Many other researchers and clinicians began a similar journey around the same time, examining the problems and stressors that families encountered and developing services and interventions for them.

EARLY INTELLECTUAL INFLUENCES

Families had always been a focus in social gerontology. Before the 1970s, much of the family-oriented research addressed the extent to which older people maintained ties with children and grandchildren or became socially isolated (e.g., Shanas, 1968). There was, however, little explicit focus on caregiving. Clinical work with older people likewise emphasized the "patient" and rarely mentioned the role of family.

The one area where family caregivers received attention was in the community mental health field. Robert L. Kahn, a clinical psychologist who was my mentor at the University of Chicago, drew on community mental health principles to develop a model for treatment of older people and their families. In the process, he introduced several important concepts to the gerontological literature. Kahn (1975) emphasized that keeping people at home increased their autonomy and quality of life. However, when older people had chronic mental health problems or dementia, physicians and other professionals often made the mistake of focusing on the symptoms that could not be treated. Seeing the illness as unrelenting, professionals would frequently urge the family to institutionalize the person. Providing too much help would lead to "excess disabilities," a term that Kahn (1965) introduced to indicate a greater dependency than warranted by the person's condition. Kahn (1975) argued that we should view dementia and similar problems as a biopsychosocial phenomenon, and that whereas the underlying biological factors might resist treatment, it was often possible to modify psychological or social aspects of the care situation. He recognized that home care could place considerable burden on the family, so he advocated helping caregivers manage the demands placed on them more effectively. He believed that caregivers could learn to tolerate common behavior problems, such as repetitive questions, and also benefit from respite services such as adult day care and overnight respite.

In developing this model, Kahn drew on the experiences of early clinical demonstrations that suggested the value of supporting the family. A British physician, Duncan Macmillan, developed a model mental health program for older people that emphasized home care (Macmillan, 1968). Families were supported with consultation about care and management and with "holiday relief," that is, short-term care for the patient in a hospital. Macmillan also assured continuity of care by integrating inpatient and outpatient staff. Another important early influence on the caregiving field was Benjamin Pasamanick (e.g., Pasamanick et al., 1967), who emphasized the role of the family in helping maintain people with schizophrenia in the community. In an evaluation of an innovative community program, Pasamanick and colleagues found that a visiting nurses program reduced symptoms of the person with schizophrenia and also rates of reinstitutionalization. The nurses worked with both the patient and the family, and this support of the family appeared to be a crucial element in lowering the incidence of rehospitalization.

The development of studies of family caregiving coincided with the emergence of sociological and psychological theories of stress. In particular, work by Richard Lazarus (1966) and by Leonard Pearlin and Carmi Schooler (1978) provided new perspectives on the stress process. Rather than using mechanistic models that focused only on underlying biological processes, this work showed that people engaged in active appraisal and coping processes modified the impact of stressors. These adaptational processes, along with the psychosocial context in which stressors occurred, influenced the extent of impact that stressors had on an individual's life. Growing directly from this work, one of the earliest and most enduring findings in the caregiving literature was that whether caregivers experience a negative outcome when faced with stressors depends on the influence of these appraisal and coping processes, as well as the availability of social support and resources (e.g., Pruchno and Resch, 1989; Zarit, Reever, and Bach-Peterson, 1980).

THE FIRST PHASE OF CAREGIVING RESEARCH: CONSTRUCTS AND DEFINITIONS

Caregiving research in the 1980s was dominated by two intertwined questions: what were the effects of caregiving and what was the optimal way of defining and measuring these effects. In our early study (Zarit, Reever, and Bach-Peterson, 1980), we developed a measure of subjective burden that drew on the work of Marjorie Fiske Lowenthal and colleagues (Lowenthal, Berkman, and Associates, 1967). In a study of mentally ill elders in the community, they characterized home care as affecting the psychological, physical, and financial resources of family caregivers (Lowenthal, Berkman, and Associates, 1967). We incorporated those dimensions in our concept of burden and added two others, the effect that providing care has on the caregiver's social and leisure activities and on his or her relationship with the care receiver. We believed that the additive effects of impact in these domains would be a useful indicator of how well a caregiver was managing the demands of care and his or her likelihood of continuing in the role. This definition of burden was also consistent with the work of Grad and Sainsbury (1963, 1968), who used burden as a measure of the effectiveness of a home-based intervention for families of mentally ill elders.

In that early study, we were also concerned with measurement of the stressors that caregivers experienced. Because we were working with caregivers of people with dementia, we focused on two domains—behavior problems, which had been found to be particularly troublesome for caregivers in previous studies (Lowenthal,

1964; Sainsbury and Grad de Alarcon, 1970), and assistance with activities of daily living, which placed tangible demands on caregivers. For our 1980 study, we developed the Memory and Behavior Problems Checklist, a measure of sixteen common problems that occurred with dementia, and assessed the frequency with which they had happened in the past week. A subsequent revision of the measure included caregivers' appraisals of the stressfulness of each problem (Zarit and Zarit, 1982; Zarit, Todd, and Zarit, 1986). This approach was derived from stress theory (e.g., Lazarus, 1966) that suggested that an important determinant of the impact of a particular stressor was the degree to which a person appraises it as a threat. This measure also drew from the work of Sanford (1975), who found that caregivers varied in their ability to tolerate problems associated with care. Teri and her colleagues (Teri et al., 1992) developed a revised and expanded version of this measure, and other investigators had taken a similar approach (e.g., Vitaliano et al., 1991).

The use of the term *burden* became a major focus of contention in this early period. In mental health research on the effects of deinstitutionalization, a distinction had been made between objective burden, that is, the changes that providing care imposes on the roles and resources of the family, and subjective burden, the caregiver's emotional response (e.g., Hoenig and Hamilton, 1966; Thompson and Doll, 1982). This conceptualization had been made partly to explain findings that suggested that some families reported little or no emotional distress, despite apparently difficult circumstances (Thompson and Doll, 1982). Montgomery, Gonyea, and Hooyman (1985) used this distinction in developing a measure for objective and subjective burden of caregivers of older people. In their framework, objective burden was a rating of the adequacy of the caregiver's resources (time, money, energy), and subjective burden was assessed with measures of perceived changes in the relationship with the care receiver as well as the emotional impact on the caregiver.

Taking an approach consistent with stress theory, Poulshock and Deimling (1984; see also Deimling and Bass, 1986) defined burden as the appraisal of stressful events, such as assisting with activities of daily living or managing symptoms of cognitive loss. Vitaliano and colleagues (Vitaliano, Maiuro, Ochs, and Russo, 1989; Vitaliano et al., 1991) expanded this approach in their measure of appraised burden. This scale assesses the frequency with which a variety of stressful events occur and how stressful caregivers rate them. The events are predominantly behavior and cognitive problems but also include the social impact on caregivers. Burden is defined as the degree to which caregivers find these events stressful. Also drawing on stress theory, Kinney and Stephens (1989a, 1989b) developed a measure of caregiving hassles, consisting of common behavior problems and other difficulties that caregivers frequently encountered.

Multidimensional approaches to burden were also developed. Lawton and colleagues (1989) proposed five dimensions of burden: subjective burden, impact of caregiving, mastery, satisfaction, and reappraisal. Novak and Guest (1989) developed a burden measure consisting of five dimensions: time dependence, developmental burden, physical burden, social burden, and emotional burden; they suggested that caregivers might vary on which dimensions they found problematic. Stommel, Given, and Given (1990) defined burden as the impact caregivers report arising from caregiving situations, and they proposed five dimensions: impact on finances, impact on health, impact on schedule, feeling of being abandoned by family, and sense of entrapment. Several other measures of caregiver burden were also developed.

As these varying definitions and measures indicate, the term *burden* was used in so many different ways that its meaning became obscured. The use of caregiver-specific measures was itself criticized by George (1994; George and Gwyther, 1986). She argued that caregiving research should use standardized measures that could be administered to a general population of noncaregivers, as well as to caregivers. In that way, it would be possible to identify the relative burden caregivers experience as compared to an age-and-gender-matched sample of people who were not caregivers. According to George, measures of burden and other caregiver-specific indices do not provide any point of reference, and so the meaning of high or low subjective burden cannot be interpreted. Use of normed measures that showed that caregivers were relatively worse off in some domains than noncaregiving samples would be useful for making the argument that people need services and other assistance. George also argued that caregiver-specific measures implied attribution of cause, that is, that one's distress was due to caregiving, and that these kinds of attributions may not be accurate.

Both of George's arguments have merit, and research that demonstrates the relative disadvantage of caregivers compared to other populations has had a valuable impact. Caregiver-specific measures, however, provide useful information that cannot be obtained from more general assessments. The thoughts and feelings that caregivers have about their situation are critical and affect the decisions they make. It does not matter if a caregiver is more or less distressed than the average person his or her age, or if that caregiver has misattributed his or her distress to caregiving rather than to other causes. Rather, the perception of distress as burdensome and due to caregiving will influence that person's important decisions, such as whether to use social services or to institutionalize a relative.

Despite these debates over definitions, a consensus gradually emerged about the effects of caregiving. Caregivers generally reported subjective distress or burden, as well as experiencing decreases in well-being compared to normative populations (e.g., Anthony-Bergstone et al. 1988; Gallagher et al., 1989; George and Gwyther, 1986; Pruchno and Resch, 1989; Schulz, Visintainer, and Williamson, 1990). There were also some indications that caregivers' health might suffer, although the results tended to be mixed (e.g., Schulz et al., 1990). Consistent with early research, the findings generally supported the notion that there were considerable individual differences in how caregivers responded to stressors. Some experienced high levels of distress despite caring for an elder with fairly minimal problems, while others reported low levels of distress despite facing very high care demands. Clearly, the steps that caregivers took in managing specific stressors made a difference in these outcomes (Zarit, Todd, and Zarit, 1986).

Another aspect of caregiving that began receiving attention was that many caregivers had positive experiences in the course of their activities, such as uplifts and satisfaction from providing care (e.g., Kinney and Stephens, 1989a, 1989b; Lawton et al., 1989). These positive feelings could serve as an incentive for caregivers to carry on in the role despite its many stressors.

Other studies examined who within the informal network became a caregiver. The media-driven focus was on the sandwich generation, daughters caught in the middle of responsibilities to parents and children, but the reality was more complex. In a landmark study, Stone, Cafferata, and Sangl (1987) used Medicare records to identify a sample of caregivers who were helping older relatives with one or more activities of daily living. The largest group of caregivers was spouses, accounting for 36 percent of all primary caregivers. After spouses, daughters and daughters-in-law were the most likely helpers. Some daughters could be characterized as being "sandwiched" between responsibilities for children and a parent, but many were older themselves, and their children were grown. Whether spouses or daughters, many caregivers were coping with their own aging. Horowitz (1985) showed that sons also became caregivers, but only when no parent or sister was available, and they frequently turned over responsibility for day-to-day care to a wife or to formal service agencies. Matthews (1987; Matthews and Rosner, 1988) identified other factors that influenced which sibling would provide the primary assistance to a parent, including affectional ties, birth order, and competing roles.

Although care takes place within a family system, much of the early work viewed caregivers as individuals without considering the context in which they carried out their activities. Cantor (1983) was one of the first people to study the broader social network of disabled older people, including kin and nonkin. She hypothesized that the closer the relationship, the more distressing was the caregiving role. Spouses generally report greater levels of distress than other caregivers, although this difference is at least partly due to living arrangements. Spouse caregivers, of course, almost always share a household with their husbands or wives, while daughters or other caregivers may live in a separate household. In comparing spouses to daughters who share a household with a parent they are caring for, no differences in distress are found (Townsend et al., 1989).

Cohler and colleagues (1989) contributed an early theoretical piece that examined how the care experience emerged from the relationship between care receiver and giver. They posited that affection and obligation were critical mediators that affected how caregivers experienced stressors. People who felt a responsibility for providing care and who had a positive relationship with the care recipient would function with less distress, though also being prone to feelings of loss. Williamson and colleagues (e.g., Williamson and Schulz, 1990) also began exploring how the quality of the relationship affected caregiving.

Overall, however, the significance of the type and quality of relationship for caregiving outcomes has not been fully explored. Moreover, most of what we know about caregiving concerns spouses and daughters. The other people who become caregivers, including sons, siblings, grandchildren, and other kin and nonkin, constitute 23 percent of all primary caregivers (Stone, Cafferata, and Sangl, 1987), a sizable group about whom very little is known.

One of the perspectives that did not receive much attention during this period was that of the people receiving care. An exception was the work of Brody and colleagues (Brody et al., 1983, 1984), who explored the expectations that people held about helping and being helped. Brody and colleagues found that many older people did not want to be a burden to their children and did not want to share a household with them (Brody et al., 1984). Older women were more accepting of using formal help, while, surprisingly, their granddaughters approved the least of using formal services and preferred drawing on informal sources (Brody et al., 1983).

THE FIRST PHASE OF CAREGIVING RESEARCH: INTERVENTIONS

In many cases, the grassroots movement that led to the formation of the Alzheimer's Association as well as other caregiver organizations grew from community-based support groups, where people with commons problems came together to learn from one another and share coping strategies. Much of the early intervention research focused on these groups. When compared to control conditions, people in support groups were found to have modest or no benefit (e.g., Haley, Brown, and Levine, 1987; Toseland, Rossiter, and Labrecque, 1989). Several factors contributed to these disappointing findings. First, sample size was often too small to demonstrate a reliable difference. Second, the studies typically employed global outcome measures rather than more specific dimensions of the caregiving experience (e.g., feeling supported or learning new coping strategies) that are likely to change with group participation. There was also a problem of dosage, that is, of how much exposure to an intervention was needed to produce change (see Zarit, 1990, and Zarit and Leitsch, 2001, for a discussion of these methodological issues).

Our group took a different approach. We had found that family support was associated with less subjective burden (Zarit, Reever, and Bach-Peterson, 1980). In thinking about these findings, we considered that it might be possible to intervene directly with families to increase the help they were providing. Compared to formal paid services, family help could be flexible, delivered when caregivers need it most, and at little or no cost. We also built on psychoeducational approaches that helped primary caregivers understand the changes their relatives were experiencing and learn to use behavioral strategies for managing specific stressors. These strategies were combined into a seven-session structured counseling intervention. One of the sessions was a family meeting to which the primary caregiver invited his or her extended family and other informal support persons. In a randomized trial, this program of individual and family counseling (IFC) was compared to a support group and a wait list control. People in IFC had better outcomes for subjective burden and well-being than did participants in the other two conditions (Whitlatch, Zarit, and von Eye, 1991). In retrospect, it seems that the greater intensity of IFC compared to support groups, as well as its specific focus on family support, may have led to its effectiveness.

THE MATURING OF THE FIELD

Studies from 1990 on are probably more familiar, so here I highlight a few contributions that I believe had the greatest impact. In doing so, of course, it is necessary to omit other important work, which would be included in a more comprehensive review.

Perhaps the most important and most cited paper of the decade was a conceptual piece by Leonard Pearlin and associates (Pearlin, Mullan, Semple, and Skaff, 1990). This paper presented a compelling model of the stress process of caregiving, as well as measures that operationalized the major components of the model. There were several key features of the model that are now quite familiar to the field. First is the distinction between primary stressors, which are embedded in caregiving, and secondary stressors, which represent the impinging of primary stressors on other areas of the person's life. Second, primary and secondary stressors are conceptualized as having objective and subjective dimensions. Similar to the earlier distinction of objective and subjective burden, objective stressors include the events or changes that occur, while subjective stressors focus on appraisals and emotional impact. Third, Pearlin and colleagues emphasized that there were considerable individual differences in the effects of caregiving on outcomes such as health and well-being. Outcomes were the result of stressors acting in conjunction with processes that led to their proliferation or containment. Personal and social resources were believed to contain the impact of primary onto secondary stressors, and both types of stressors on health and well-being. Proliferation occurred, in turn, when there was an absence of resources or when stressors were too demanding for the available resources.

The stress process model was tested in a large-scale longitudinal study of people caring for someone with dementia, and support was found for the many of the hypothesized relationships (Aneshensel et al., 1995). In particular, the study reported that individual differences in outcome could be explained by the proliferation or containment of stress.

One effect of the stress process model was clarification of the definitional disputes around burden and other constructs that characterized early caregiving research. The various definitions of burden can be mapped onto different dimensions of the stress process—primary objective stressors, primary subjective stressors, secondary stressors, and even outcomes. Rather than arguing over the semantics of what is or is not burden, it is more productive to think about what processes in which one is interested and to find the best ways of assessing those processes.

Another important contribution was made by Schulz and Beach (1999), who examined the effects on the health of caregivers. As noted, many studies had conflicting findings on this matter, in part because of varying strategies of measuring health, which ranged from subjective reports to assessment of immune system functioning. Using a large, longitudinal panel of people being followed in a health study, Schulz and Beach compared people who had become caregivers for a spouse with participants who did not experience caregiving. After adjusting for sociodemographic factors and preexisting health conditions, those caregivers who reported strain in their roles had significantly higher risk of mortality compared to other participants. This study provides the clearest evidence of the harmful consequences of caregiving and the need for interventions that help families manage the stresses placed on them.

Studies of interventions to assist caregivers lagged considerably behind other research, but there were some notable contributions. Two early pioneers in providing clinical services to caregivers were Gert Steinberg and Emma Shulman, who were social workers at New York University. Their work led to development of an enhanced treatment program that incorporated training caregivers in the management of behavior problems and other stressors and an emphasis on building family support. Caregivers in the program participated in several individual counseling sessions and at least two family meetings. At the completion of the intensive phase of the intervention, caregivers received ongoing support through groups. This intervention was evaluated in a series of studies by a research team headed by Mary Mittelman. The results indicated that people in the treatment group had lower subjective burden, lower depression, and a lower rate of institutionalizing their elders compared to a usual treatment control group (Mittelman et al., 1995, 1996). Unlike many unsuccessful trials, this treatment provides sufficient time and resources to address the complexity and chronicity of care-related stressors (Zarit and Leitsch, 2001).

The most ambitious intervention trial to date has been the REACH (Resources for Enhancing Alzheimer's Caregiver Health) study (Gitlin et al., 2003; Schulz et al., 2003). This study conducted a randomized clinical trial to examine the effects of caregiver interventions delivered at six different sites. Interventions and populations served varied across the sites. A major advance was the inclusion of significant numbers of minority caregivers. Overall, caregivers in the treatment groups reported less upset or distress over behavior problems (which the researchers called "burden"), and one intervention that combined family treatment and use of communications technology showed a decrease in depression. There was also an indication that subgroups of caregivers responded better to some interventions compared to others. This finding highlights the fact that caregivers are quite varied and that standard interventions that offer a fixed protocol might not address the main problems or concerns of a particular family. Studies that target specific problems or that use a flexible protocol that matches treatment modules to need may be more successful in improving outcomes for caregivers.

The type of help that most caregivers use is respite services. At the end of the 1980s, M. Powell Lawton and colleagues (1989) described the results of a randomized trial of respite services, in which some caregivers received help from a care manager to match them with respite services and others were given a list of community resources to find help on their own. Although Lawton et al. reported positive outcomes, their paper was strongly criticized by Callahan (1989), who argued that the findings were minimal and that respite was not helpful. Despite the limited findings, the study was a step forward in the caregiving literature because of its attempt to conduct a large-scale field trial of respite.

The results of a large multisite trial, the Medicare Alzheimer's Disease Demonstration (MADDE) (Newcomer, Fox, and Harrington, 2001), were similar to those reported by Lawton and colleagues (1989). In MADDE, care managers implemented a social model of care that linked caregivers to community services, including respite. Care management did result in greater use of community services but had no effect on caregivers' reports of distress or on institutionalization.

Although the results from the Lawton et al. (1989) study did not provide strong support for the value of respite, the study provided directions for more effective strategies for evaluating services. In reviewing that study, my colleagues and I identified problems that may have restricted the likelihood of finding a treatment effect (Zarit, 1990; Zarit, Stephens, Townsend, and Greene, 1998). A careful examination of the findings from Lawton et al. indicates that many participants received only small amounts of respite, which might not have been sufficient to lower distress. Some people in the control group also used respite services during the course of the study, which further reduced differences between the groups. Another problem is that the outcome measures were not targeted well to assess the likely effects of respite.

Building on these observations, my colleagues and I (Zarit, Stephens, Townsend, and Greene, 1998) undertook a study of the effects of adult day care on caregivers of people with dementia. We specifically sought to overcome some of the difficulties that Lawton and colleagues (1989) as well as other investigators had encountered. One step we took was to control exposure to the treatment. We felt that an adequate test of adult day care or other respite services would involve participants receiving enough service to produce beneficial effects. In other words, caregivers would need to receive a therapeutic dosage of the treatment. This notion of how much treatment is needed has rarely been considered in intervention studies with caregivers. Based on input from participating day care programs, we set a minimum amount of use that we felt could be expected to produce positive effects (two days a week for three months) and excluded people who did not meet that threshold. We also thought that the treatment and control group had to differ in exposure to the treatment or to comparable treatments in order to test the effects of day care. We did not think that a control group that included people who also used day care or comparable respite services that freed up their time would provide an appropriate comparison. We therefore eliminated participants in the control group who used services likely to have similar effects to day care in freeing up the caregiver's time. Finally, we identified the most likely aspects of the stress process to be affected by adult day care and focused on those dimensions as possible outcomes of treatment. Using the Pearlin stress process model (Pearlin et al., 1990), we hypothesized that adult day care was likely to have its most direct effect on primary subjective stressors such as feelings of overload and strain, rather than on more global constructs such as well-being. Our findings confirmed that caregivers experienced significant decreases in primary subjective stressors, but we also found generalized effects on two measures of well-being, depression, and anger.

A major development in the 1990s was the pioneering work of Tom Kitwood (1997). Kitwood called attention to the dehumanizing ways that people with dementia are often treated and proposed a "person-centered approach." Specific elements of this approach include respecting the past preferences of people with dementia, respecting their personal and cultural identity, giving them a voice in the decisions that affect their daily lives, shaping decisions based on a concern for quality of life as they might define it, and responding to their emotional and spiritual side, rather than just to cognition (Woods, 1999).

Attention to the needs of people with dementia has been growing, fueled in part by an emphasis on early diagnosis. Yale (1989, 1999) developed protocols for early stage support groups that involve people with dementia at a point when they can still make decisions about how they want to live and about their future care. Feinberg and Whitlatch (2001) examined decision-making abilities of people with early dementia, with a goal of helping caregivers identify the needs and preferences of the person with dementia.

In an intriguing study, Linda Teri and colleagues (Teri, Logsdon, Uomoto, and McCurry, 1997) demonstrated the possible gains for psychosocial treatment of people in the middle to later stages of dementia, as well as for their caregivers. People with dementia who had comorbid depression and their caregivers were randomly assigned into one of four treatment groups. The first treatment, based on Lewinsohn's (Lewinsohn, Muñoz, Youngren, and Zeiss, 1992) behavioral therapy for depression, instructed caregivers in strategies for increasing the patient's engagement in pleasant activities. The second treatment used problem-solving approaches to help caregivers manage depressive symptoms and other problem behaviors. These two active treatments were contrasted with a control condition involving treatment as usual, that is, support and referral to community agencies and to a waiting list control. People with dementia in the two active treatments, pleasant events and problem solving, showed decreased depressive symptoms compared to the control conditions. Caregivers in those conditions also improved significantly compared to controls. The study remains the best evidence to date that treatment that helps people with dementia also helps caregivers, and vice versa. In further work that builds on this study, Teri and colleagues (2003) showed that caregivers can implement a program of exercise and behavior management for their relatives, with the result that persons with dementia improve their daily functioning and have lower depression than do controls.

CONCLUSION

The dramatic growth in research and practice on family caregivers reflects the demands placed on contemporary families and the need to develop effective programs and policies that help families meet the challenges that they face. This review of the development of the field has necessarily been selective, and many important contributions to the field have been omitted. I hope, however, that this brief history has identified the converging social forces that led to the emergence of caregiving as a major social issue, as well as the intellectual traditions that influenced the development of the field. As "past is prologue," I end with a few suggestions of future directions that might be fruitful.

1. *Focus on the whole family.* Most of what we know about "family" caregiving comes from one person, the primary caregiver. We know other people are often involved in helping and that increasing the involvement of other family members as well as nonkin can be very helpful. Expanding our focus to include the perspectives and involvement of the whole family would be very useful in clarifying how family members can support one another, as well as for developing better family-focused interventions. New statistical approaches that allow us to model families make this a timely line of inquiry.

2. *Conduct longitudinal studies, particularly at the earliest points of providing care.* Much of the research on caregiving still involves cross-sectional or very short-term longitudinal panels. We capture, in effect, the people who have selected to stay involved in caregiving and know very little about those individuals who have already given up the role, or the reasons why. Cross-sectional studies can also obscure the sequence of events that lead to the evolution of caregiver distress or other important outcomes. For example, we often postulate that social support may moderate the effects of stressors on outcomes such as depression, but caregivers may only seek out informal and formal support when they experience higher levels of depression. In a cross-sectional analysis, it may appear that support is related to higher depression. Longitudinal studies that begin near the onset of caregiving could help us more fully understand how people make decisions and how their involvement and experiences change over time.

3. *Conduct intervention research.* There is a continuing need for intervention research. Intervention research can lead to practical benefits for caregivers, but it can also be used to test theories about stressors and the processes that contain them. The findings of the REACH program (e.g., Schulz et al., 2003) underscore the complexity

of interventions, particularly the need for more individually tailored treatments that take into account a person's care situation, care relationship, and cultural and ethnic background.

4. *Involve the person with dementia or other disability.* The growing interest in the person with dementia and other care recipients is a positive trend. With early diagnosis of dementia, there is an opportunity to involve people with dementia in research and to examine how they along with their families are coping with the illness. There are also opportunities to intervene early so that people with dementia can express their preferences about the type of care they want to receive.

5. *Involve diverse populations.* Despite promising research on minority populations by Dilworth-Anderson (Dilworth-Anderson, Williams, and Cooper, 1999), Haley (Haley et al., 1996), the REACH program (Schulz et al., 2003), and others, most research remains focused on white middle-class caregivers. Inclusion of diverse groups as well as cross-cultural comparisons can enrich our understanding of the variety of approaches to caregiving and the needs of families that are not addressed by current programs and services.

6. *Research and practice on family caregiving needs to continue to consider the social and policy implications.* Caregiving is one of the unexpected and still unplanned for consequences of an aging population. Although policy advocates and policy makers are well aware of caregiving issues, it remains one of many competing demands on the public's and government's attention. A national caregiving benefit that makes real and sufficient resources available to families is clearly needed. Yet even modest proposals such as making adult day care reimbursable through Medicare remain unlikely to be realized in the near future. Research that at its core is concerned with the well-being of caregivers must inevitably address these kinds of policy issues.

REFERENCES

Aneshensel, C., Pearlin, L. I., Mullan, J. T., Zarit, S. H., and Whitlatch, C. J. 1995. *Profiles in caregiving: The unexpected career.* New York: Academic Press.

Anthony-Bergstone, C. R., Zarit, S. H., and Gatz, M. 1988. Symptoms of psychological distress among caregivers of dementia patients. *Psychology and Aging* 3:245–48.

Brody, E. M. 1985. Parent care as normative family stress. *Gerontologist* 25:10–29.

Brody, E. M., Johnsen, P. T., Fulcomer, M. C., and Lang, A. M. 1983. Women's changing roles and help to the elderly: Attitudes of three generations of women. *Journal of Gerontology* 38:597–607.

Brody, E. M., Johnsen, P. T., and Fulcomer, M. C. 1984. What should adult children do for elderly parents? Opinions and preferences in three generations of women. *Journal of Gerontology* 39:736–46.

Callahan, J. J. 1989. Play it again Sam—There is no impact. *Gerontologist* 29:5–6.

Cantor, M. H. 1983. Strain among caregivers: A study of experience in the United States. *Gerontologist* 23:597–604.

Cassel, C. K., Rudberg, M. A., and Olshansky, S. J. 1992. The price of success: Health care in an aging society. *Health Affairs* 11:87–99.

Cohler, B. J., Groves, L., Borden, W., and Lazarus, L. 1989. Caring for family members with Alzheimer's disease. In E. Light and B. Lebowitz (Eds.), *Alzheimer's disease treatment and family stress: Directions for research* (pp. 50–105). Washington, D.C.: U.S. Government Printing Office.

Deimling, G., and Bass, D. M. 1986. Symptoms of mental impairment among elderly adults and their effects on family caregivers. *Journal of Gerontology* 41:67–82.

Dilworth-Anderson, P., Williams, S. W., and Cooper, T. 1999. Family caregiving to elderly African Americans: Caregiver types and structures. *Journal of Gerontology: Psychological Science and Social Science* 54(4):S237–41.

Feinberg, L. F., and Whitlatch, C. J. 2001. Are cognitively impaired adults able to state consistent choices? *Gerontologist* 41:374–82.

Fox, P. 1989. From senility to Alzheimer's disease: The rise of the Alzheimer's disease movement. *Milbank Quarterly* 67(1):58–102.

Gallagher, D., Rose, J., Rivera, P., Lovett, S., and Thompson, L. W. 1989. Prevalence of depression in family caregivers. *Gerontologist* 29:449–56.

George, L. K. 1994. Caregiver burden and well-being: An elusive distinction. *Gerontologist* 34:6–7.

George, L. K., and Gwyther, L. P. 1986. Caregiver well-being: A multidimensional examination of family caregivers of demented adults. *Gerontologist* 26:253–59.

Gitlin, L. N., Belle, S. H., Burgio, L. D., Czaja, S. J., Mahoney, D., Gallagher-Tompson, D., et al. 2003. Effect of multicomponent interventions on caregiver burden and depression: The REACH multisite initiative at 6-month follow-up. *Psychology and Aging* 18(3):361–74.

Grad, J., and Sainsbury, P. 1963. Mental illness and the family. *Lancet* 1:544–47.

Grad, J., and Sainsbury, P. 1968. The effects that patients have on their families in a community care and control psychiatric service—a two-year follow up. *British Journal of Psychiatry* 114 (508): 265–78.

Haley, W. E., Brown, S. L., and Levine, E. G. 1987. Experimental evaluation of the effectiveness of group intervention for dementia caregivers. *Gerontologist* 27:376–82.

Haley, W. E., Roth, D. L., Coleton, M. I., Ford, G. R., West, C. A., Collins, R. P., and Isobe, T. L. 1996. Appraisal, coping, and social support as mediators of well-being in black and white family caregivers of patients with Alzheimer's disease. *Journal of Consulting and Clinical Psychology* 64(1):121–29.

Hetzel, L., and Smith, A. 2001. *The 65 years and over population: 2000—Census 2000 brief.* Washington, D.C.: U.S. Census Bureau.

Hoenig, J., and Hamilton, M. 1966. The schizophrenic patient in the community and his effect on the household. *International Journal of Social Psychiatry* 12:165–76.

Horowitz, A. 1985. Sons and daughters as caregivers to older parents: Differences in role performance and consequences. *Gerontologist* 25:612–17.

Kahn, R. L. 1965. Excess disabilities in the aged. In *Proceedings of the York House Institute on the Mentally Impaired Aged.* Philadelphia: Philadelphia Geriatric Center.

Kahn, R. L. 1975. The mental health system and the future aged. *Gerontologist* 15:24–31.

Kinney, J. M., and Stephens, M. A. P. 1989a. Caregiving Hassles Scale: Assessing the daily hassles of caring for a family member with dementia. *Gerontologist* 29:28–32.

Kinney, J. M., and Stephens, M. A. P. 1989b. Hassles and uplifts of giving care to a family member with dementia. *Psychology and Aging* 4:402–8.

Kitwood, T. 1997. *Dementia reconsidered: The person comes first.* Bristol, Pa.: Open University Press.

Lawton, M. P., Brody, E., and Saperstein, A. R. 1989. A controlled study of respite services for caregivers of Alzheimer's patients. *Gerontologist* 29:8–16.

Lazarus, R. S. 1966. *Psychological stress and the coping process.* New York: McGraw-Hill.

Lazarus, R. S., and Folkman, S. 1984. *Stress, appraisal, and coping.* New York: Springer.

Lewinsohn, P. M., Muñoz, R. F., Youngren, M. A., and Zeiss, A. M. 1992. *Control your depression* (rev. ed.). New York: Simon & Schuster.

Lowenthal, M. F. 1964. *Lives in distress.* New York: Basic Books.

Lowenthal, M. F., Berkman, P., and Associates. 1967. *Aging and mental disorder in San Francisco.* San Francisco: Jossey-Bass.

Macmillan, D. 1968. Problems of a geriatric mental health service. *British Journal of Psychiatry* 113:175–81.

Matthews, S. H. 1987. Provision of care to old parents: Division of responsibility among adult children. *Research on Aging* 9:45–60.

Matthews, S. H., and Rosner, T. 1988. Shared filial responsibility: The family as the primary caregiver. *Journal of Marriage and the Family* 50:185–95.

Mittelman, M. S., Ferris, S. H., Shulman, E., Steinberg, G., Ambinder, A., Mackel, J., and Cohen, J. 1995. A comprehensive support program: Effect on depression in spouse-caregivers of AD patients. *Gerontologist* 35:792–802.

Mittelman, M. S., Ferris, S. H., Shulman, E., Steinberg, G., et al. 1996. A family intervention to delay nursing home placement of patients with Alzheimer disease: A randomized controlled trial. *Journal of the American Medical Association* 276(21):1725–31.

Montgomery, R. J. V., Gonyea, J. G., and Hooyman, N. R. 1985. Caregiving and the experience of subjective and objective burden. *Family Relations* 34:19–26.

Neugarten, B. L. 1979. The middle generations. In P. K. Ragan (Ed.), *Aging parents.* Ethel Percy Andrus Gerontology Center: University of California Press.

Newcomer, R. J., Fox, P. J., and Harrington, C. A. 2001. Health and long-term care for people with Alzheimer's disease and related dementias: Policy research issues. *Aging and Mental Health* 5(1):S124–37.

Novak, M., and Guest, C. 1989. Application of multidimensional caregiver burden inventory. *Gerontologist* 29:798–803.

Pasamanik, B., Scarpitti, R. P., and Dinitz, S. 1967. *Schizophrenics in the community: An experimental study in the prevention of hospitalization.* New York: Appleton-Century Crofts.

Pearlin, L. I., Mullan, J. T., Semple, S. J., and Skaff, M. M. 1990. Caregiving and the stress process: An overview of concepts and their measures. *Gerontologist* 30:583–94.

Pearlin, L. I., and Schooler, C. 1978. The structure of coping. *Journal of Health and Social Behavior* 19:2–21.

Poulshock, D. W., and Deimling, G. T. 1984. Families caring for elders in residence: Issues in the measurement of burden. *Journal of Gerontology* 39:230–39.

Pruchno, R. A., and Resch, N. L. 1989. Aberrant behaviors and Alzheimer's disease: Mental health effects on spouse caregivers. *Journal of Gerontology: Social Sciences* 44:S177–82.

Sainsbury, P., and Grad de Alarcon, J. 1970. The psychiatrist and the geriatric patient: The effects of community care on the family of the geriatric patient. *Journal of Geriatric Psychiatry* 1:23–41.

Sanford, J. F. A. 1975. Tolerance of debility in elderly dependents by supports at home: Its significance for hospital practice. *British Medical Journal* 3:471–73.

Schulz, R., Visintainer, P., and Williamson, G. 1990. Psychiatric and physical morbidity effects of caregiving. *Journal of Gerontology: Psychological Sciences* 45:181–91.

Schwartz, A. N. 1979. Psychological dependency: An emphasis on the later years. In P. K. Ragan (Ed.), *Aging parents*. Ethel Percy Andrus Gerontology Center: University of California Press.

Shanas, E., and others. 1968. *Old people in three industrial societies*. New York: Atherton Press.

Shulz, R., and Beach, S. R. 1999. Caregiving as a risk factor for mortality: The Caregiver Health Effects Study. *Journal of the American Medical Association* 282(23):2215–19.

Shulz, R., Burgio, L., Burns, R., Eisdorfer, C., Gallagher-Thompson, D., Gitlin, L. N., and Mahoney, D. F. 2003. Resources for Enhancing Alzheimer's Caregiver Health (REACH): Overview, site-specific outcomes, and future directions. *Gerontologist* 43:514–20.

Stommel, M., Given, C. W., and Given, B. 1990. Depression as an overriding variable explaining caregiver burdens. *Journal of Aging and Health* 2(1):81–102.

Stone, R., Cafferata, G. L., and Sangl, J. 1987. Caregivers of the frail elderly: A national profile. *Gerontologist* 27:616–26.

Teri, L., Gibbons, L. E., McCurry, S. M., Logsdon, R. G., Buchner, D. M., Barlow, W. E., et al. 2003. Exercise plus behavioral management in patients with Alzheimer disease: A randomized controlled trial. *Journal of the American Medical Association* 290(15):2015–22.

Teri, L., Logsdon, R. G., Uomoto, J., and McCurry, S. M. 1997. Behavioral treatment of depression in dementia patients: A controlled clinical trial. *Journal of Gerontology: Psychological Sciences* 52B(4):159–66.

Teri, L., Truax, P., Logsdon, R., Uomoto, J., Zarit, S. H., and Vitaliano, P. P. 1992. Assessment of behavioral problems in dementia: The revised memory and behavior problems checklist. *Psychology and Aging* 7:622–31.

Thompson, E. H., and Doll, W. 1982. The burden of families coping with the mentally ill: An invisible crisis. *Family Relations* 31:379–88.

Toseland, R. W., Rossiter, C. M., and Labrecque, M. S. 1989. The effectiveness of peer-led and professionally led groups to support family caregivers. *Gerontologist* 29:465–71.

Townsend, A., Noelker, L., Deimling, G., and Bass, D. 1989. Longitudinal impact of interhousehold caregiving on adult children's mental health. *Psychology and Aging* 4:393–401.

U.S. Census Bureau. 2000. Population by Sex by Age by Group. Census 2000 Summary File.

Vitaliano, P. P., Maiuro, R. D., Ochs, H., and Russo, I. 1989. A model of burden in caregivers of DAT patients. In E. Light and B. Lebowitz (Eds.), *Alzheimer's disease: A report of progress in research* (pp. 267–91). Washington, D.C.: Government Printing Office.

Vitaliano, P. P., Russo, J., Young, H. M., Becker, J., and Maiuro, R. D. 1991. The Screen for Caregiver Burden. *Gerontologist* 31:76–83.

Whitlatch, C. J., Zarit, S. H., and von Eye, A. 1991. Efficacy of interventions with caregivers: A reanalysis. *Gerontologist* 31:9–14.

Williamson, G. M., and Schulz, R. 1990. Relationship orientation, quality of prior relationship, and distress among caregivers of Alzheimer's patients. *Psychology of Aging* 5(4):502–9.

Woods, B. 1999. The person in dementia care. *Generations* 23(3):35–39.

Yale, R. 1989. Support groups for newly-diagnosed Alzheimer's clients. *Clinical Gerontologist* 8:86–89.

Yale, R. 1999. Support groups and other services for individuals with early-stage Alzheimer's Disease. *Generations* 23(Fall):57–61.

Zarit, S. H. 1979. Organic brain syndrome and the family. In P. Ragan (Ed.), *Aging parents*. Los Angeles: University of Southern California Press.

Zarit, S. H. 1990. Interventions with frail elders and their families: Are they effective and why? In M. A. P. Stephens, J. H. Crowther, S. E. Hobfoll, and D. L. Tennenbaum (Eds.), *Stress and coping in later life families* (pp. 241–65). Washington, D.C.: Hemisphere Publishers.

Zarit, S. H., and Leitsch, S. A. 2001. Developing and evaluating community based intervention programs for Alzheimer's patients and their caregivers. *Aging and Mental Health* 5(Suppl.):S84–98.

Zarit, S. H., Reever, K. E., and Bach-Peterson, J. 1980. Relatives of the impaired elderly: Correlates of feelings of burden. *Gerontologist* 20:649–55.

Zarit, S. H., Stephens, M. A. P., Townsend, A., and Greene, R. 1998. Stress reduction for family caregivers: Effects of day care use. *Journal of Gerontology: Social Sciences* 53B:S267–77.

Zarit, S. H., Todd, P. A., and Zarit, J. M. 1986. Subjective burden of husbands and wives as caregivers: A longitudinal study. *Gerontologist* 26:260–70.

Zarit, S. H., and Zarit, J. M. 1982. Families under stress: Interventions for caregivers of senile dementia patients. *The hidden victims of Alzheimer's disease: Families under stress*. New York: New York University Press.

PART 2

Individual Aspects of Caregiving

In chapter 2 Sharon K. Ostwald defines the term *caregiver* and categorizes caregivers into two groups: formal and informal. Dr. Ostwald is well acquainted with both formal and informal caregivers in a variety of professional roles, including direct patient care, care of the caregiver, and social advocacy for caregivers at the institutional, state, and regional levels. Her research centers on psychosocial interventions and caregiving. Dr. Ostwald discusses caregiving using a fictional couple, the Nyquists, and their daughter Janet, who gradually assumes primary responsibility as caregiver for an aging mother and a father who is developing dementia. Dr. Ostwald provides many compelling statistics on caregivers and caregiving, including the demographics of caregivers, minority caregiving, and the role of caregivers in Alzheimer disease. Table 2.3 is particularly informative: it shows the characteristics of informal and formal caregivers in various work settings and in the provision of long-term care. Dr. Ostwald recommends partnerships between the interdisciplinary team, patients, and their caregivers. She suggests that the health care team assist caregivers in improving their access to resources needed for optimal care. Finally, she suggests that concerned professionals promote public policies that provide incentives for home care for persons with dementia.

In chapter 3, Irving Hellman describes transitions along an ascending continuum of levels of care, which are yoked to the progression of dementia through the various stages. He discusses acute medical and long-term care services and the housing, psychosocial, and legal/financial services needed in the care of patients with dementia. He lists the guiding principles that determine appropriate care, including the right to safety with the least restrictions and self-determination. Optimal care is the least restrictive care, permitting aging in place with dignity and allowing transitions to appropriate levels of care that are in the patient's best interest. It is often hard for caregivers to take care of themselves while honoring all the rights and principles of caregiving for others. The clinician's role is empathic listening and helping the caregiver negotiate a response, which may necessitate a compromise between meeting the needs of the caregiver and preserving the dignity of the patient. Dr. Hellman creatively applies Prochaska's Transtheoretical Model of Change to coping with dementia. Each stage is presumed to follow the other in a linear progression, as the caregiver and care recipient successfully overcome difficulties in coping with dementia. He provides a deeper understanding and application of this model in his vignette about Joe and Carol and their daughter Monica. As Joe's dementia worsens, the family must make use of a variety of progressively restrictive long-term care options including home care, then assisted living, and finally nursing home placement.

Victor A. Molinari starts chapter 4 with a description of caregiver burden, including the physical, emotional, social, vocational, and financial tolls of caregiving. He briefly describes the scales used in the assessment of caregiver burden, including the Burden Inventory, the most widely used scale. He then identifies the benefits of caregiving, some of which include pleasure in the happiness and safety of the parent, fulfilling family and moral obligations, showing appreciation to one's parents, feelings of accomplishment in meeting a challenge, and maintaining a sense of life's purpose. Dr. Molinari makes a plea for theory-driven research in caregiving. In doing so, he draws on the considerable body of work described by Dr. Zarit in the first chapter and identifies directions for future research. One area that may be of special interest is caregiver resiliency in the face of adversity, which enables some caregivers to successfully adapt while others become overwhelmed. This and other areas of caregiving research will help furnish the data for evidence-based guidelines on how to provide optimal care to this frail population with dementia.

Dementia

D . ,   R . N . ,   G N P ,   F G S A

Caregivers, literally those who provide assistance to another person, are increasingly in demand. The term *informal caregiver,* the focus of most of this book, is often used interchangeably with the term *family caregiver.* An informal caregiver is defined as "one who provides care without pay and whose relationship to the care recipient is due to personal ties (rather than to the service system): family, friends, or neighbors, who may be primary or secondary caregivers, provide full time or part time help, and live with the person being cared for or separately" (Feinberg and Pilisuk, 1999, p. 3). Although this is a generally accepted, comprehensive definition, each agency or program has its own definition, which may act to limit services based on age, illness, geographic location, amount of income, or other characteristic of the caregiver or care recipient.

The term *caregiver* may also refer to professionals or paraprofessionals who provide care in exchange for money. Nurses, nursing assistants, home health aides, and personal care workers are the major groups of formal caregiver. Volunteers with a church or voluntary organization are also sometimes considered formal caregivers, whereas friends and neighbors are considered informal caregivers. A commonly accepted definition of formal caregiver is "professionals, paraprofessionals, or volunteers associated with a service system who provide care at home, in community agencies, or to institutions or residential facilities" (Family Caregiver Alliance [FCA], March 1998, p. 3).

Although individuals, traditionally women, have always provided care to family members and friends, the recognition of this phenomenon has increased over the last decade. As evidence of this increase, the number of occurrences of the word *caregiver* in the newspapers and media tripled between 1990–1994 and 1996–2001. In 2001, the American Association of Retired Persons (AARP) hired a research firm to conduct telephone interviews of a nationally representative sample of 4,037 adults to determine how many people identified themselves as caregivers. In this sample, 69 percent defined a caregiver as a person providing care for someone, and only 10 percent had no idea who a caregiver was (AARP, 2001).

Although caregiving encompasses the provision of care to individuals of all ages with multiple diseases, research on caregiving inevitably includes those caring for family members with Alzheimer disease (AD) because of the long-term, unrelenting commitment necessary to provide care to these persons. Approximately 4 million people currently have AD, and this number is expected to triple by 2050. In total, an estimated 13.1 to 15.5 million Americans have some type of dementia. This includes those with AD, stroke, Parkinson disease, Huntington disease, and traumatic brain injury (FCA, 2003).

> The Nyquists, married for 62 years, are an elderly couple who have lived for forty years in a small two-story bungalow in a St. Paul neighborhood. Mr. Nyquist, now 86, was a salesperson for a small retail men's clothing store that closed about fifteen years ago. His wife, age 82, was primarily a homemaker, although she supplemented the family income by doing some alterations for the clothing store where he worked. He retired at age 65 and they lived carefully on his Social Security and small pension. The Nyquists had two children and they were active in their local Lutheran church when the children were young. They socialized primarily with a small circle of neighbors and her older sister and her husband. Their son was killed in the Vietnam War, and their daughter, Janet, now age 50, lives with her husband and three children in Indianapolis.
>
> The Nyquists enjoyed their retirement until about six years ago, when Mr. Nyquist began showing signs of dementia—getting lost when driving and making errors in the checkbook. Five years ago during a visit home, Janet noticed that her father was confused much of the time, and on questioning her mother she learned that he had been getting more confused during the last year, but that she had not sought any help. With the daughter's urging, Mr. Nyquist was seen by a neurologist and diagnosed with dementia of the Alzheimer type (DAT). Mrs. Nyquist was resistant to seeking any help, saying that it was her responsibility to care for him. Janet began flying home once a month to assess the situation and provide some respite

last decade. As evidence of this increase, the number of occurrences of the word *caregiver* in the newspapers and media tripled between 1990–1994 and 1996–2001. In 2001, the American Association of Retired Persons (AARP) hired a research firm to conduct telephone interviews of a nationally representative sample of 4,037 adults to determine how many people identified themselves as caregivers. In this sample, 69 percent defined a caregiver as a person providing care for someone, and only 10 percent had no idea who a caregiver was (AARP, 2001).

Although caregiving encompasses the provision of care to individuals of all ages with multiple diseases, research on caregiving inevitably includes those caring for family members with Alzheimer disease (AD) because of the long-term, unrelenting commitment necessary to provide care to these persons. Approximately 4 million people currently have AD, and this number is expected to triple by 2050. In total, an estimated 13.1 to 15.5 million Americans have some type of dementia. This includes those with AD, stroke, Parkinson disease, Huntington disease, and traumatic brain injury (FCA, 2003).

The Nyquists, married for 62 years, are an elderly couple who have lived for forty years in a small two-story bungalow in a St. Paul neighborhood. Mr. Nyquist, now 86, was a salesperson for a small retail men's clothing store that closed about fifteen years ago. His wife, age 82, was primarily a homemaker, although she supplemented the family income by doing some alterations for the clothing store where he worked. He retired at age 65 and they lived carefully on his Social Security and small pension. The Nyquists had two children and they were active in their local Lutheran church when the children were young. They socialized primarily with a small circle of neighbors and her older sister and her husband. Their son was killed in the Vietnam War, and their daughter, Janet, now age 50, lives with her husband and three children in Indianapolis.

The Nyquists enjoyed their retirement until about six years ago, when Mr. Nyquist began showing signs of dementia—getting lost when driving and making errors in the checkbook. Five years ago during a visit home, Janet noticed that her father was confused much of the time, and on questioning her mother she learned that he had been getting more confused during the last year, but that she had not sought any help. With the daughter's urging, Mr. Nyquist was seen by a neurologist and diagnosed with dementia of the Alzheimer type (DAT). Mrs. Nyquist was resistant to seeking any help, saying that it was her responsibility to care for him. Janet began flying home once a month to assess the situation and provide some respite

CHAPTER TWO

The Caregiver in Dementia

SHARON K. OSTWALD, PH.D., R.N., GNP, FGSA

Caregivers, literally those who provide assistance to another person, are increasingly in demand. The term *informal caregiver,* the focus of most of this book, is often used interchangeably with the term *family caregiver.* An informal caregiver is defined as "one who provides care without pay and whose relationship to the care recipient is due to personal ties (rather than to the service system): family, friends, or neighbors, who may be primary or secondary caregivers, provide full time or part time help, and live with the person being cared for or separately" (Feinberg and Pilisuk, 1999, p. 3). Although this is a generally accepted, comprehensive definition, each agency or program has its own definition, which may act to limit services based on age, illness, geographic location, amount of income, or other characteristic of the caregiver or care recipient.

The term *caregiver* may also refer to professionals or paraprofessionals who provide care in exchange for money. Nurses, nursing assistants, home health aides, and personal care workers are the major groups of formal caregiver. Volunteers with a church or voluntary organization are also sometimes considered formal caregivers, whereas friends and neighbors are considered informal caregivers. A commonly accepted definition of formal caregiver is "professionals, paraprofessionals, or volunteers associated with a service system who provide care at home, in community agencies, or to institutions or residential facilities" (Family Caregiver Alliance [FCA], March 1998, p. 3).

Although individuals, traditionally women, have always provided care to family members and friends, the recognition of this phenomenon has increased over the to her mother. It was clear that Mrs. Nyquist had little relief from caregiving and was becoming increasing exhausted. Two years ago, despite her mother's reluctance, Janet arranged for her father to attend an Alzheimer day care program at a local church three days a week. The Nyquists were able to pay part of the cost by dipping into their savings and Janet picked up the remaining cost.

About six months ago, Mr. Nyquist become increasingly resistant to leaving the house. His wife was not able to get him dressed to be transported by bus to the day care. Their bedroom was on the second story and the bathroom was downstairs. Mr. Nyquist wandered at night, had lost weight, and was incontinent. Janet insisted that her mother hire a home health care aide to stay with Mr. Nyquist two nights a week so she could get some rest, and Janet helped pay the cost. Last night he slipped on some urine on the stairs and broke his hip. Janet has now returned to St. Paul to assess the options for caring for her father when he is discharged from the hospital in approximately one week.

The Nyquists represent a typical elderly couple with a small social network and limited economic resources who are faced with trying to manage when one of them develops dementia. Mrs. Nyquist, although suspicious that her husband may have been developing dementia, did not share her concerns with anyone, not even her daughter. She was embarrassed by his behavior and was determined to not bring shame on the family or to "wash their dirty laundry" in public. She was committed to caring for her husband herself without involving any "outsiders." The neighborhood had changed over the last 40 years, so they no longer had close relationships with neighbors, and most of their friends and relatives had died or moved away. Their only remaining daughter lives in another state with her family. They did not have close ties with a church or other civic club.

The daughter, a long-distance caregiver, increased her visits and telephone calls in an effort to monitor the situation. Finally, seeing her mother's increasing exhaustion, she arranged for formal services, an Alzheimer adult day care with transportation. This arrangement provided respite for her mother and lasted for about 18 months. When Mr. Nyquist needed more assistance, she helped her mother find home care for two nights a week, which, while not enough, was all that they could afford. Janet continued to contribute financially to the costs, which now included incontinence pads, food supplements, and paraprofessional care—about $500 per month.

In addition to helping pay for health care costs, she also incurred the additional costs of air travel between Indianapolis and St. Paul and long-distance phone calls.

To manage the increasing visits to Minnesota, Janet was forced to cut her work hours from full time to part time. The situation finally reached a crisis point when Mr. Nyquist fell and fractured his hip. The hospital was eager to discharge him after a week, and it was clear that Mrs. Nyquist could not care for him at home without daily help. The family is now faced with quickly finding a nursing home placement. The Nyquists' life savings will be exhausted after approximately three months in a nursing home, and thus they are advised to seek a nursing home that accepts Medicaid reimbursement.

CHARACTERISTICS OF INFORMAL CAREGIVERS

Informal caregivers have often been referred to as the "backbone" of our long-term care (LTC) system because of the hours of assistance that they provide to family members (Feinberg and Pilisuk, 1999). The U.S. Department of Health and Human Services (USDHHS) (1998) predicted that about one in three Americans, or about 52 million persons, provides care each year for a family member. Wagner (1997) estimates that by the year 2007 the number of caregiving households could reach 39 million in the United States.

The National Alliance for Caregiving (NAC) and the American Association of Retired Persons (AARP) (1997) conducted the first telephone survey with oversampling of minorities to provide nationwide information on the magnitude, intensity, and types of caregiving. Caregiving was defined broadly as "providing unpaid care to a relative or friend who is aged 50 or older to help them take care of themselves." This definition included activities of daily living (ADLs) and instrumental activities of daily living (IADLs), as well as arranging for outside services and visiting regularly.

NAC/AARP (1997) developed an Index of Care based on a factor analysis of five questions that were designed to assess different aspects of the amount of care, intensity of care, or degree of difficulty of care involved in informal caregiving. The factor that emerged measured intensity of care and included the number of hours of care provided each week and the type of care provided. The five levels of care are shown in table 2.1.

The main results of the NAC/AARP (1997) survey of caregivers for elderly persons are shown in table 2.2. More than 20 percent of the caregivers said that they took care of someone with AD, confusion, dementia, or forgetfulness. This translates to an average of 5,020,000 households caring for persons with dementia. African American caregivers (28%) were most likely to report dementia in their care recipients, compared to Caucasians (22%), Hispanics (20%), and Asian caregivers at only 3 percent. Increased numbers of caregivers providing Level 4 and 5 care re-

TABLE 2.1
Levels of Informal Care Index

Level	Hours of Care Per Week	Type of Care
1	0–8	0 ADLs and ≤ 2 IADLs
2	9–20	0 ADLs and 2+ IADLs
3	21–40	0 ADLs and 2+ IADLs
4	41 or more	0–1 ADL with or without IADLs
5	41 hours to "constant care"	2+ ADLs with or without IADLs

SOURCE: Adapted from the National Alliance for Caregiving/AARP, 1997.

TABLE 2.2
NAC/AARP (1997) Survey of Caregivers of Elderly Persons

Caregivers caring for those with dementia	22%
Mean age of caregiver	45 years
Mean age of care recipient	78 years
Female	72%
Married	62%
Adult daughters	29%
Wives	23%
Husbands	14%
Sons	7%
Employed	64%
Average length of time caregiving	4.5 years
Provide care for more than five years	20%
Provide care for more than ten years	10%
Average number of hours caregiving	17.9 hours per week
Care for more than one person	31%
Sole caregiver	34%

ported that the care recipients had dementia as either a primary or a secondary problem.

It is generally accepted that women provide most family caregiving, regardless of the age of the care recipient or the cause of the disability. Approximately three-quarters of caregivers are women, mostly wives and daughters (NAC/AARP, 1997; Wagner, 1997). Reasons vary why women continue to provide the majority of family care, in spite of their heavy entry into the workplace. Gilligan (1982), in her book *In a Different Voice,* reported that women identified caring as a moral ideal. However, Wuest (2001), in her article on women's caring, points out that various social trends that emerged in the later part of the twentieth century help explain this phenomenon and its impact on women's lives. These include feminization of the labor force with increasing numbers of women assuming jobs as formal caregivers while continuing as informal caregivers at home (a double burden of caring), a shift toward personal responsibility for health while still holding women responsible for maintaining the health of their children and spouse (nutrition, preventative care appointments, etc.), and cost-cutting efforts that strive to replace formal care with informal care with little concern for the impact of these efforts on the family.

Wives are the caregivers of choice when they are available and able. In many instances, however, the care recipient is unmarried; in others the spouse is also frail and in need of care. Therefore, 29 percent of the caregivers are adult daughters, followed closely by wives (23%) (Stone, Cafferta, and Sangl, 1987). Fewer men have traditionally taken on the responsibility of caregiving (husbands 14% and sons 9%), although this is beginning to change. Siblings, grandchildren, aunts and uncles, nieces and nephews, friends and neighbors make up the remaining 26 percent (Stone, Cafferta, and Sangl, 1987). Adult children account for 42 percent of all caregivers of unmarried care recipients (McGarry, 1998). Spouses and adult children are the primary caregivers for persons with dementia because of the intensive, long-term commitment. Most caregivers provide care for one to four years. However, at least 20 percent provide care for five years or more. Of these, 10 percent have provided care for more than 10 years (NAC/AARP, 1997; Stone, Cafferta, and Sangl, 1987).

As the population ages and more women continue in the workplace, the number of male caregivers has been increasing. The percentage of men reporting in the National Long Term Care Survey that they were caregivers increased 50 percent between 1984 and 1994 (Spillman and Pezzin, 2000). Kramer (2002) reports that, in the general population, approximately one out of three caregivers is male. In an online survey of almost 1,400 caregivers at three Fortune 500 companies, Metlife Mature Market Institute (2003) found that men were almost as likely as women to be caregivers, and men were more likely to be long-distance caregivers (more than one hour from home). Men were as involved as women in providing instrumental activities of daily living (IADLs), such as providing transportation, doing grocery shopping, and managing medications. However, women were more likely to be involved in providing other IADLs, such as house cleaning, cooking, and laundry, and providing all activities of daily living (ADLs), including bathing, dressing, feeding, and toileting.

Caregiving typically occurs during middle age. In the NAC/AARP (1997) survey, 64 percent of the care recipients were over age 75, and 24 percent were over the age of 85: the mean age was 78 years. Caucasian caregivers provide care for the oldest individuals (x = 77.6 years), followed closely by African Americans, Hispanics, and Asians. While the average age of caregivers is 43, spousal caregivers average 55 years of age (USDHHS, 1998). Among caregivers of the frail elderly, the average age is 57 years, but 25 percent are between 65 and 75 years, and 10 percent are over age 75 (Stone, Cafferta, and Sangl, 1987). In the NAC/AARP (1997) study, caregivers over the age of 65 were more likely to be caring for a spouse and to be providing the highest level of care. Seventy percent of the caregivers who provided assistance with two or more ADLs and provided care for 40 or more hours per week reported living in the same house as the care recipient. This is the group of caregivers most likely to be caring for persons with dementia, and husbands were well represented among this group of caregivers (Fitting, Rabins, Lucas, and Eastham, 1986).

In the NAC/AARP (1997) survey, approximately two-thirds of the caregivers were married; African American caregivers were least likely to report being married (51%). More than 50 percent of the African American, Hispanic, and Asian caregivers reported having children under the age of 18 in their households, compared to 38 percent of the Caucasian caregivers. "Sandwich generation" is a term used to refer to caregivers who provide care to an older family member while still having responsibility for a child under the age of 18 (Spillman and Pezzin, 2000). Approximately 20 to 40 percent of caregivers fall into this category. Sixty-nine percent of the caregivers in the NAC/AARP (1997) study cared for only one person; the Asian and African American caregivers were more likely to provide care for more than one family member.

Caregivers cross the entire income distribution. The survey by the Lewin Group found that approximately one-quarter of the caregivers have family incomes of less than $20,000; two out of five have moderate incomes ($20,000 to $50,000); about one-third have annual incomes above $50,000 (Alecxih, Zeruld, and Olearczyk, 1998). However, one study concluded that the caregiving time burden fell more heavily on women with incomes at or below the national median of $35,000; 52 percent of these women caregivers spent 20 hours or more each week providing care (The Commonwealth Fund, 1999).

Minority families are more likely to be engaged in caregiving than Caucasian families (NAC/AARP, 1997). However, although minority caregivers may proportionally provide more care in the home than Caucasian families, they may be more reticent to acknowledge that their family member has dementia. In some cultures, dementia carries a stigma and may bring shame to the family (Yeo and Gallagher-Thompson, 1996). Asian and Hispanic families may avoid talking about aberrant behaviors or identifying their caregiving role as burdensome (Mahoney, 2003). In many languages, such as Italian, there is no word for burden at all.

THE ROLE OF INFORMAL CAREGIVERS

Caregivers fill many roles: care provider, treatment monitor, care manager, advocate, friend and counselor, homemaker, and information seeker and communicator. What caregivers do is frequently measured by the number of ADLs with which they assist, the number of hours that they report providing care, their ability to leave the care recipient for periods of time, the presence or absence of other caregivers, and the length of time that they have provided care (Kasper, Steinbach, and Andrews, 1994). On average, caregivers report spending 17.9 hours per week providing care. Women report spending, on average, 18.8 hours per week in caregiving activities, in contrast to 15.5 hours per week for men. However, this varies from less than one hour to "constant care." Twenty percent (4.5 million out of 22.4 million) of caregivers providing care for very impaired older adults spend more than 40 hours per week (NAC/AARP, 1997). The average number of hours spent providing care for care recipients with complex and dementia-related needs is 56.5 hours per week.

Feinberg (2002) notes that one of the neglected areas of caregiver assessment is that of the actual tasks performed by family caregivers beyond personal care functions (i.e., ADLs). Eighty-one percent of the caregivers reported assisting with three or more IADLs, including transportation, grocery shopping, household chores, meals, finances, medications, and arranging and supervising outside services. Men and women generally report doing these IADLs in similar numbers, but women were more likely to do the housework and prepare meals (Metlife Mature Market Institute, 2003). Family income does appear to influence who does IADLs. Caregivers with annual incomes under $15,000 were more likely to do housekeeping and prepare meals, while caregivers with incomes over $50,000 were more likely to hire and supervise outside help and to help with finances (NAC/AARP, 1997).

The actual tasks that caregivers perform for persons with AD vary according to the stage of the disease. In the early phase, the caregiver's tasks may be related to learning more about the disease, planning for future needs, providing supervision, and organizing the legal, financial, and household responsibilities. As the disease progresses, these important parts of family life will be able to continue uninterrupted. During the middle phase of the disease, caregivers assume increasing responsibilities for managing the household, arranging for medical and personal care, and ensuring that the environment is safe. During this stage, the family caregivers must assume responsibility for all IADLs and increasingly supervise or assist with ADLs, such as bathing, dressing, grooming, toileting, and feeding. Caregivers also carry out medical procedures that require specialized techniques and equipment, such as administering oxygen, giving tube feedings, and administering injections. They are often the only person available to monitor the care recipient's response to treatment and to report changing health conditions. During the final phase of AD, the care recipient is totally dependent on the caregiver for all daily needs. In their study, Kasper and colleagues (1994) found that providing assistance with three to six ADLs and not being able to leave the care recipient alone was associated with the termination of informal caregiving at home, although longer-term caregivers and, especially spouses, were more likely to continue to provide care even in overwhelming situations. Cognitive impairment of the care recipient was a major underlying reason for needing assistance and supervision with more than three ADLs, and for not being able to leave the person alone.

Other major roles of informal caregivers are those of information seekers and care managers; they arrange for the purchase, delivery, and payment of special supplies and equipment, hire and manage home care workers, and arrange for services like adult day care or other social services. They act as patient advocates by seeking second opinions, pushing to have problems addressed, making decisions about treatment options and living arrangements. In one research study, 51 caregivers (primarily wives and daughters) and 51 care recipients with cognitive impairment living in the community were interviewed regarding their choices of care for everyday assistance (Feinberg, Whitlatch, and Tucke, 2000). More than 80 percent of the caregivers reported using some paid services since the memory problems had begun. The most used services were illness information (65%), support groups (55%), and help with IADLs (53%). The least used services were Internet information (14%), caregiver education classes (25%), and help managing financial and legal issues (22%). These findings are consistent with a follow-up telephone survey of baby boom women that reported 82 percent had sought information on caregiving during the preceding year, particularly if there had been a change in the care recipient's condition. The most valuable information that they received was related to the care recipient's illness, treatment, care, ADLs, comfort and safety, drug administration and side effects. Forty-five percent of the women said that the most valuable information came from doctors, nurses, or hospitals, 14 percent from friends, relatives, and other caregivers, and 12 percent from health and human services agencies (NAC, 1998). To carry out their caregiving duties, more than 70 percent of the caregiving women said that information on dealing with the stresses of caregiving, finding and evaluating in-home health-related services and services related to daily care, practical "hands on" training, and balancing caregiving with family and work were important (NAC, 1998).

Caregiver vigilance is a term that describes much of what informal caregivers for persons with dementia do in their caregiving role. Some researchers have reported that caregiver tasks include surveillance, control, and vigilance to prevent those with AD from harming themselves or others (Aneshensel et al., 1995). Mahoney (2003) used an Internet chat room to obtain descriptions of caregiver vigilance. When the analysis of 566 messages between caregivers had been analyzed, she found that while tasks varied according to the stage of the disease, vigilance threaded through all stages. Data were reduced into the following five categories: (1) watchful supervising, (2) protective intervening, (3) anticipating, (4) being on duty, and (5) being there.

The definition that emerged was, "Vigilance in AD caregiving is defined as the caregiver continually overseeing the CR's (care recipient's) activities" (Mahoney, 2003, p. 28). When caregivers are vigilant, they are supervising, anticipating, managing disruptive behaviors, and initiating protective measures, many of the tasks mentioned by other authors.

To help understand the process by which caregivers manage caregiving tasks and marshal resources, Wuest (2001) developed a middle range theory of "precarious ordering," which she defines as "a process of setting limits on caring demands, altering environmental conditions, and reorganizing caring activities such that fraying connections are minimized" (p. 189). In her theory, she suggests ways that women negotiate with the formal system by using strategies such as reframing their responsibility, harnessing resources, and becoming an expert. By learning about the formal system and networking with the informal system, caregivers try to understand and maximize the assistance available to them and their care recipients.

Although most caregivers report that they share caregiving tasks with another family member, 34 percent of those who provide the most intensive, time-consuming care for persons with complex and dementia-related problems report that no one else helps them (NAC/AARP, 1997). Sixty-one percent of Asian caregivers and 54 percent of Hispanic caregivers feel that other relatives do their "fair share," compared to only 49 percent of Caucasian and 43 percent of African American caregivers. Only 35 percent of caregivers who help with three or more ADLs use any formal home care and only 5.4% rely solely on formal care (USDHHS, 1998).

WORK FORCE PARTICIPATION OF INFORMAL CAREGIVERS

About two-thirds (64%) of family caregivers are employed outside of the home (USDHHS, 1998). The number of older women, traditionally the family caregivers involved, continues to increase. Caregivers who are working women age 55 and older are projected to increase by 52 percent between 2000 and 2010, from 6.4 million to 10.1 million (Francese, 2003). About 14.4 million full and part-time caregivers juggle caregiving and job responsibilities at any given time (Metropolitan Life Insurance, 1999). The literature on the relationship between caregiving and labor supply has been mixed. Johnson and Lo Sasso (2000) investigated this question using longitudinal data from the Health and Retirement Study (HRS). They found that 60 percent of the women between the ages of 53 and 63, with at least one living parent, were working for pay, and 26 percent of them provided help to a parent. However, the work-force participation did decrease to 40 percent among women whose parents could not be left alone. Johnson and Lo Sasso (2000) found that men were much less likely to provide assistance to parents, with only 15 percent of men reporting that they had helped with ADLs, errands, or chores. However, this percent increased for men older than 55 years of age whose parents needed help with personal care. In contrast to women, there were significant differences in the percentage of working men and nonworking men who provided care to parents (14% versus 20%). Between the HRS panels in 1992 and 2000, the percentage of men and women who reported helping their parents increased.

Johnson and Lo Sasso's (2000) findings that the provision of care for elderly parents may compromise men and women's ability to work full-time during their mid-life years (53–63) is consistent with the findings from the NAC/AARP (1997) survey and the Metropolitan Life Insurance Company report (1999). When women or men spent 100 hours per year (average 2 hours per week) helping their parents with ADLs or errands or chores, they reduced their labor supply by 460 hours per year. The NAC/AARP (1997) survey also demonstrated a significant correlation between the level of care provided by the caregiver and work-related modifications, including altering the daily schedule, taking a leave of absence, or giving up work entirely. Thirty percent of caregivers providing 40 or more hours of care per week reported quitting work entirely due to caregiving responsibilities, and 26 percent took a leave of absence. Caring for a person with dementia who lived in the same household was associated with high levels of caregiving and work-related adjustments (Feinberg and Whitlatch, 1995). The NAC/AARP (1997) survey reported that about 10 percent of retired caregivers took early retirement or quit work altogether because of caregiving responsibilities; 32 percent of caregivers providing intensive care on a daily basis were retired. Employed caregivers who were caring for elders who had long-term care insurance were almost twice as likely to stay in the workplace than those caring for uninsured elders (Metropolitan Life Insurance, 1997). These caregivers did not provide less time in caring, but they reported more "quality time" and less need to do hands-on care like bathing and grooming. The caregivers of elders with LTC insurance reported that caregiving interfered less with their emotional and social health.

Johnson and Lo Sasso (2000) reported that adult children were more likely to help their parents if the parents were in poor health and if the parents lacked alternative sources of social support, like a spouse or other children. The adult children's competing time demands did not appear to deter them from providing caregiving support to their parents. In summary, they found that "the provision of care appears to be determined primarily by the needs of the parents, while the ease with which children can fulfill those needs plays only a secondary role" (p. 27). While relatively few caregivers report family conflicts about caregiving responsibilities, employed caregivers (24%) are more likely to experience family conflict over caregiving than unemployed caregivers (16%) (FCA, 1998).

THE COST OF INFORMAL CAREGIVING

The availability of a family caregiver is often the determining factor in whether or not persons with dementia will be maintained in their own homes or be placed in nursing homes. In fact, 50 percent of the elderly persons who need LTC but have no available family are in nursing homes, compared to only 7 percent who have a family caregiver (U.S. Administration on Aging, 2000). In recent years, some policy makers have begun to realize that family caregiving for disabled elders can save public dollars that might be spent on nursing home care (Feinberg, Newman, and Von Steenberg, 2002). In the United States, most LTC is provided by informal caregivers at no cost to the public (Arno, Levine, and Memmott, 1999; NAC, 1997; Tennstedt, Crawford, and McKinlay, 1993). The value of informal care has been estimated at $257 billion nationally, compared to home care ($32 billion) and nursing home care ($92 billion) (Arno, 2002). Direct and indirect costs of caregiving for AD are estimated at $100 billion, with the average lifetime cost for an individual with AD estimated at $174,000 (FCA, 2003). Max, Webber, and Fox (1995) estimated the cost of caring for a person with AD at home at $47,083 per year (1990 dollars). Institutionalizing a person with dementia, however, does not mean that the cost to the family disappears. Nursing home residents and their families finance, on average, about 31 percent of all nursing home expenditures, and the expectation is that by 2030 their share will grow to be about 48 percent (Friedland and Summer, 1999). However, when families are able to prolong the length of time that the frail elder is cared for at home, there are substantial savings to the formal health care system. Leon, Cheng, and Neumann (1998) estimated that an annual savings of $1.12 billion in formal costs could be achieved by delaying the placement of people with AD into a nursing home by just one month.

Studies continue to show that the cost of caregiving can be higher than previously recognized for informal caregivers (Max, Webber, and Fox, 1995; Metlife Mature Market Institute, 2003). The loss of 459 annual work hours for women translates into a loss of $7,800 in actual wages (1994 dollars) (Johnson and Lo Sasso, 2000). Because families of persons with AD often care for their family members over many years, their financial burden is particularly heavy. The Metlife Study (2003) of working caregivers reported that 48 percent of the men and 42 percent of the women contributed financial support—an average of $273 per month or nearly $3,300 per year in out-of-pocket expenses—to the care recipient. Caregivers who cut back on their work-force participation lose not just current wages but also retire-ment savings because they contribute fewer credits toward future Social Security and private pension benefits. Women, in particular, often sacrifice future economic security because of caregiving responsibilities. According to the Social Security Ad-ministration (2002), women caregivers are likely to spend an average of 12 years out of the work force raising children and caring for an older relative or friend. Infor-mal caregivers are estimated to lose an average of $25,494 in Social Security bene-fits, $67,202 in pension benefits, and an average of $656,000 in lost wages, pensions, and Social Security benefits (Metropolitan Life Insurance, 1999). While policy mak-ers have expressed concern about the costs of caring for frail elderly persons, their focus has been on the costs to the formal system, not the costs that families are bearing or the threat to their present and future economic stability.

FORMAL CAREGIVERS

Changes in reproductive and family patterns during the last two decades, com-bined with the feminization of the work force in the late twentieth century, have led to smaller nuclear and extended families, increasingly mobile families, and more working women (Alecxih, Zeruld, and Olearczyk, 1998), thus increasing the demand for formal caregivers. The need for adequately trained LTC health care providers is urgent. At present no health care profession has enough geriatric-trained personnel to adequately address the unique health care needs of persons with functional limi-tations, AD, or other dementias (USDHHS, 1998).

Formal caregivers are an essential component of the LTC system, assisting infor-mal caregivers to provide quality care in the home and assuming the major caregiv-ing role in residential settings when informal caregivers are not available or are over-whelmed with the increasing demands of care. Most formal caregiving for persons with dementia occurs in nursing homes. While figures vary widely, the U.S. Centers for Medicare and Medicaid Services (2001) estimate the U.S. work force in nursing homes to be 137,000 registered nurses (RNs), 22,000 to 27,000 licensed practical nurses (LPNs), and 181,000 to 310,000 nursing assistants (USDHHS, 2002). The average num-ber of RNs per nursing home bed is 0.06; for-profit homes have the lowest average at 0.05. Total employees per bed equals 0.88, with the highest percentage being nursing assistants (0.41) (AHCA, 1991; Health Care Compensations Services, 1994).

Nurses make up the largest formal health care work force. In March 2000, ap-proximately 2.7 million persons were estimated to have licenses to practice as RNs in this country; it is estimated that 82 percent of nurses with active licenses are ac-tually employed in nursing (USDHHS, 2002). Of all RNs employed in nursing in

2000, 6.9 percent worked in nursing homes and extended care facilities. The RN population is aging, with an average age of 45.2 in the year 2000; an estimated 5.4 percent of the RN population are men (USDHHS, 2002). The aging RN work force reflects fewer young nurses entering the RN population, large cohorts of the RN population moving into their fifties and sixties, and women entering basic nursing education programs at a later age. Among all nursing employment settings, RNs in nursing homes receive the lowest annual wage and report the lowest level of overall job satisfaction (USDHHS, 2002).

Licensed practical (vocational) nurses (LPNs) held about 700,000 jobs in 2000. The U.S. Bureau of Labor Statistics (2001) estimated that about 29 percent of LPNs (208,000) worked in nursing homes and about 43,000 were employed in the home health care industry. The need is expected to grow through 2010, and nursing homes are expected to offer the most new jobs for LPNs.

Paraprofessionals perform the most direct, intimate tasks in nursing homes and private homes. There are approximately two million of these front-line workers (home health aides, nursing aides, orderlies and attendants, and personal and home care aides); approximately 750,000 nursing assistants work in nursing homes (U.S. Bureau of Labor Statistics, 2001). The typical paraprofessional caregiver is a single mother with a high school degree, or less, living near the poverty line. Approximately 35 percent of paraprofessionals are African American and at least 10 percent are from socioeconomically disadvantaged backgrounds; 20 percent do not have a high school education (Paraprofessional Healthcare Institute, 2003). Wuest (2001) found that when the women's culture is different from the culture of the person for whom they care, the women were marginalized by the difference in ethnicity, race, sexual orientation, and socioeconomic status. These cultural differences are often at play in our long-term care settings, where Caucasian care recipients are still the majority. Indeed, many of these workers are also stigmatized by the type of work that they do (Stone and Wiener, 2001).

Primarily women, these workers are largely confined to nonunionized, low-paying, low-status jobs with no career advancement (Wuest, 2001). They do physically heavy and emotionally draining work at near minimum wage. In 2000, the median wage of home care workers was $8.23 per hour, leaving "many women working, yet impoverished" (Paraprofessional Healthcare Institute, 2003, p. 1). The median annual income of all nursing home paraprofessionals in 2000 was $13,287 and the median for home care paraprofessionals was only $12,265 per year (U.S. General Accounting Office, 2001). The rate for being uninsured is as high as 70 percent among these workers (Stone and Weiner, 2001; Konrad and Morgan, 2002). Many paraprofessionals are themselves informal as well as formal caregivers, with insufficient money to hire domestic help for themselves, suggesting that they experience a double burden of caregiving.

Given the realities of the work environment, it is no surprise that LTC providers are reporting record-level vacancies and turnover rates of 45 to more than 100 percent for paraprofessional jobs (Stone and Weiner, 2001). Konrad and Morgan (2002) reported that annual turnover rates for nursing assistants in the year 2000 for residential facilities were more than twice as high as for nonresidential settings. They reported turnover rates for nursing homes of 100 percent and for adult care homes of 119 percent, compared to home health care agencies of 53 percent and hospices of 40 percent.

THE CRISIS IN CAREGIVING

Socioeconomic and demographic trends are placing increasing stress on our informal and formal care system. Declining mortality rates have led to increases in the elderly population, particularly the oldest old. In addition, although the rates of disability are decreasing (Manton, Corder, and Stallard, 1993), the actual number of individuals with disability continues to rise. The incidence of AD increases with age, rising to as high as 45 percent after the age of 85. The population over the age of 85 is now 33 times larger than in 1900. By 2040, there will be almost four times as many people over 85 as there were in 1999 (U.S. Bureau of Census, 1999).

Just as the demand for help is rising dramatically, the supply of available caregivers is shrinking (Brown, 2002). Coincidentally, the fertility rates have fallen, producing fewer new family caregivers. In 1990 there were 11 informal caregivers for every older person receiving care, but by 2030 the ratio will be 6:1 (FCA, 2000). At the same time, increasing numbers of women, the traditional informal caregivers, have returned to work (Johnson and Lo Sasso, 2000; Stone and Kemper, 1990).

As the population ages and LTC becomes one of the major issues facing the country, policy makers have expressed concerns that funding more programs to assist families will result in families abandoning their responsibilities and relying totally on the formal care system. This has been referred to as the "out of the woodwork" phenomenon, which implies that even families who would have ordinarily cared for a sick family member at home will now in large numbers resort to placement, thus overwhelming formal systems of care. Research, however, has not supported the existence of this phenomenon (Institute for Health and Aging, 1998; Montgomery and Borgatta, 1989; Tennstedt et al., 1993; Whitlatch, Feinberg, and Sebesta, 1997). To the contrary, Feinberg (1999) and others have reported that informal caregivers tend to use formal services only as a last resort. As shown in table 2.3, large numbers of family

TABLE 2.3
*Characteristics of Informal and Formal Caregivers in Long-term Care (LTC)
and Their Work Settings*

Variable	Family Caregivers	Paraprofessionals	Registered Nurses
Supply (in numbers)	22.4 million[a]	2,000,000[b]	258,000[b]
Proportion women	75%[a]	>90%[b]	>94%[c]
Proportion minority	24%	45–50%[e]	12%[c]
	27% Hispanic		
	29% African American		
	32%[d]		
Mean age	46 years[a]	37–41 years[b]	45.2 years[c]
Annual salary	0	$13,287[b]	$43,779[c]
Health insurance benefits	0	32%[f]	97%[c]
Retention rate	average 4.5 years[a]	0–50%/year[g]	50–80%/year[b]
Vacancy rate	NA	11.7%[h]	13–20%[e]
Projected new caregivers needed by 2010	17 million[i]	780,000[b]	561,000[b]

NOTE: Includes caregivers in private homes, group homes, adult day care programs, assisted living facilities, and nursing homes.

[a]National Alliance for Caregiving and American Association for Retired Persons, 1997

[b]Paraprofessional Healthcare Institute, 2003

[c]USDHHS, 2002

[d]Family Caregiver Alliance, 2001

[e]U.S. General Accounting Office, 2001

[f]Konrad and Morgan, 2002

[g]Stone and Wiener, 2001

[h]American Health Care Association, 1991

[i]Wagner, 1997

members provide care without compensation for long periods of time. The supply of informal and formal caregivers, traditionally drawn from a pool of women aged 25 to 54, is falling after decades of steady growth (U.S. Bureau of Census, 1999). These shortages in formal and informal caregivers are expected to increase and are widely acknowledged by the media, by state and federal policymakers, and by the LTC industry to threaten the quality of life for older Americans (Family Caregiver Alliance, 2000; Institute for Health and Aging, 1996; Select Committee on Aging, 1993; Paraprofessional Healthcare Institute, 2003; USDHHS, 1998).

Difficulty in recruiting and retaining qualified personnel to provide LTC remains a critical problem, as seen in the retention and vacancy rates for the major direct-care providers in table 2.3. In a recent assessment of the adequacy of health care personnel in various states, the U.S. Department of Health and Human Services (USDHHS, 1990) identified nursing as one of four occupations that most frequently posed supply problems. The major reason for the dearth of RNs in nursing homes is economic, with federal and state regulations requiring very few RNs and with salaries of nursing home nurses always lagging behind the salaries of other nurses, typically at least a $4 hourly discrepancy (AHCA, 1991; USDHHS, 1987).

The low pay, poor training, and meager prospects for advancement are largely responsible for the alarming retention and vacancy rates shown in table 2.3 for paraprofessionals. However, Brannon and colleagues (2002) also demonstrated a relationship between management strategies, environment, and turnover rates. Low turnover among nursing assistants was significantly associated with facilities that had low RN turnover, supervisors trained in management, administrators with fewer middle managers to supervise, and union organizations for nursing assistants.

IMPLICATIONS FOR CLINICAL PRACTICE

1. *Develop partnerships between the health care team, individuals with dementia, and their informal caregivers.* Informal caregivers, particularly family members, provide the majority of personal care to persons with dementia in our society. They can provide the health care team with valuable information about care recipients' health status, their behaviors, and their responses to treatments. Unfortunately, caregivers often feel that their input is not welcome, or worse yet, they feel discounted by the health care system. Persons with dementia will receive optimal care when the informal caregivers understand the disease, work closely with the providers to adapt their approaches to the stage of the disease, and modify the environment to meet the individuals' needs. This is most likely to happen when the caregivers receive education from the provider, feel valued for their unique perspective, and are encouraged to share their observations with the team. This may require separate meetings with the informal caregivers, identifying a consistent staff member to triage telephone calls, or referring informal caregivers to special educational groups hosted by organizations, such as the Red Cross or the Alzheimer's Association.

2. *Monitor the changing course of the disease and help the informal caregiver access the resources needed to provide optimal care through the different stages of the disease.* Dementia is a dynamic and changing disease, requiring different skills and resources at different times. Most family members have not had previous experience with a person with dementia and so are not well prepared to anticipate their changing needs. The health care team can provide valuable assistance by including an assessment of the caregivers' health status, skills, emotional well-being, informal network, financial resources, and preferences for care at least twice a year. The professionals should provide written information on local resources, such as support groups, in-home services, and adult day care services, as well as assisted living and nursing home services when appropriate. If the caregiver does not bring up the

topic, professionals need to be sensitive to the time when these topics need to be discussed, and give caregivers permission to seek help.

3. *Promote public policies that generate incentives for family members to provide comprehensive home care for elders with dementia, grants and scholarships to educate geriatric professionals and paraprofessionals, and a fair wage with benefits for nurses and nursing assistants who provide direct care to persons with dementia.* The high turnover in the health care system causes discontinuity in relationships between care recipients and informal and formal caregivers, increases the costs of recruitment and training, and negatively impacts the quality of care provided to the most vulnerable elders needing care. Formal and informal caregivers provide care that is physically exhausting and emotionally draining with few financial incentives. The United States is on the verge of a national shortage of informal and formal caregivers of epidemic proportions that will require a long-term, broad-based, public and private commitment to LTC financing reform (Paraprofessional Healthcare Institute, 2003). Assuring quality of care for all of our citizens will involve making educational programs for professionals and paraprofessionals who care for the vulnerable elderly a priority, reducing the wage and benefit discrimination that currently exists between LTC and acute care, and providing incentives for family members to provide LTC for their relatives at home.

REFERENCES

AARP. 2001. AARP Caregiver Identification Study (www.RESEARCH.AARP.org).

Alecxih, L. M. B., Zeruld, S., and Olearczyk, B. 1998. *Characteristics of caregivers based on the survey of income and program participation.* NFCSP: Selected Issue Briefs.

American Health Care Association (AHCA). 1991. *AHCA issue and data book for the United States Congress.* Washington, D.C.: American Health Care Association.

Aneshensel, C. S., Pearlin, L., Mullan, J., Zarit, S., and Whitlatch, C. 1995. *Profiles in caregiving: The unexpected career.* San Diego: Academic Press.

Arno, P. S. 2002. The economic value of informal care U.S. 2000. Updated figures. Presented at the American Association for Geriatric Psychiatry Meeting, Orlando, Fla., February 24, 2002. (In Feinberg, Newman, and Von Steenberg, 2002).

Arno, P. S., Levine C., and Memmott, M. M. 1999. The economic value of informal caregiving. *Health Affairs* 18:182–88.

Brannon, D., Zinn, J., S., Mor, V., and Davis, J. 2002. An exploration of job, organizational, and environmental factors associated with high and low nursing assistant turnover. *Gerontologist* 42:159–68.

Brown, N. P. 2002. A crisis in caregiving: Longer-range solutions for long term care. *Harvard Magazine* 104(3):24A.

Family Caregiver Alliance. 1998. *Analysis of caregiver resource center statewide assessment database, January–June 1997.* San Francisco: Family Caregiver Alliance.

Family Caregiver Alliance. March 1998. *Selected caregiver statistics: Fact sheet.* San Francisco: Family Caregiver Alliance.

Family Caregiver Alliance. 2000. *An invitational state policy conference proceedings.* San Francisco: Family Caregiver Alliance.

Family Caregiver Alliance. 2003. *Fact sheet: Alzheimer's disease.* www.caregiver.org/factsheets/alzheimersC.html. Accessed 8/24/2003.

Feinberg, L. F. August 1997. *Options for supporting informal and family caregiving: A policy paper.* San Francisco: American Society on Aging.

Feinberg, L. F. September 2002. *The state of the art: Caregiver assessment in practice settings.* San Francisco: Family Caregiver Alliance.

Feinberg, L. F., Newman, S. L., and Van Steenberg, C. 2002. *Family caregiver support: Policies, perceptions, and practices in ten states since passage of the national family caregiver support program.* San Francisco: Family Caregiver Alliance.

Feinberg, L. F., and Pilisuk, T. L. October 1999. *Survey of fifteen states' caregiver support programs: Final report.* San Francisco: Family Caregiver Alliance.

Feinberg, L. F., and Whitlatch, C. J. August 1995. *A study of pre-and post-placement family caregiving for individuals with Alzheimer's disease and related disorders: Final report.* San Francisco: Family Caregiver Alliance.

Feinberg, L. F., Whitlatch, C. J., and Tucke, S. May 2000. *Making hard choices: Respecting both voices: Final report.* San Francisco: Family Caregiver Alliance.

Fitting, M., Rabins, P., Lucas, M. J., and Eastham, J. 1986. Caregivers for dementia patients: A Comparison of husbands and wives. *Gerontologist* 26:248–52.

Francese, P. March 2003. Trend ticker: Investing in demographics. *American Demographics.*

Friedland, R. B., and Summer, L. January 1999. *Demography is not destiny.* Washington, D.C.: National Academy on an Aging Society.

Gilligan, C. 1982/1993. *In a different voice.* Cambridge, Mass.: Harvard University Press.

Health Care Compensations Services. 1994. *A graphic comparison of registered and licensed practical nurses in nursing homes, home care agencies and hospitals.* Oakland, N.J.: HCS.

Health Resources and Services Administration, USDHHS. 1998. *Full national agenda for geriatric education: White papers.* Rockville, Md.: Health Resources and Services Administration.

Institute for Health and Aging, University of California at San Francisco. August 1996. *Chronic care in America: A twenty-first century challenge.* Princeton, N.J.: The Robert Wood Johnson Foundation.

Institute for Health and Aging, University of California at San Francisco. October 1998. *Medicare Alzheimer's disease demonstration evaluation.* San Francisco: University of California–San Francisco.

Johnson, R. W., and Lo Sasso, A. T. February 7, 2000. *The trade-off between paid employment and time assistance to elderly parents at midlife.* Washington, D.C.: The Urban Institute.

Kasper, J. D., Steinbach, U., and Andrews, J. 1994. Caregiver role appraisal and caregiver tasks as factors in ending caregiving. *Journal of Aging and Health* 6(3):397–414.

Konrad, T. R., and Morgan, J. C. 2002. *Workforce improvement for nursing assistants: Supporting training, education, and payment for upgrading performance.* Chapel Hill, N.C.: North Carolina Department of Health and Human Services, Division of Facility Services, and the North Carolina Institute on Aging.

Kramer, B. J. 2002. Men caregivers: An overview. In B. J. Kramer and E. H. Thompson (Eds.), *Men as caregivers: Theory, research and service implications* (pp. 3–19). New York: Springer Publishing Co.

Leon, J., Cheng, C., and Neumann, P. J. December 1998. Alzheimer's disease care: Costs and potential savings. *Health Affairs* 17:206–16.

Mahoney, D. F. 2003. Vigilance: Evolution and definition of caregivers of family members with Alzheimer's disease. *Journal of Gerontological Nursing* 29(8):24–30.

Manton, K. G., Corder, L., and Stallard, L. 1997. Chronic disability trends in elderly United States populations 1982–1994. *Proceedings of the National Academy of Sciences* 94(6):2593–98.

Max, W., Webber, P., and Fox, P. 1995. Alzheimer's disease: The unpaid burden of caring. *Journal of Aging and Health* 7:179–99.

McGarry, K. 1998. Caring for the elderly: The role of adult children. In D. A. Wise (Ed.), *Frontiers in economics of aging* (pp. 133–63). Chicago: University of Chicago Press.

Metlife Mature Market Institute. 2001. *The Metlife study of employed caregivers: Does long term care insurance make a difference.* Westport, Conn.: Mature Market Institute MetLife.

Metlife Mature Market Institute. 2003. *The Metlife study of sons at work: Balancing employment and eldercare.* Westport, Conn.: Mature Market Institute MetLife.

Metropolitan Life Insurance Company. 1997. *The Metlife study of employer costs for working caregivers.* New York: Metropolitan Life Insurance Company.

Metropolitan Life Insurance Company. 1999. *The Metlife juggling act study: Balancing caregiving with work and the costs involved.* New York: Metropolitan Life Insurance Company.

Montgomery, R. V. J., and Borgatta, E. F. 1989. The effects of alternative support strategies on family caregiving. *Gerontologist* 29:457–64.

National Alliance for Caregiving (NAC). 1998. *The caregiving boom: Baby boomer women providing care.* San Francisco: NAC.

National Alliance for Caregiving (NAC) and AARP. 1997. *Family caregiving in the US: Findings from a national survey.* Washington, D.C.: NAC.

Paraprofessional Healthcare Institute. 2003. *Long-term care financing and the long-term care workforce crisis: Causes and solutions.* Washington, D.C.: Citizens for Long Term Care.

Select Committee on Aging. 1993. *Shortage of health care professionals caring for the elderly: Recommendations for change.* Washington, D.C.: Government Printing Office (Comm. Pub. No. 102–915).

Spillman, B. C., and Pezzin, L. C. 2000. Potential and active family caregivers: Changing networks and the "sandwich generation." *Milbank Quarterly* 78:347–74.

Stone, R. I., Cafferta, G. I., and Sangl, J. 1987. Caregivers of the frail elderly: A national profile. *Gerontologist* 27:616–26.

Stone, R. I., and Kemper, P. 1990. Spouses and children of disabled elders: How large a constituency for long-term care reform? *Milbank Quarterly* 67(3):485–96.

Stone, R. I. and Wiener, J. M. 2001. *Who will care for us? Addressing the long-term care workforce crisis.* Washington, D.C.: Urban Institute.

Tennstedt, S. L., Crawford, S. O. L., and McKinlay, J. B. 1993. Is family care on the decline? A longitudinal investigation of the substitution of formal long-term care for informal care. *Milbank Quarterly* 71:601–24.

The Commonwealth Fund. May 1999. *Informal caregiving* (Fact Sheet). New York: The Commonwealth Fund.

U.S. Administration on Aging. Fall 2000. *America's families care: A report on the needs of America's family caregivers.* Washington, D.C.: U.S. Administration on Aging.

U.S. Bureau of the Census. 1999. *Population division, international programs center, international data base.* Washington, D.C.: Government Printing Office.

U.S. Bureau of Labor Statistics. 2001. *National occupational employment and wage estimates for 2000.* Washington, D.C.: Bureau of Labor Statistics.

U.S. Centers for Medicare and Medicaid Services. Winter 2001. *Appropriateness of minimum nurse staffing ratios in nursing homes: Phase II final report.* Cambridge, Mass.: Abt Associates.

U.S. Department of Health and Human Services (USDHHS). 1987. *Analysis of the environment for the recruitment and retention of registered nurses in nursing homes.* Rockville, Md.: Health Resources and Services Administration.

U.S. Department of Health and Human Services (USDHHS). 1990. *States' assessment of health personnel shortages: Issues and concerns.* Rockville, Md.: Health Resources and Services Administration (DHHS No. HRS-'P-OD 90-6).

U.S. Department of Health and Human Services (USDHHS). 1998. *Informal caregiving: Compassion in action.* Washington, D.C.: Office of the Assistant Secretary for Planning an Evaluation and The Administration on Aging (data sources: 1987 and 1992 National Surveys of Families and Households).

U.S. Department of Health and Human Services (USDHHS). 2002. *The registered nurse population: Findings from the national sample survey of registered nurses.* Rockville, Md.: USDHHS, Public Health Service, Bureau of Health Professions.

U.S. General Accounting Office. 2001. *Nursing workforce: Recruitment and retention of nurses and nurse aides is a growing concern,* GAO-01-750T. Washington, D.C.: U.S. General Accounting Office.

U.S. Social Security Administration. February 2002. *Women and social security* (Fact Sheet). Washington, D.C.: U.S. Social Security Administration.

Wagner, D. June 1997. *Comparative analysis of caregiver data for caregivers to the elderly: 1987 and 1997.* Bethesda, Md.: National Alliance for Caregiving.

Whitlatch, C. J., Feinberg, L. F., and Sebesta, D. S. 1997. Depression and health in family caregivers: Adaptations over time. *Journal of Aging and Health* 9:222–45.

Wuest, J. 2001. Precarious ordering: Toward a formal theory of women's caring. *Health Care for Women International* 22:167–93.

Yeo, G., and Gallagher-Thompson, G. (Eds.). 1996. *Ethnicity and the dementias.* Washington, D.C.: Taylor & Francis.

CHAPTER THREE

From Home to Nursing Home

A Continuum of Care for Persons with Dementia

IRVING HELLMAN, PH.D.

> Old people just grow lonesome,
> Waiting for someone to say,
> Hello in there, Hello . . .
>
> —*John Prine*

The process of aging and caregiving involves transitions along a continuum of higher levels of care. In the case of persons with dementia, these transitions typically follow predictable stages that require action and coping on the part of the patients and their caregivers. Persons with dementia, their families, and health care professionals struggle with a relentless, irreversible, and progressive neurological syndrome. As our population ages, the incidence and prevalence of various dementias will increase in the absence of new methods for preventing or reversing this disease. Alzheimer disease (AD), the most frequent cause of dementia in developed Western countries, can last from 2 to 20 years. Over time, adults with dementia invariably develop both cognitive and functional impairments that predispose them to behavioral symptoms and the loss of intellectual capacity, personality functioning, and the ability to communicate their wishes.

The impact of making and implementing decisions to provide higher levels of care is often subtle but profound for the elder patient, family members, and formal caregivers. For elders, these transitions dictate the final chapter of their lives and shape where and how they live, what they do, whom they see, and their relationships. There is a growing consumer literature providing guidance and tools for coping with such transitions effectively (Hipskind and Brown, 1999; Mace and Rabins, 1999; McLeod, 1999; Morris, 1996). There is also a growing professional literature to guide health care providers in assisting persons with dementia and their loved ones through the phases of the disease, preparing them for its relentless progression, and supporting them in accessing the resources for the continuum of care (Aneshensel et al., 1995; Cantor, 1994; Coon et al., 2003; Molinari, 2000; Schulz, 2000).

THE CONTINUUM OF CARE

The continuum of care available to older people with dementia involves both formal (often paid by public or private funds and specialized) and informal (often unpaid and unspecialized) caregiving resources. Management of dementia in older adults requires an individualized and multimodal approach that involves use of acute medical, long-term care, housing, psychosocial, financial, and legal services, in addition to patient and family education. The typical continuum of dementia care includes acute medical services (e.g., outpatient, emergency, primary, specialty, inpatient, rehabilitative, and skilled nursing care); long-term care services (e.g., geriatric care managers), home care providers (e.g., homemaker care, home-delivered meals, home health aides, personal care assistants, in-home therapists, and nurses), recreational, educational, treatment, and respite care senior centers, and institutional nursing home care); housing services (e.g., independent congregate housing, apartments with congregate meals and services, subsidized housing, board-and-care, assisted living, continuing care retirement communities [CCRC]); psychosocial services (e.g., telephone reassurance, elder companions, transportation services, support, psychoeducation, socialization groups, and counseling services); and legal/financial services (e.g., Medicare and Medicaid assistance, estate and financial planning).

THE CRISIS IN CAREGIVING

The backbone of the dementia care system is family caregiving. Currently, family caregiving is provided to 1.5 million persons aged 65 and older in the United States (U.S. Department of Health and Human Services, 1999). The caregiver crisis has been established by data indicating that family members provide 90 percent of the long-term care in this country; this has profound emotional and physical consequences for elders and their caregivers (Stone et al., 1987; National Survey of Caregivers, 1997). In general, 75 percent of frail community-dwelling elders rely solely on informal resources (e.g., family/friends) for support, while the other 25 percent rely on a combination of family care and paid assistance (Cohen et al., 2001).

In the search for high-quality, compassionate, and affordable care of persons with dementia, the demand for caregiving is dramatically increasing, while the supply of capable caregivers is decreasing. Americans are facing a caregiving crisis, fueled by such demographic trends as the rapid growth in the oldest segment of our population, increased incidence and early detection of dementia, and reduction in the birth rate resulting in fewer children to care for aging parents (Blazer, 1990). In addition, financial and sociopolitical trends have prompted more women to enter the work force, thereby further eroding the pool of available caregivers. These demographics will collide to create a social emergency in which families and persons with dementia will become progressively at risk.

DEMENTIA CARE

Health care providers can assist persons with dementia and their loved ones through all phases of dementia by preparing them for the relentless progression of the disease and by supporting them through the intellectual and emotional conflicts accompanying this condition. Multidisciplinary dementia care professionals require ongoing education to enable them to best serve this population and to help them take advantage of a range of services to optimize the quality of their care. On conducting a review of the literature in this area, I uncovered the following overarching principles of dementia care. They have been adopted by many professionals in the field (Hellman, 2001):

— the best interest of the elder
— the right of self-determination
— safety with the least restrictions
— aging in place with dignity
— transitions that are least disruptive to lifestyle.

These principles are particularly relevant to the quality of the continuum of care for persons with dementia. The medical literature has repeatedly described the availability of meaningful activities, optimal management of medical issues, and appropriate treatment of psychiatric/behavioral problems as contributing factors in improving quality of care of older patients (Volicer, 2001). Such factors were expanded by Kane (2001) to include the following domains: security, comfort, meaningful activity, relationships, enjoyment, dignity, autonomy, privacy, individuality, spiritual well-being, and functional competence. The American Academy of Neurology developed quality standards for the management of dementia which include the following educational and nonpharmacological recommendations: short-term educational programs for caregivers and care receivers about dementia, intensive long-term education and support services for caregivers to delay nursing home placement, dementia education for staff of long-term care facilities, and care environment alterations (Doody et al., 2001). Comprehensive care also includes case management, legal and financial planning, and family consultation (Keady and Gilliard, 1999).

THE STAGES OF DEMENTIA CAREGIVING

Dementia is a disease that significantly affects the life not only of the individual afflicted but also the lives of the entire family who must mobilize their resources to provide increasing levels of care to the person as the disease progresses. Any discussion of the stages of dementia should therefore be embedded within an appreciation of the circumstances of caregiving. Woods et al. (1985, p. 19) delineated the stages of dementia within a social context as follows: "Family members of the afflicted individual tend to pass through various phases of reaction as the disease progresses. These include (1) initial recognition of the problems; (2) clarification and emotional acceptance of the diagnosis, sometimes including extensive seeking of alternate opinions and potential cures; (3) establishment of appropriate expectations; (4) grieving; (5) problem-solving and coping with respect to deteriorating behavior; and (6) decision-making regarding appropriate care." Management of dementia in older adults requires an individualized and multimodal approach that involves use of somatic, psychological, social, financial, and legal treatments and tools, in addition to patient and family education. Dementia is an acquired disorder characterized by multiple impairments of cognition (distinct elements of intellectual processing such as memory, abstraction, judgment, and language) occurring in an individual who is fully alert and attentive (Rabins, 2001). The progressive nature of dementia and the invariable presence of comorbidity complicate the management tasks, although symptoms characteristic of the various phases of dementia can provide helpful clinical clues to guide evolving care (Schindler and Cucio, 2000).

Progressive dementias such as Alzheimer disease cause the repeated experience of grief and loss in the patient and family members through the different phases of the disease process. Bearing witness, for example, to the gradual "death" of a loved one's memory and personal identity from AD brings a unique form of grief associated with current and anticipated losses before bodily death (Meuser and Marwit, 2001). In her personal account of caregiving, Beth McLeod (1999) states, "Being a caregiver means having your heart broken over and over again."

MODELS OF CHANGE

The career of caregiving traverses various stages that are consistent with a variety of theoretical stage models of change. While caregiving has typically been viewed as a specific activity, Pillemer et al. (2003) view the process of becoming a dementia caregiver as a "status transition" similar to other transitions in the life course, such as becoming a new parent, a widow, or a retiree. The transtheoretical model of behavior change already has successfully been adapted to clinical work in the treatment of alcohol dependence and substance abuse (Prochaska et al., 1997), and in this chapter we make similar application for addressing the needs of caregivers. Using this framework also serves a heuristic conceptual purpose, suggesting five distinct transitional stages of caregiving: precontemplation, contemplation, preparation, action, and maintenance. Each stage is presumed to follow the other in a linear progression as the caregiver and care receiver successfully overcome difficulties in coping with dementia.

Consistent with these stages of change, Hipskind and Brown (1999) suggested four stages of caregiving. In the first stage, there is some loss and variability in the ability to perform instrumental activities of daily living (IADLs) (e.g., the elder requires help with money and medication management, transportation, meal preparation, shopping, and/or housework). Although there is no immediate crisis, caregiving is inevitable, and more vigilant and consistent monitoring by the expectant caregiver is initiated. In the second stage, the care receiver is typically in the early stage of dementia and the level of involvement by the freshman caregiver increases beyond monitoring to hands-on assistance with IADLs. In the third stage, the elder's dementia progresses to the middle stage and the level of assistance by the entrenched caregiver is daily or constant, with assistance needed with most IADLs and many activities of daily living (ADLs) (e.g., the elder requires help with transferring, bathing, dressing, eating, and toileting). The final stage is the caregiver in loss, when the elder is in the final stage of dementia and requires constant care. These authors also described common blocks to coping and offered action plans and keys for successful coping with each stage.

These stages are best illustrated by clinical vignettes that are typical of the caregiving career. In the following example, an aging couple, one with Alzheimer disease and the other with vascular dementia, progressively deteriorate, requiring a variety of adjustments in their care. Both the principles of care and the models of change (i.e., the stages of caregiving model and the transtheoretical model of behavioral change), will be applied in further explaining the transition of adjustments in the care of this typical aging couple. These naturally occurring transitions to different stages of dementia require that a continuum of medical, long-term care, housing, psychosocial, and legal/financial services be accessed at the corresponding stages of the caregiver career.

The Expectant Caregiver

Joe and Carol, both in their early eighties, live in their suburban neighborhood in Los Angeles where they raised their three children. Monica, their oldest child, lives 20 minutes away, while her siblings live outside of California. Joe, a 30-year cigarette smoker, has several chronic illnesses (diabetes, cardiovascular disease, emphysema), while Carol, who is active and relatively healthy, is showing signs of mild cognitive impairment. She has often lost her way in the neighborhood, left the water running in the kitchen sink, and missed appointments with her family and health care providers. Monica is now anticipating her parents' decline and has begun discussing her concerns with her parents, siblings, and friends. She has begun to accompany her parents to their professional appointments (e.g., medical, legal).

Following recognition of dementia symptoms by the elder and his or her family, mildly impaired persons and their families often begin planning for and adapting to the disorder. Family members gather information about the dementing process, talk with others who have had similar experiences, and determine potential service options based on the best interests of the person and the available family resources. Family meetings including siblings, healthy spouse, and patient are helpful at this stage in assisting family members in defining the level to which they will be involved in caregiving and the role that they will play over time. Hellman (2000) summarizes a variety of concerns that need to be addressed in developing an action plan for caregiving at this early stage of the caregiving career (see table 3.1).

The Freshman Caregiver

Joe and Carol continue living in their home. Joe's chronic conditions progress to the point that he requires a walker for mobility and daily oxygen treatment. Carol's cognitive problems progress. Their daughter Monica installs hand bars and rails in the bathroom and bedroom, and seats to enable her parents' ease of transfer when attending to their activities of daily living. Monica, painfully aware of her parents' needs, has begun to assist

TABLE 3.1
Minimizing Caregiver Stress while Maximizing Elder Independence

Getting Organized / Assessing Your Loved One's Needs
    Psychological: Decision-making capacity; delirium / depression / dementia
    Health: Health care providers / medications / disease-specific prognosis
    Financial: Assets, income, liabilities, insurance, and tax planning
    Legal: Estate planning / durable power of attorney
    Social: Activities / services / resources / continuum of housing options
Defining One's Role as Caregiver
    Family meetings with parents and siblings to negotiate specialized roles
    Distribute specialized roles among family and extended social network
Developing an Extended Care Plan
    Caregiving from a distance: frequent visiting, care manager, relocating
    Use formal support: consultants / care coordinators / in-home services
    Housing options: relocating to a continuum of higher levels of care
Surviving the Stresses of Caregiving
    Balancing work and family: competing demands, changing roles and routines
    Refining your caregiving skills: education / hands-on training / practice
    Preventing physical, social, and emotional burnout
Death and Dying
    Preparing for death: emotionally / financially / logistically / spiritually; hospice
    Grief and bereavement of the elder and the survivors

them with their IADLs (e.g., financial and medical management, shopping, cooking, and cleaning). They have also consulted attorneys and financial planners to establish durable powers of attorney and a living trust. She also helps her parents hire a homemaker for several hours daily to assist with meals and household chores. Finally, she continues in her attempts to engage her siblings about their parents, but they have little interest in getting involved until there is a "true need."

Older persons developing difficulties performing basic IADLs are often able to overcome such difficulties through brief organizational assistance. Often, however, disabled elderly persons need help from others (personal assistance) to perform some of these activities. Most of the initial IADL assistance that community-dwelling elderly persons receive is provided informally by family caregivers; in some instances this care is supplemented by formal services. Formal care may substitute for some, but not most, informal care and the two systems appear to work in tandem to meet long-term care needs (Cohen et al., 2001). An older person's difficulties performing basic ADLs (e.g., walking, dressing, bathing) can often be overcome through the use of assistive devices and environmental modifications (Hartke, Prohaska, and Furner, 1998). But it is important to note that too much "assistance" can create excess dependency and thereby conflict with the person's right of self-determination. Individuals with dementia must be allowed to have input into decision making in accord with their remaining cognitive functions.

The Entrenched Caregiver: Aging in Place

Joe had a sudden, debilitating stroke while on a trip with Carol for their fiftieth wedding anniversary. Joe now has left-sided paralysis and requires substantial assistance with ADLs (e.g., transferring, toileting, bathing, and dressing). Carol continues to provide most of the simple tasks for her husband's care, and she has brought in formal assistance for some of the heavier and time-intensive duties. Monica has reduced her work schedule to half time in order to provide what has become daily care for and monitoring of her parents. She is a devoted daughter, and she is uncomfortable with the possibility of their living in a "home." She is determined to have them "age in place" under her supervision, as long as possible. However, she has begun to consider relocating them to an assisted living facility. She has also convened several family meetings, although her siblings continue to be reluctant to get involved.

Long-term care (LTC) is a mixture of personal care and assistance that enables persons with disabilities to flourish as much as possible; these tasks are sometimes arduous, time-consuming, and tedious, and often unpredictable and inimical to scheduling (Kane et al., 1998). These services are typically needed when a person has an ongoing, long-term disability as indicated by increases in physical and cognitive impairments which diminish the ability to perform ADLs. Embedded in formal LTC services is the overarching principle of providing the best quality of life that is consistent with health and safety. "LTC is intimate care, and how it is given, when it is given, and by whom it is given shapes the biography of the LTC consumer and, by extension, the biography of family caregivers and the collective biography of the whole family (Kane, 2001, p. 294). Nursing home care is obviously LTC, but so is care that people receive while living in a variety of other settings, including private homes and apartments and a wide array of congregate living settings with many services.

The Entrenched Caregiver: Assisted Living

Carol progressively wears herself out caring for Joe. While assisting him in transferring to his wheelchair she falls and breaks her hip. Following reparative surgery, Carol is placed in rehabilitative skilled-nursing facility for a month. Joe, who continues to require ongoing care, moves in with his daughter, Monica. Monica is now caregiving full time for her father and visiting her mother daily. Her father is unable to use his walker and has become wheelchair bound, while her mother's cognitive impairment has progressed. Monica is encouraged by her caregiver support group to immediately move her parents to an assisted living facility, where they can be more adequately provided with the intensive care they need, and she can enjoy more quality time with them.

Institutionalization of an elderly relative with dementia is a key transition in the caregiving career. Increased caregiver burden and level of elder disability often precipitates the transition from community living to institutionalization. An element of successful aging is a person's ability to age in place in a stable living environment. Assisted living (AL) sometimes functions as an intermediate step in the long-term care continuum. It emphasizes a residential setting with services on a 24-hour (or unscheduled) basis and a high degree of consumer choice and control (Kane and Wilson, 1993). AL settings provide supervision and safety in less restrictive environments where dignity and freedom are more likely to be preserved.

Central to the philosophy of AL is greater resident control of his or her environment, including what services are received, when, and how. Such flexibility is compatible with the overarching principle of "aging in place," in which the facility adjusts its service provision and level of care criteria to meet residents' changing needs and to avoid having to discharge individuals to a higher level of care prematurely.

At least half of the estimated 1 million AL residents have dementia or cognitive impairment, with many AL facilities offering specialized dementia services. Dementia-specialized AL facilities occupy a unique position in the LTC continuum and are distinct from home-care and nursing facilities. Such facilities typically provide intermediate care for the longest period of time, thus postponing admission to a nursing facility (Zimmerman et al., 2003).

The Caregiver in Loss: The Nursing Home

Joe's condition deteriorates after another stroke and he now requires full-time care best provided by a skilled nursing facility. Carol's dementia has progressed to the middle stage (e.g., severe difficulty with memory, sleeping, and agitation). After years, Monica's caregiving is taking a toll on her and her family. She moves her parents to a continuum of care facility that has both skilled nursing and dementia care assisted living. She continues to visit them several times a week and to get support from her caregiver support group. Her siblings become more involved in their care, convinced that their parents are deteriorating, which has required their relocation to institutional living.

Nursing home placement is commonly considered the final transition in the continuum of care and it is a critical event for the elder and caregiver. The decision to institutionalize a person with dementia is complex, and is based on patient and caregiver characteristics and the sociocultural context of patients and caregivers (Haley, 1997; Yaffe et al., 2002). The decision must be made with an understanding of the various causes of frailty in older adults and with an understanding of the full range of residential and home care services available. In addition, the decision is influenced by the communication patterns of the family; the family's ability to tolerate the stress of caregiving; the availability of emotional support for caregivers; and the ability of service providers to comprehend the interplay of values, emotions, and decades of family history in the making of this decision (Frazer, 1999).

Once an older adult is too frail physically and cognitively to make the decision to move, the family often assumes control over the decision of where and when to move. The loss of control over the decision to move can affect older adults' satisfaction with services as well as their emotional well-being. Relocation can also cause stress, isolation, grieving, and an overall decline in physical and psychological functioning in older adults (Chapin and Dobbs-Kepper, 2001). There is a direct interplay between problematic behavior, caregiver emotional stress, diminishing functional status, and nursing home placement of older adults with dementia.

Numerous individual factors have been identified as predictors of nursing home placement, including age, functional impairment, Alzheimer disease, marital status (i.e., unmarried), socialization, and ethnicity (Borrayo et al., 2002; Greene and Ondrich, 1990). A variety of family factors have been associated with nursing home placement (Naleppa, 1996). High levels of involvement from family members lower the risk for nursing home placement. Spouse caregivers are more likely to provide higher levels of care for prolonged periods than are children. Ethnic background is predictive of placement, with African American and Latino families using nursing homes significantly less than Caucasian families (Wallace, Levy-Storms, Kington, and Andersen, 1998). Gaugler et al. (2003) found that institutionalization decisions lie heavily with the family member who provides the bulk of assistance at home, and those who have emotional difficulty adapting to care demands will likely seek residential LTC options for disabled elderly relatives.

There is a misconception that nursing home residents are abandoned by relatives. In fact, family members and friends stay in contact, retain close emotional ties, and continue to contribute to basic care needs of residents (Naleppa, 1996). Continued family involvement has the potential to positively influence the transition to the nursing home setting and to reduce disruption in the lives of nursing home residents by retaining personal continuity with known loved ones. The personal and societal consequences are improved psychological well-being of residents, reduced care burden of staff, and increased public involvement in the concerns of America's enlarging elderly population.

ISSUES OF SPECIAL INTEREST
Financial and Legal Planning

Persons with cognitive impairment may verbalize to family and friends their preferences for care. A person in the early stage of dementia who is disoriented to time and place may still be capable of making choices and expressing preferences about many aspects of care (Feinberg and Whitlach, 2001). As disabilities progress, it becomes more difficult for the care receiver to voice preferences for care. During the later stages, the family caregivers face the critical task of determining what services are available to keep their loved ones at home, or whether another living arrangement is appropriate. Formulation of an advance proxy plan and powers of attorney are important to ensure that the elder's previous wishes or best interests are considered when care decisions are made. In some cases, elders become so mentally incapacitated that the caregiver may be required to become a surrogate decision maker (i.e., conservator) (Moye, 1999). Even when a caregiver makes decisions that reflect the care recipient's clearly stated wishes, the family may experience considerable anguish and conflict. The lack of guidelines to help identify values and care preferences integral to the decision-making process, as well as the high costs of care, can amplify the family's distress.

Elders who require paid LTC are likely to rely on out-of-pocket payments to fund such care. Private long-term care insurance, which helps to bring formal caregivers into the home or to access institutional care, typically reimburses the costs of care provided in nursing homes and AL facilities as well as in-home personal care services such as home health aides, personal care services, therapies and nursing services. In the absence of such benefits, state-subsidized institutional alternatives would likely be required.

Caregiver Stress

Much of the caregiving literature emphasizes the importance of minimizing caregiver stress while maximizing care receiver independence. As elders' dependence on assistance increases, the level of caregiver strain rises. The caregiver may develop feelings of anger, grief, loneliness, and resentment, and the health and well-being of most caregivers are often affected. Potential burdens associated with family caregiving are numerous and can include managing behavioral disturbances, attending to physical needs, and providing constant vigilance. The effects of these stressors on family caregivers can include increased levels of depression and anxiety, higher use of psychoactive medications, decline of physical health, compromised immune function, and increased mortality (Light et al., 1994).

The Family Caregiving Stress Process Model, first described by Zarit et al. (1985), suggests a variety of ways for elders and their caregivers to successfully adapt to caregiving over time through their appraisal of the level of difficulty, through coping techniques that are problem oriented and emotionally focused, and through social support that is both emotional and task focused. Over the past 25 years, a plethora of psychosocial interventions aimed at alleviating distress associated with dementia caregiving have included intensive personalized counseling, supportive group counseling, psychoeducational programs, specific therapeutic skills training, enhancing problem-solving skills, and teaching basic caregiving skills and behavior management techniques (Bourgeois et al., 1996; Gallagher-Thompson et al., 1998; Schulz et al., 2002).

Maximizing care recipients' sense of independence was first discussed by Rodin and McAvay (1992), who suggested that, as people age, a sense of control may become progressively important and that opportunities for control are an essential element of well-being later in life. Recognizing the interdependence of caregivers' well-being on persons with dementia, Pruchno et al. (1997) found that patients who perceived that they contributed to other family members in multigenerational households experienced more personal control and psychological well-being. Yale (1995) reported the utility of early-stage Alzheimer support groups in the management of persons with dementia.

Elder Abuse

Elder abuse is a multidimensional phenomenon that encompasses the infliction on older people of physical abuse, abandonment, emotional or psychological abuse, financial abuse, or neglect (National Center on Elder Abuse [NCEA], 1998). Researchers have identified a wide range of factors associated with increased risk of elder abuse (Lachs et al., 1997). These include age, gender, race, poverty, disability, cognitive impairment, and isolation (Wolf and Pillemer, 2000). If the need for assistance is unmet, older adults may be at risk for a variety of adverse outcomes, including increased use of health services, depression, institutionalization, or the most common type of elder abuse, self-neglect (Hellman et al., 2001).

The causes of mistreatment include the following dimensions: (1) the degree of the victim's dependency; (2) the effect of caregiver stress; (3) a unique family pathology of solving problems by intimidation and violence; (4) psychopathology of the abuser; (5) ageism, sexism, and discrimination against the disabled; and (6) greed (Quinn and Tomita, 1997). The caregiver who is not skilled in behavior management and has not learned appropriate methods to cope with his or her own stress will not respond in a manner conducive to the best interest of the elder and may resort to abusive behavior. Considerable evidence also suggests that abusers have common personality characteristics, such as poor mental or physical health, alcohol or drug dependence, financial dependence on the elder, poor empathy skills, and social isolation. Abuse is more likely to occur during the later stages of the disease, as the care recipient becomes more dependent and the caregiver experiences more and more demands.

Caregiving occurs within a societal context especially capable of bringing out the best and worst of the parties involved. Anetzberger (2000) suggested that caregiver stress and burden is not the primary cause of elder abuse. Rather, it is a context for interaction from which the potential to commit abuse evolves. Abuse may result when the worst comes to the fore and when there are no measures in place to prevent the abuse from occurring.

IMPLICATIONS FOR CLINICAL PRACTICE

Clinicians working with dementia patients and their caregiving families can provide more comprehensive services with a knowledge of the continuum of care for persons with dementia, the standards for such care, and the subtle and profound impact at different stages of dementia on patients, family members, and formal caregivers. Offering persons with dementia and their loved ones detailed information on the relentless progression and the predictable stages of the caregiving career (e.g., expectant caregiver, freshman caregiver, entrenched caregiver, and the caregiver in loss), and supporting them in accessing multiple formal and informal resources for a continuum of care (e.g., acute medical services; LTC services; housing services; psychosocial service; legal and financial services) would be most beneficial.

Multiple and complex interventions for elders and their caregivers should be consistent with the following overarching principles of dementia care reviewed in this chapter: (1) the best interest of the elder; (2) the right of self-determination; (3) safety with the least restrictions; (4) aging in place with dignity; (5) transitions that are least disruptive to lifestyle. Identifying the specific caregiving transitional stage (e.g., precontemplation, contemplation, preparation, action, and maintenance), and addressing the possibility of caregivers' and care receivers' needing to transition through other stages will maximize their chances of successfully overcoming difficulties in coping with dementia. Minimizing caregiver stress while maximizing elder independence can best be achieved by following the steps described in table 3.1 (e.g., getting organized / assessing your loved one's needs; defining your role as caregiver; developing an extended care plan; surviving the stresses of parent caregiving; preparing for and accepting death and dying). Practitioners can provide additional benefits to their clients by addressing the special issues described in this chapter, including the need to proactively address financial and legal planning, reduction of caregiver stress, and the prevention of elder abuse.

CONCLUSION

The transitions along a continuum of care for persons with dementia typically follow predictable stages that require action and coping on the part of care recipients and caregivers. The geometric rise in the aging population, particularly those with dementia, coupled with the erosion in the pool of available caregivers will collide to create a social emergency in the next 50 years. Comprehensive quality care will require an ongoing proactive and vigilant approach to access appropriate medical, long-term care, housing, psychosocial, and legal and financial services at each stage of dementia caregiving. Implementing such changes will require an adherence to the standard of minimizing caregiver stress while maximizing independence of the care recipient.

REFERENCES

Aneshensel, C. S., Pearlin, L. I., Mullan, J. T., Zarit, S. H., and Whitlach, S. J. 1995. *Profiles in caregiving: The unexpected career.* San Diego: Academic Press.

Anetzberger, G. J. 2000. Caregiving: Primary cause of elder abuse? An alternative explanatory model. *Generations* (Summer): 46–51.

Blazer, D. 1990. What should the federal government do about Alzheimer's disease? *Journal of Gerontology: Medical Sciences* 45(1): M1–M2.

Borrayo, E. A., Salmon, J. R., Polivka, L., and Dunlop, B. D. 2002. Utilization across the continuum of long-term care services. *Gerontologist* 42:603–12.

Bourgeois, M. S., Schulz, R., and Burgio, L. 1996. Intervention for caregivers of patients with AD. *International Journal of Aging and Human Development* 43:35–92.

Cantor, M. 1994. *Family caregiving: Agenda for the future.* San Francisco: ASA.

Chapin, R., and Dobbs-Kepper, D. 2001. Aging in place in assisted living: Philosophy versus policy. *Gerontologist* 41:43–50.

Cohen, M. A., Miller, J., and Weinrobe, M. 2001. Patterns of informal and formal caregiving among elders with private long-term care insurance. *Gerontologist* 41:180–87.

Coon, D. W., Gallagher-Thompson, D., and Thompson, L. W. (Eds.). 2003. *Innovative interventions to reduce dementia caregiver distress*. New York: Springer.

Doody, R. S., Stevens, J. C., Beck, C., Dubinsky, R. M., Kaye, J. A., Gwyther, L., Mohs, R. C., Thal, L. J., Whitehouse, P. J., DeKosky, S. T., and Cummings, J. L. 2001. Management of dementia (an evidence-based review). *Neurology* 56:1154–66.

Feinberg, L. F., and Whitlatch, C. J. 2001. Are persons with cognitive impairment able to state consistent choices? *Gerontologist* 41:374–82.

Frazer, D. W. 1999. Understanding and treating the effects of dementia onset and nursing home placement. In M. Dufy (Ed.), *Handbook of counseling and psychotherapy with older adults* (pp. 281–93). New York: John Wiley and Sons.

Gallagher-Thompson, D., Coon, D. W., Rivera, D., Povers, D., and Zeiss, A. M.. 1998. Family caregiving: Stress, coping, and intervention. In M. Hersen and V. B. Hasselt (Eds.) *Handbook of clinical geropsychology* (pp. 469–93). New York: Plenum Press.

Gaugler, J. E., Kane, R. L., Kane, R. A., Clay, T., and Newcomer, R. 2003. Caregiving and institutionalization of the cognitively impaired. *Gerontologist* 43:219–29.

Greene, V. L., and Ondrich, J. I. 1990. Risk factors for nursing home admissions and exits. *Journal of Gerontology: Social Sciences* 45: S250–S258.

Haley, W. E. 1997. The family caregiver's role in AD. *Neurology* 48: S25–S29.

Hartke, R. J., Prohaska, T. R., and Furner, S. E. 1998. Older adults and assistive devices: Use, multiple-device use, and need. *Journal of Aging and Health* 10:99–116.

Hellman, I. D. 2000. Minimizing caregiver stress and maximizing parent independence. Presentation for CWDA adult services annual conference, Asilomar, California.

Hellman, I. D. 2001. Standards of eldercare work and advanced risk assessment. Presentation for NAAPSA annual conference, Palm Springs, California.

Hipskind, M. G., and Brown, D. M. 1999. *The four stages of caregiving*. Parkridge, Ill.: Tad.

Kane, R. A. 2001. Long-term care and a good quality of life: Bringing them closer together. *Gerontologist* 41:293–304.

Kane, R. A., Kane, R. L., and Ladd, R. C. 1998. *The heart of long-term care*. New York: Oxford University Press.

Kane, R. A., and Wilson, K. 1993. *Assisted living in the United States: A new paradigm for residential care for older persons?* Washington, D.C.: AARP.

Keady, J., and Gilliard, J. 1999. The early experience of Alzheimer's disease: The implications for partnership and practice. In T. Adams and C. Clarke (Eds.). *Dementia care: Developing partnerships in practice*. London: B. Tindall.

Lachs, M. S., Williams, C., O'Brien, S., Hurst, L., and Horowitz, R. 1997. Risk factors for reported elder abuse and neglect. *Gerontologist* 37:469–74.

Light, E., Nierderhe, G., and Lebowitz, B. (Eds.). 1994. *Stress effects on family caregivers of Alzheimer's patients: Research and interventions*. New York: Springer.

Mace, N. L., and Rabins, P. V. 1999. *The 36-Hour day*. Baltimore: Johns Hopkins University Press.

McLeod, B. W. 1999. *Caregiving: The spiritual journey of love, loss, and renewal*. New York: John Wiley and Sons.

Meuser, T. M., and Marwit, S. J. 2001. A comprehensive, stage-sensitive model of grief in dementia caregiving. *Gerontologist* 41:658–70.

Molinari, V. (Ed.) 2000. *Professional psychology in long-term care.* New York: Hatherleigh.

Morris, V. 1996. *How to care for aging parents.* New York: Workman Publishing.

Moye, J. 1999. Evaluating competency and decision-making capacity. In P. Lichtenberg (Ed.), *Handbook of assessment in clinical gerontology* (pp.488–528). New York: Wiley.

Naleppa, M. 1996. Families and the institutionalized elderly: A review. *Journal of Gerontological Social Work* 27(1/2):87–111.

National Center on Elder Abuse (NCEA). 1998. *The national elder abuse incident study: Final report.* Prepared for the Administration on Aging: U.S. Department of Health and Human Services.

National Survey of Caregivers. 1997. Final report. Washington, D.C.: National Alliance for Caregiving and American Association of Retired Persons.

Pillemer, K., Suitor, J. J., and Wethington, E. 2003. Two case studies from caregiving research. *Gerontologist* 43:19–28.

Prochaska, J. O., Redding, C. A., and Evers, K. E. 1997. The transtheoretical model and stages of change. In K. Glanz, F. M. Lewis, and B. K. Ricen (Eds.), *Health behavior and health education.* San Francisco: Josey-Bass.

Pruchno, R. A., Burant, C. J., and Peters, N. D. 1997. Coping strategies of people living in multigenerational households. *Psychology and Aging* 12:115–24.

Quinn, M. J., and Tomita, S. K. 1997. *Elder abuse and neglect: Causes, diagnosis, and intervention strategies* (2nd ed.). New York: Springer.

Rabins, P. V. 2001. Dementia and Alzheimer's disease: An overview. In Symposium: Joint conference on legal/ethical issues in the progression of dementia. *Georgia Law Review* 35(2):451–65.

Rodin, J., and McAvay, G. 1992. Determinants of changes in perceived health in a longitudinal study of older adults. *Journal of Gerontology* 47:373–84.

Schindler, R. J., and Cucio, C. P. 2000. Late life dementia: Review of the APA guidelines for patient management. *Geriatrics* 55(10):55–60.

Schulz, R. (Ed.). 2000. *Handbook on dementia caregiving: Evidence-based interventions for family caregivers.* New York: Springer.

Schulz, R., O'Brien, A., Czaja, S., Ory, M., Norris, R., Martire, L. M., et al. 2002. Dementia caregiver intervention research. *Gerontologist* 42:589–602.

Stone, R., Cafferata, G. L., and Sangl, J. 1987. Caregivers of the frail elderly: A national profile. *Gerontologist* 27:616–26.

U.S. Department of Health and Human Services. 1999. Health and aging chartbook. DHHS Publication No. (PHS) 99–1232–1. Washington, D.C.: Government Printing Office.

Volicer, L. 2001. Management of severe Alzheimer's disease and end-of-life issues. *Clinical Geriatric Medicine* 17(2):377–91.

Wallace, S. P., Levy-Storms, L., Kington, R. S., and Andersen, R. M. 1998. The persistence of race and ethnicity in the use of long-term care. *Journals of Gerontology: Psychological Sciences and Social Sciences* 53(2): S104–12.

Wolf, R. S., and Pillemer, K. 2000. Elder abuse and case outcome. *Journal of Applied Gerontology* 19:203–20.

Woods, A. M., Niederehe, G., and Fruge, E. 1985. Dementia: A family systems perspective. *Generations* (Fall): 19–23.

Yaffe, K., Newcomer, R., Sands, L., Lindquist, K., Dane, K., and Covinsky, K. E. 2002. Patient and caregiver characteristics and nursing home placement in patients with dementia. *Journal of the American Medical Association* 287(16):2090–97.

Yale, R. 2001. *Developing support groups for individuals with early-stage Alzheimer's disease.* Baltimore: Health Professions Press.

Zarit, S. H., Orr, N., and Zarit, J. 1985. Understanding the stress of caregiving. In S. H. Zarit, N. Orr, and J. Zarit (Eds.), *Hidden victims of AD* (pp. 69–86). New York: NYU.

Zimmerman, S., Gruber-Baldini, A. L., Sloane, P. D., Eckert, J. K., Hebel, J. R., Morgan, L. A., Sterans, S. C., Wildfire, J., Magaziner, J., Chen, C., and Konrad, T. R. 2003. Assisted living and nursing homes. *Gerontologist* 43:107–17.

CHAPTER FOUR

Caregiver Burden

VICTOR A. MOLINARI, PH.D., ABPP

This chapter is not meant to be an exhaustive review of all the studies on caregiver burden, but will focus on the main findings of the empirical literature and how they might assist professionals in providing support to caregivers. First, I present a composite vignette to highlight the personal side of caregiving. I next address the research on the psychological, physical, social, vocational, and financial aspects of burden for those caring for persons with dementia and how these affect placement decisions. This is followed by a discussion on the assessment of burden. I then summarize the benefits of caregiving and the resilience of caregivers in the face of their burden. Practice implications are then examined. I conclude with a plea for theory-driven research and suggest areas for future investigation.

Mrs. A. is a 45-year-old woman who recently became a member of the Alzheimer Day Center support group. She has been taking care of her 85-year-old father for the last three years and her blood pressure has recently significantly increased. She has always been very attached to her father because he had "always been there for her" when she needed him. She is beginning to feel overwhelmed. She has found herself waking up in the middle of the night, unable to return to sleep, and sobbing about her predicament. Since she began caregiving, and particularly since her father moved into her house one year ago, she has had to reduce the time she spends attending the school functions of her two teenage daughters. Her husband has been supportive, but has had to work later hours to make up for their diminished income and depleted savings. This was caused by some of her father's unexpected medical expenses and her cutting back on the number of hours she spends as a bank officer, a job she always enjoyed and for which she had been in line for a promotion (which she turned down because it involved additional work-related responsibilities). Mrs. A has always prided herself on her family's self-sufficiency, and she has been reluctant to ask for support from her friends. She has not been able to continue with the dance classes, which kept her in good physical condition and where she had nurtured some long-standing friendships. She has also begun arguing with her sister over not "pitching in" to help with the financial strain of their father's care and not offering to take care of him on alternate weekends. Worst of all, her brother from the West Coast has been opposed to the idea of placement in an assisted living facility, saying that he will pay for more help in the home but that she needs to bear the brunt of the caregiving because she was their father's favorite child. After her father "struck out" at her a month ago, an employee of the local Alzheimer Association recommended respite care so that she could attend her own medical appointments and spend some leisure time to promote her own well-being and quality of life.

This vignette illustrates the many facets of caregiver burden, including emotional upheaval, medical morbidity, reduced social contacts, family conflict, vocational challenges, and financial strain.

CAREGIVER BURDEN

Caregiver burden can be defined rather simply as the amount of difficulty a caregiver experiences in the day-to-day conduct of caregiving. The "objectification" of such a complex concept by professionals may not render full justice to its multiple facets and to the diverse personal reactions of family members to the caregiving enterprise, but defining the term serves the heuristic purpose of targeting a specific negative feature of caregiving for closer scientific scrutiny. Analyzing data from a survey of 1,509 family caregivers, Ory et al. (1999) found that caregiving for a person with dementia is uniquely stressful. Compared with other types of caregivers, dementia caregivers spend more time providing care and report more employment difficulty, strain, mental and physical health problems, family conflict, and less leisure time for themselves or family members. Burdened caregivers overestimate the extent of the care recipients' impairment (Hadjistavropoulos, Taylor, Tuokko, and Beattie, 1994), which may negatively affect the course of the disease (Dunkin and Anderson-Hanley, 1998). More than 20 years ago, there was already a budding literature on caregiver burden for relatives of persons with dementia. The development of the most widely used scale to assess caregiver burden, the Burden Inventory (Zarit, Reever, and Bach-Peterson, 1980), initiated a vast research program on the stresses of caregiving. Investigators documented the (1) psychological (anger, depression, guilt), (2) physical (chronic fatigue), (3) social (family conflict, isolation), and (4) vocational (loss of employment) tolls that caregivers of persons with dementia encountered.

Psychological Toll

We know that caregivers are more likely to become depressed and/or anxious than noncaregivers. In their review of the mental health literature, Ory, Yee, Tennstedt, and Schulz (2000) noted that a variety of studies using self-report measures provide evidence for increased depressive and anxiety symptoms. Adult caregivers also feel resentful, angry, and guilty at times (Cavanaugh, 1999). Less emotional investment in the spouse is predictive of depression for both husband and wife caregivers (Pruchno and Resch, 1989), while positive parental bonding is related to reduced emotional distress for caregiving sons (Daire, 2002). Meshefedjian, McCusker, Bellavance, and Baumgarten (1998) investigated variables associated with severity of depressive symptoms for 321 informal caregivers living in a Canadian community. They found three caregiver characteristics (being a spouse or adult child of care recipient, ethnicity other than English/French Canadian, lower education) and two care recipient characteristics (more behavior problems, moderate/severe functional impairment) to be related to depression. Depression also appears to be linked to ethnic status, with Hispanic caregivers experiencing more depression than African American caregivers (Knight, Silverstein, McCallum, and Fox, 2000).

It appears that there is a reciprocal and ever-spiraling association between the behaviors of care recipients and the feelings of caregivers. Intense care recipient behavior problems and caregiver role entrapment are associated with role overload, depression, and adaptation over time (Gaugler, Davey, Pearlin, and Zarit, 2000). Burden and depression, together with patient behavior problems, are associated with family caregivers' lower global ratings of Alzheimer disease (AD) relatives' quality of life compared with what caregivers believe care recipients would rate themselves (Karlawish, Casarett, Klocinski, and Clark, 2001). Caregivers who exhibit higher levels of expressed emotion make more patient-causal attributions for negative events and have higher levels of caregiver distress and strain (Tarrier et al., 2002). When caregivers exhibit low personal resiliency and engage in conflicted relationships with care recipients, their affect is poor and minor psychiatric symptoms are elevated (Braithwaite, 2000).

Physical Toll

Caregiver burden is a significant predictor of death or institutionalization of persons with AD both in the United States and Japan (Hirono et al., 2002; Yaffe et al., 2002). Caregivers believe themselves to be less healthy and may have less time to care for their own medical problems. Objective and subjective indices of burden were found to be associated with poorer health-related quality of life among a large group of caregivers of veterans who qualified for formal health care (Hughes et al., 1999). Psychoneuroimmunological studies of caregivers reveal poorer immune response (Glaser and Kiecolt-Glaser, 1997), lower T-cell counts (Pariante et al., 1997), increased cardiovascular risk factors (Vitaliano, Young, and Russo, 1991), and increased systolic blood pressure (Moritz, Kasl, and Ostfeld, 1992). Caregivers also report greater use of psychotropic medications (Schulz, O'Brien, Bookwala, and Fleissner, 1995). Ory et al. (2000) noted that poor finances, high levels of neuroticism, low levels of mastery, and limited social support are associated with negative self-rated health. Vitaliano, Maiuro, Ochs, and Russo (1990) sampled 63 caregiver-patient dyads and found that 34 percent of them reported that a health problem had bothered them within the last month.

Nonetheless, a review of this literature by Dunkin and Anderson-Hanley (1998) suggests that negative health-related effects of caregiving are more consistently detected for self-reported than objective health indices. A study of 64 white family caregivers of community-dwelling persons with AD (Harwood, Barker, Ownby, and Duara, 2000) may help explain why there are diverse findings depending on self-reported versus objective measures of caregiver health. These authors discovered that poorer self-rated physical status was more strongly related to caregiver variables than to care recipient factors. In particular, these authors found that depression and older age of the caregiver were related to self-reported health problems. Subclinical depressive symptomatology may adversely affect self-reported health ratings, perhaps reflecting psychological morbidity more than objective health impairment. Ethnicity may also be related to health status, with a significant proportion of both African American and Hispanic caregivers reporting deterioration in their health (Harwood et al., 1998).

Social Toll

Because of the frequent all-consuming nature of caregiving, caregivers have less leisure time to spend with others. They are frequently embarrassed by the behavior of their loved one and may try to keep people from knowing that the person has dementia. Unfortunately, a main factor associated with burden is lack of support (Coen, O'Boyle, Coakley, and Lawlor, 2002), so a cycle is initiated in which the individual may become more and more mired in caregiving tasks leading to further social isolation. In the Alameda County longitudinal study, Seeman et al. (1987) found clear evidence that isolation and reduced social networks are linked to limited physical functioning, frailty, and mortality in older adults. In their review of the social network literature of family caregivers, Pillemer, Suitor, and Wethington (2003) contend that caregiving causes constricted social networks, lower social participation, and elevated interpersonal stress from family and friends, resulting in an overall negative effect on well-being. Clyburn, Stones, Hadjistavropoulos, and Tuokko (2000) studied 613 Canadian caregivers and found that, in addition to behavior problems, caregiver burden was related to low informal support. Poignantly, caregivers of those patients exhibiting more disturbing behavior and greater functional limitations receive less informal support. Overburdened caregivers perceive a lack of informal support, experience family conflict and poorer mental health, and say that they need more time away from the person with dementia (Coen, O'Boyle, Coakley, and Lawlor, 2002). Correspondingly, a larger social network and satisfaction with social support is associated with diminished burden (Vitaliano et al., 1991) and less depression (Pillemer and Suitor, 1996).

For participants caring for a loved one for at least eight years, qualitative analysis has revealed social support is an important variable in finding relief (Karlin, Bell, and Noah, 2001). In their exploration of the benefits of European day center programs which provide support to informal caregivers, Calvez, Joel, Ponton-Sanchez, and Roper (2002) concluded that the main benefit was reduction in feelings of social isolation. However, the time that caregivers spend with others must be positive for improved well-being to occur (Ingersoll-Dayton, Morgan, and Antonucci, 1997). In her introduction to a special series of articles on negative interactions in close relationships, Lachman (2003) notes that verbal discord may lead to poor psychological and physical consequences. Chronic strain may result from relationships that involve negative interactions with individuals who also provide some social support. Increasing positive contacts with other like-minded caregivers who can commiserate concerning their plight is the underlying theory behind support groups (Pillemer, Suitor, and Wethington, 2003). Finally, in a thought-provoking study, Chappell and Reid (2002) found social support to be strongly related to caregiver well-being (but surprisingly not burden), suggesting conceptual distinctiveness between the two concepts. The authors cogently argue that caregivers can enjoy well-being despite instrumental burden, and that caregivers' quality of life can be enhanced even when burden continues.

Vocational Toll

There is a sizable literature documenting caregiving conflicts stemming from ambivalence over how much time to spend on labor force participation versus provision of informal care (Doty, Jackson, and Crown, 1998). "Women in the middle" may be caught between trying to fulfill a traditional "career" of raising children while also caring for their demented parents. Under such conditions, work-related ambitions will almost surely suffer (Stephens and Franks, 1999). Early studies recognized that being a caregiver interfered with work performance (Moeller and Shuell, 1988) and kept many women from engaging in paid labor (Nissel, 1984). More than half of the caregivers of persons with dementia report that they have had to go to work late, leave work early, or take time off from their jobs. Twelve percent say that they had to take a leave of absence, and 13.4 percent had to work less time or take a less demanding job. Even compared with caregivers of persons without dementia, more caregivers of persons with dementia report taking less demanding jobs, early retirement, losing job benefits, and giving up work (Ory et al., 1999).

Financial Toll

AD is the third most expensive disease in the United States (ADRDA, 1994), adding billions of dollars in cost to the economy (Huang, Cartwright, and Hu, 1988). It has been shown to have a major economic impact on family caregivers in Europe as well (Cavallo and Fattore, 1997). Medical work-ups, medications, and day care can be expensive. The average lifetime cost per patient has been approximated at $174,000 (ADRDA, 1994), though such determinations may be underestimates because it is so difficult to place a monetary value on the myriad hidden costs related to caregiving sacrifices. Caregivers frequently get hit with a "double whammy" in terms of loss of income of the person with dementia along with loss of the caregivers' own salary when full or part-time caregiving responsibilities are assumed. More than 60 percent of the formal services to persons with dementia are financed "out-of-pocket" by family caregivers (Rice et al., 1993). Chiriboga, Yee, and Weiler (1992) found that lower income generated additional stress in adult child caregivers.

Coen, O'Boyle, Coakley, and Lawlor (2002) studied the social/psychological characteristics and quality of life in high- and low-burdened caregivers and determined that
financial constraints are major contributory factors to poor quality of life among
highly burdened caregivers.

> Mrs. A. joined a support group to discuss the emotional stress of witness-
> ing her revered father deteriorate mentally despite her best efforts. She grad-
> ually became aware that her psychological problems were compounded by
> hypertension that was inadequately treated due to inability to take time off
> for herself, by family friction and decreased contact with friends leading to re-
> duced social support, by loss of self-esteem associated with no longer being
> gainfully employed as a bank officer, and by financial woes due to her father's
> medical expenses and loss of income from her job. Freeing up time for her-
> self and commiserating with peers in the support group also allowed her to
> recognize that she wanted to continue caregiving for as long as possible, be-
> cause she was proud of herself for paying back a debt to her generous father
> and for serving as a role model for her children by honoring family elders.

Nursing Home Placement

Caregiver health and well-being do not necessarily improve with nursing home
placement, and emotional burden on family caregivers of persons with AD continues after institutionalization. Lieberman and Fisher (2001) conducted a two-year longitudinal study that compared test scores on physical symptomatology, psychological symptomatology, and well-being between caregivers who did and did not place
their loved ones in a nursing homes. They found no differences between caregivers
and concluded that although instrumental burden may be reduced with nursing
home placement, emotional dysphoria and somatic complaints may continue. Tornatore and Grant (2002) studied the burden of 276 female caregivers of AD victims
in nursing homes. Older age, shorter caregiver experience before placement, more
hands-on care in nursing home, and lower caregiver expectations (suggesting a loss
of confidence in institutional care) are associated with more burden. The authors indicate that caregiver experiences, both before and after placement, affect adaptation. Likewise, Yeh, Johnson, and Wang (2002) report that four months after nursing home placement, global burden on caregivers decreased due to improvements
in family support, scheduling, and physical health. However, self-esteem problems
and concern over finances continued. In a more qualitative analysis of in-depth
interviews with ten relatives who placed their loved ones in a nursing home, Ryan

and Scullion (2000) found that many caregivers experienced ambiguous feelings. They felt relief that the burden of instrumental care had been lifted but felt guilty that they could not fulfill their perceived familial obligations. Lieberman and Fisher (2001) note that the overall family context of care is most important for the psychological well-being of relatives who have placed loved ones in nursing home settings.

ASSESSMENT OF BURDEN

It is beyond the scope of this chapter to review in detail all the instruments that have been developed to measure aspects of caregiver burden. Five major considerations should suffice concerning general assessment of caregivers.

First, the Burden Inventory (Zarit, Reever, and Bach-Peterson, 1980) used in conjunction with the Behavior Problem Checklist (Zarit and Zarit, 1982) is the most widely used scale to assess burden. The Burden Inventory was originally developed as a 29-item scale with four Likert-style choice points (never to always), but it was later reduced to a 22-item scale. It has good reliability and validity, but has been criticized because it was initially developed as a unidimensional scale (Novak and Guest, 1989) and for not including caregiver-centered problems, such as the degree of disruption in family and social life (Vitaliano, Young, and Russo, 1991).

Second, all of the scales that measure caregiver burden have been developed primarily for research rather than clinical purposes, and extrapolations to clinical practice therefore should proceed with caution (Dougherty and Chamblin, 1999).

Third, assessment of caregiver burden must be conducted across multiple dimensions (psychological, social, and biological) and should include an evaluation not only of the caregiver but also of the care recipient, and of both formal and informal mechanisms of support. The stage of the disease process and the length of caregiving time must also be identified (Dougherty and Chamblin, 1999).

Fourth, assessment should always include evaluations of the caregivers' knowledge base about dementia, ethnic/cultural issues, overt and covert family conflict, and perhaps potential for abuse (Dunkin and Anderson-Hanley, 1998).

Fifth, Vitaliano, Young, and Russo (1991) present a more detailed review of specific caregiver scales, and Lawton et al. (1989) provide a discussion of the conceptual issues involved in caregiver burden scale development.

THE BENEFITS OF CAREGIVING

Although the negative effects of caregiving have rightly received a great deal of clinical and research attention, it has been only more recently that the positive aspects of caregiving have been investigated. Motenko (1989) conducted lengthy interviews with spousal caregivers of males with dementia. The meaning of caregiving vis-à-vis continuity of marital closeness was more related to wives' well-being than the amount of care provided. Farran et al. (1999) promote an existential approach to improving our understanding of caregiving by delineating day-to-day meaning-finding (proximal meaning) and philosophical/religious/spiritual meaning-finding (ultimate meaning).

Although qualitative analyses suggest that caregivers may have limited opportunity to engage in activities that might facilitate a broader sense of self-identity (Acton, 2002), caregivers are quite resourceful. Cohen, Colantonio, and Vernich (2002) questioned 289 caregivers and found that 73 percent of them could identify at least one positive feature of caregiving. Positive feelings about caregiving were associated with lower depression, lower burden, and higher self-assessed health. Stephens and Franks (1999) interviewed adult caregivers and discovered that more than half of them endorsed the following items reflecting rewards of caregiving: knew parent was well cared for; fulfilled family obligation; spent time in the company of parent; gave care because wanted to not because had to, saw parent enjoy small things; parent showed affection or appreciation; helped parent with personal care; parent was cooperative or not demanding; parent's good side came through despite the illness; parent was calm or content; relationship with parent became closer; parent's health improved. Waldman (1998) and Haley et al. (2001) noted similar positive aspects for caregivers of dementia and dying patients: feelings of accomplishment in meeting a challenge despite the odds, fulfilling moral obligations to someone who has cared for them, maintaining a helpful function, enjoying little moments of pleasure with the loved one, promoting a role model for children, and maintaining a sense of life's purpose.

It would be a mistake to conceptualize the majority of caregivers in a reactive role buffeted by stressors. Perhaps more accurately, we can view many caregivers as choosing this difficult role, bringing to bear a wealth of personal resources to the task, and coping reasonably well (Chappell, 2001). Despite the psychological, physical, social, vocational, and financial hazards, caregivers tend to use their coping skills to meet the task, at times spurring their own spiritual and psychological development. Research does not support a simple "wear and tear" (inexorable stress-related decline in caregiver ability) hypothesis regarding long-term caregiving, but instead points to variability in caregiver stress levels over time and diverse adaptation to caregiving based on sundry internal and external resources (Lawton, Moss, Hoffman, and Perkinson, 2000).

There are low correlations between the severity of a care recipient's dementia and the amount of psychological burden a caregiver experiences. Caregivers who appraise stressors as benign, use appropriate coping skills, and have good social support report better mental health (Goode, Haley, Roth, and Ford, 1998). More than half of spousal caregivers believe that they have some control over the major stressor in their lives (Vitaliano, Maiuro, Ochs, and Russo, 1990). Boss, Caron, Horbal, and Mortimer (1990) interviewed 70 persons with dementia and their caregivers. Low ambiguity over the afflicted individual's role in the family is associated with feelings of mastery in the caregiving situation, leading to less depression. Although the severity of behavior problems is associated with physical morbidity of the caregiver (Moritz, Kasl, and Ostfeld, 1992), it appears that caregiver psychological and social resources are more important than care recipient characteristics in maintaining mental health.

IMPLICATIONS FOR CLINICAL PRACTICE

It appears that, as in much of gerontology, the literature on caregiver burden generally yields methodologically rigorous data, but without much theoretical sophistication. Grounding in general psychological theory would assist researchers in lending interpretive clarity to research findings and serve as a heuristic mechanism for future work that has clinical relevance. Dougherty and Chamblin (1999) observe that thus far caregiver burden research has been guided by theories of stress and adaptation. They argue that one of these theories, the Stress Process Model (Pearlin, Mullan, Sample, and Skaff, 1990) has helped organize some of the literature's overall findings by conceptually separating stress into primary stressors (negative events caused by the direct provision of care) and secondary (noncaregiving life hassles), as well as subjective (emotional impact) and objective (actual activities performed) stressors. Primary subjective stressors appear to predict caregiver burden better than primary objective stressors (Dougherty and Chamblin, 1999). This theory may have far-reaching clinical consequences. Delineating the details of how the emotional impact of a care recipient's disruptive behavior is mediated by the nature of the prior relationship with the caregiver may guide preventative as well as ameliorative intervention efforts.

Mrs. W. is a caregiver for her husband, who has mild vascular dementia. He was a former drill sergeant in World War II and a career military man. The staff is confused about why Mrs. W. and her son are having such a difficult time dealing with what appears to be Mr. W.'s minor forgetfulness and lapses of judgment. However, when their marital history is probed, it is discovered that the care recipient had always been a dominant, rigid man who did things the "military" way, had sided with his family against his wife's relatives who lived in another country, and had a long-standing feud with the son over the latter's prior delinquent behavior and misuse of finances. The stroke mellowed Mr. W.'s personality (the current personality that the staff perceives), but the family continued to relate to the "tyrant" of the past. Separation from Mrs. W. to be cared for by another son with a more positive history with Mr. W. was then regarded as a viable, if not fully satisfactory, option. Another spouse with a more positive history with a demented care recipient who exhibited similar behaviors may have managed much more easily at home.

Vitaliano, Maiuro, Ochs, and Russo (1990) also developed a sophisticated model of caregiving that make sense of some of the findings on caregiver burden. Caregiver distress is quantified as exposure to stressors (e.g., care recipient's cognitive status and behavior problems, financial problems) plus vulnerability (e.g., health status and personality) divided by psychological (e.g., self-efficacy, coping style) and social (e.g., informal support) resources. Many of the variables in the caregiver burden literature fit neatly into one of these four domains. Conceptually driven studies can yield results that are interpretable within a broader psychological framework. One such study was conducted by Chiriboga, Yee, and Weiler (1992), who employed a caregiver stress model to guide interviews of 385 adult caregiving children. This study was planned with the recognition that stress is multifaceted and that caregiving for older adults can be more or less stressful depending on the context of the individual doing the caregiving. Their results highlight the importance of the life context in the caregiver's appraisal of their burden. Greater burden was associated with exposure to more stressors as exemplified by being the primary caregiver and being the provider of greater amounts of "hands-on" care. Interestingly, general noncaregiving hassles showed the strongest association with depression. These authors aptly note that researchers who solely focus on their own specific topic of interest may exclude more highly relevant variables related to the caregiving enterprise. They recommend the use of comprehensive and global inventories of stress conditions in addition to assessing the specific caregiving variable of most relevance to the researcher.

The above conceptual work of Vitaliano, Maiuro, Ochs, and Russo (1990) and Chiriboga, Yee, and Weiler (1992) may yield a wealth of practical hypotheses that could guide clinical applications. For example, when evaluating a caregiving spouse's ability to continue to handle the stress of a demented husband's aggressive behavior in the community, a working algorithm that recognizes that there is no one-to-one correspondence between severity of behavior problems and institutional placement can guide clinical decision making. This more complex practitioner-relevant model recognizes that the interaction of caregiver personality, coping style, social support, and other sources of stress in the caregiver's life gives a more realistic assessment of the total picture.

Unfortunately, theoretical formulations, informed by life-span developmental concerns, are also lacking to clarify intervention-based research findings. Researchers might familiarize themselves with Baltes's Selection, Optimization, and Compensation model (SOC) (Baltes, 1997) to direct interventions with spousal caregivers. This model provides a framework for understanding change across the life span and incorporates the tenets of selecting goals from limited resources, optimizing resources, and compensating for limitations in order to achieve those goals. Of particular relevance to caregiving, the SOC model suggests that older spouses need to be encouraged to select very specific and realistic caregiving goals, and that strategies for achieving these goals should be based on an analysis of caregiver internal/external strengths and limitations.

The earlier vignette serves as an example of SOC theory's clinical relevance. Mrs. A. may select continued home care for her spouse as her primary caregiving goal despite the burden. She may have external/internal strengths (e.g., financial, no major medical problems, inner-directed coping skills) and also external/internal limitations (introverted, limited informal support, difficulty expressing negative emotions). Mental health professionals could address her burden by suggesting that she hire a home health care agency to assist with the hands-on care while she continues to serve as care manager in the home. Mrs. A. thereby may still be able to attend routine medical appointments and work or volunteer to assure continued good health, adequate financial stability, and vocational happiness. Referral to support groups may not be appropriate under these circumstances, unless the focus is on teaching management skills rather that "caring and sharing."

RESEARCH DIRECTIONS

There is a confluence of thinking related to research directions in the caregiving area. As noted above, more theoretically sophisticated studies from a variety of theoretical perspectives need to be conducted. Schulz, Biegel, Morycz, and Visintainer (1990) advocate that the caregiver literature be nestled within an overarching model delineating psychological and sociological motivations for helping. They also note that the constructs of predictability, control, and self-efficacy are intimately related to caregiver outcomes and should be further studied. The absence of caregiver burden is not synonymous with positive well-being; future investigations should focus on improving the quality of the caregiver/care-recipient relationship and overall quality of life of the caregiver.

Some of the results of well-controlled empirical studies on reducing the burden on caregivers have been sobering. For example, the Medicare Alzheimer's Disease Demonstration project tested a combined case management and community care benefit for caregivers of persons with dementia (Fox, Newcomer, Yordi and Arnsberger, 2000). The additional services led to a statistically (but not clinically) significant reduction in caregiver burden and depression, and did not affect the level of services used, the number of informal caregiver hours spent helping people with dementia, or rates of nursing home placement. The authors concluded that traditional informal care networks generally function effectively, and they suggest that interventions target specific areas including 24-hour care, crisis intervention service coordination with primary care, and chronic disease management (Newcomer et al., 1999). Further, although treatment of agitation in persons with dementia makes sense as a strategy to reduce caregiver burden (Teri, Logsdon, and McCurry, 2002), a randomized control trial did not find differences in agitation reduction between psychopharmacological and behavioral management versus placebo (Teri et al., 2000). Finally, although one randomized control trial revealed that exercise combined with teaching caregivers behavioral management techniques enhanced physical health and reduced depression in persons with AD (Teri et al., 2003), another study found that teaching caregivers behavioral management techniques did not reduce long-term prescription of psychotropic medication (Weiner et al., 2002). We obviously need more creative thinking in order to identify the most potent ways of reducing caregiver stress and burden. Perhaps more researchers need to become closely aligned with the national Alzheimer's Association and the 29 Alzheimer's Disease Research Centers (ADRCs) to conduct the necessary large-sample controlled studies that are needed at this stage in the caregiving field's development. The ADRCs have added a substantial amount to the knowledge base of the neuropathology of AD, and large-scale endeavors might yield similar substantive findings in the caregiving field. The REACH study's multisite, multiproject design has already yielded valuable ethnic information (Coon et al., 2004) and promising intervention strategies (Belle et al., 2004; Burns et al., 2003), with geriatric health professionals eagerly awaiting the results of other associated clinical trials.

More follow-up studies should be conducted on the findings that gender and ethnic status are related to perceived burden, and perhaps also to varied positive benefits of caregiving. By what paths, such as performing more personal care tasks and household chores, are female caregivers more vulnerable to feeling overburdened? Do lower education, poor socioeconomic status, and less acculturation mediate perceived stress in certain ethnic groups? Studies with subgroup caregiving populations such as refugees, caregivers under the age of 21, frail elders, and the impoverished should continue to be conducted.

How some caregivers adapt and why others become overwhelmed, and the effect of extreme levels of burden on the disease course should be further explored (Dunkin and Anderson-Hanley, 1998). The beneficial effects of caregiving and the resilience of caregivers in the face of adversity are research areas worthy of more in-depth examination. Longitudinal studies should evaluate the "natural history" and diverse trajectories of caregiver burden. The relationship over time between acute and chronic stress-related immunosuppression and health consequences should continue to be conducted. Further studies on the association between the care recipient's stage of disease and caregiver burden should be explored. Finally, qualitative focus-group studies should complement quantitative ones and should serve as a catalyst to generate questions for empirical research.

CONCLUSION

Clinicians working with relatives of persons with dementia should recognize that caregiving is a uniquely stressful experience that takes an emotional, medical, social, vocational, and financial toll. They should also understand that caregiving has its benefits—resilient caregivers gain meaning and persist despite the hardship. Practitioners should labor to reduce these stressors and promote healthy adjustment by being supportive and assisting primary caregivers in harvesting individual, family, and social resources. For optimal intervention strategies, assessment of caregiving must be multidimensional and address the specific life context of the caregiver. Clinical researchers should use sophisticated psychological theory to make sense of the ever-growing body of literature. They should also promote the evolution of wide-ranging, evidence-based applications via ongoing program evaluation, so as to assist the ever-increasing number of caregivers who struggle yet persevere.

REFERENCES

Acton, G. J. 2002. Self-transcendent views and behaviors: Exploring growth in caregivers of adults with dementia. *Journal of Gerontological Nursing* 28(12):22–30.

Alzheimer's Disease and Related Disorders Association (ADRDA). 1994. *Alzheimer's disease: Statistics.* Chicago: ADRDA.

Baltes, P. 1997. On the incomplete architecture of human ontogeny: Selection, optimization, and compensation as foundation of developmental theory. *American Psychologist* 52(4): 366–80.

Belle, S. H., Zhang, S., Czaja, S. J., Burns, R., and Schulz, R. 2004. Use of cognitive enhance-ment medication in persons with Alzheimer disease who have a family caregiver; results from the Resources for Enhancing Alzheimer Caregiver health (REACH) project. *American Journal of Geriatric Psychiatry* 12(3):250–57.

Boss, P., Caron, W., Horbal, J., and Mortimer, J. 1990. Predictors of depression in caregivers of dementia patients: Boundary ambiguity and mastery. *Family Process* 29(3):245–54.

Braithwaite, V. 2000. Contextual or general stress outcomes: Making choices through care-giving appraisals. *Gerontologist* 40:706–17.

Burns, R., Nichols, L. O., Martindale-Adams, J., Graney, M. J., and Lummus, A. 2003. Primary care interventions for dementia caregivers: Two-year outcomes from the REACH study. *Gerontologist* 43:547–55.

Calvez, A., Joel, M. E., Ponton-Sanchez, A., and Roper, A. C. 2002. Health status and work burden of Alzheimer patients' informal caregivers: Comparisons of five different care programs in the European Union. *Health Policy* 60(3):219–33.

Cavallo, M. C., and Fattore, G. 1997. The economic and social burden of Alzheimer disease on families in the Lombardy region of Italy. *Alzheimer Disease and Associated Disorders* 11(4):184–90.

Cavanaugh, J. C. 1999. Caregiving to adults: A life event challenge. In I. H. Nordhus, G. R. Vandenbos, S. Berg, and P. Fromholt (Eds.), *Clinical Geropsychology* (pp. 131–35). Washing-ton, D.C.: American Psychological Association.

Cavanaugh, J. C., and Blanchard-Fields, F. 2002. *Adult development and aging* (4th ed.). Wadsworth: United States.

Chappell, N. L. 2001. Caregiving in old age. In N. J. Smelsen and P. B. Baltes (Eds.), *Interna-tional encyclopedia of social and behavioral sciences* (pp. 1479–81). Oxford, England: Perga-mon Press.

Chappell, N. L., and Reid, R. C. 2002. Burden and well-being among caregivers: Examining the distinction. *Gerontologist* 42:772–80.

Chiriboga, D. A., Yee, B. W. K., and Weiler, P. G. 1992. Stress and coping in the context of car-ing. In L. Montada, A. H. Filipp, and M. J. Lerner (Eds.), *Life crises and experiences of loss in adulthood* (pp. 95–118). Hillsdale, N.J.: Lawrence Erlbaum Associates.

Clyburn, L. D., Stones, M. J., Hadjistavropoulos, T., and Tuokko, H. 2000. Predicting care-giver burden and depression in Alzheimer's disease. *Journal of Gerontology and Psychologi-cal Sciences* 55(1):S2–13.

Coen, R. F., O'Boyle, C. A., Coakley, D., and Lawlor, B. A. 2002. Individual quality of life fac-tors distinguishing low-burden and high-burden caregivers of dementia patients. *Demen-tia and Geriatric Cognitive Disorders* 13(3):164–70.

Cohen, C. A., Colantonio, A., Vernich, L. 2002. Positive aspects of caregiving: Rounding out the caregiver experience. *International Journal of Geriatric Psychiatry* 17(2):184–88.

Coon, D. W., Rubert, M., Solano, N., Mausbach, B., Kraemer, H., Arguelles, T., Haley, W. E., Thompson, L. W., and Gallagher-Thompson, D. 2004. Well-being, appraisal, and coping in Latina and Caucasian female dementia caregivers: Findings from the REACH study. *Aging and Mental Health* 8(4):330–45.

Daire, A. 2002. The influence of parental bonding on emotional distress in caregiving sons for a parent with dementia. *Gerontologist* 42:766–71.

Doty, P., Jackson, M. E., and Crown, W. 1998. The impact of female caregivers' employment status on patterns of formal and informal eldercare. *Gerontologist* 38:331–41.

Dougherty, L. M., and Chamblin, B. 1999. Assessment as an adjunct to psychotherapy. In P. Lichtenberg (Ed.), *Handbook of assessment in clinical gerontology* (pp. 91–110). New York: John Wiley & Sons.

Dunkin, J. J., and Anderson-Hanley, C. 1998. Dementia caregiver burden: A review of the literature and guidelines for assessment and intervention. *Neurology* 51(Suppl 1):S53–60.

Farran, C. J., Miller, B. H., Kaufman, J. E., Donner, E., and Fogg, L. 1999. Finding meaning through caregiving: Development of an instrument for family caregivers of persons with Alzheimer's disease. *Journal of Clinical Psychology* 55(9):1107–25.

Fox, P., Newcomer, R., Yordi, C., and Arnsberger, P. 2000. Lessons learned from the Medicare Alzheimer Disease Demonstration. *Alzheimer's Disease and Associated Disorders* 14(2):87–93.

Gaugler, J. E., Davey, A., Pearlin, L. I., and Zarit, S. H. 2000. Modeling caregiver adaptation over time: The longitudinal impact of behavior problems. *Psychology and Aging* 15(3): 437–50.

Glaser, R., and Kiecolt-Glaser, J. K. 1997. Chronic stress modulates the virus-specific immune response to latent herpes simplex type 1. *Annals of Behavioral Medicine* 19:78–82.

Goode, K. T., Haley, W. E., Roth, D. L., and Ford, G. R. 1998. Predicting longitudinal changes in caregiver physical and mental health: A stress process model. *Health Psychology* 17: 190–98.

Hadjistavropoulos, T., Taylor, S., Tuokko, H., and Beattie, B. L. 1994. Neuropsychological deficits, caregivers' perception of deficits and caregiver burden. *Journal of the American Geriatrics Society* 42:308–14.

Haley, W. E., LaMonde, L. A., Han, B., Narramore, S., and Schonwetter, R. 2001. Family caregiving in hospice: Effects on psychological and health functioning among spousal caregivers of hospice patients with lung cancer or dementia. *Hospice Journal* 15(4):1–18.

Haley, W. E., and Pardo, K. M. 1987. Relationship of stage of dementia to caregiver stress and coping. Paper presented at 95th annual convention of the American Psychological Association, New York.

Harwood, D. G., Barker, W. W., Cantilon, M., Loewenstein, D. A., Ownby, R., and Duara, R. 1998. Depressive symptomatology in first-degree family caregivers of Alzheimer-disease patients: A cross-ethnic comparison. *Alzheimer's Disease and Associated Disorders* 12:340–46.

Harwood, D. G., Barker, W. W., Ownby, R. L., and Duara, R. 2000. Caregiver self-rated health in Alzheimer's disease. *Clinical Gerontologist* 21:19–33.

Hirono, N., Tsukamoto, N., Inoue M., Moriwaki, Y., and Mori, E. 2002. Predictors of long term institutionalization in patients with Alzheimer's disease: Role of caregiver burden. *No To Shinkei* 54(9):812–18.

Huang, L., Cartwright, W. S., and Hu, T. 1988. The economic cost of senile dementia in the United States. 1985. *Public Health Reports* 103(1):3–7.

Hughes, S. L., Gobbie-Hurder, A., Weaver, F. M., Kubal, J. D., and Henderson, W. 1999. Relationship between caregiver burden and health-related quality of life. *Gerontologist* 39: 534–45.

Ingersoll-Dayton, B., Morgan, D., and Antonucci, T. 1997. The effects of positive and negative social exchanges on aging adults. *Journal of Gerontology: Social Sciences* 52(4):S190–99.

Karlawish, J. H. T., Casarett, D., Klocinski, J., and Clark, C. M. 2001. The relationship between caregivers' global ratings of Alzheimer disease patients' quality of life, disease severity, and the caregiver experience. *Journal of the American Geriatrics Society* 49:1066–70.

Karlin, N. J., Bell, P. A., and Noah, J. L. 2001. Long-term consequences of the Alzheimer's caregiver role: A qualitative analysis. *American Journal of Alzheimer's Disease and Other Dementias* 16(3):177–82.

Kiecolt-Glaser, J. K., and Glaser, R. 1990. Caregiving, mental health, and immune function. In E. Light and B. D. Lebowitz (Eds.), *Alzheimer's disease: Treatment and family stress* (pp. 245–66). New York: Hemisphere Publishing.

Knight, B. G., Silverstein, M., McCallum, T. J., and Fox, L. S. 2000. A socio-cultural stress and coping model for mental health outcomes among African-American caregivers in southern California. *Journals of Gerontology: Psychological and Social Sciences* 55(3): 142–50.

Lachman, M. E. 2003. Negative interactions in close relationships: Introduction to a special section. *Journal of Gerontology: Psychological Sciences* 58B(2):69.

Lawton, M. P., Kleban, M. H., Moss, M., Rovine, M., and Glicksman, A. 1989. Measuring caregiver appraisal. *Journal of Gerontology: Psychological Sciences* 44(3):61–71.

Lawton, M. P., Moss, M., Hoffman, C., and Perkinson, M. 2000. Two transitions in daughters' caregiving careers. *Gerontologist* 40:437–48.

Lieberman, M. A., and Fisher, L. 2001. The effects of nursing home placement on family caregivers of patients with Alzheimer's disease. *Gerontologist* 41:819–26.

Meshefedjian, G., McCusker, J., Bellavance, F., and Baumgarten, M. 1998. Factors associated with symptoms of depression among informal caregivers of demented elders in the community. *Gerontologist* 38:247–53.

Moeller, J. W., and Shuell, H. 1988. Elder care: Caregiving in the workplace. Berkeley, Calif.: Summer Series on Aging, American Society on Aging.

Moritz, D. J., Kasl, S. V., and Ostfeld, A. M. 1992. The health impact of living with a cognitively impaired elderly spouse. *Journal of Aging and Health* 4:244–67.

Motenko, A. K. 1989. The frustrations, gratifications, and well-being of dementia caregivers. *Gerontologist* 29(2):166–72.

Newcomer, R., Yordi, C., DuNah, R., Fox, P., and Wilkinson, A. 1999. Effects of the Medicare Alzheimer's Disease Demonstration on caregiver burden and depression. *Health Services Research* 34(3):669–89.

Nissel, M. 1984. The family costs of looking after handicapped elderly relatives. *Aging and Society* 4(2):185–204.

Novak, M., and Guest, C. 1989. Application of a multidimensional caregiver burden inventory. *Gerontologist* 19:798–803.

Ory, M. G., Hoffman, R. R. 3rd, Yee, J. L., Tennstedt, S., and Schulz, R 1999. Prevalence and impact of caregiving: A detailed comparison between dementia and nondementia caregivers. *Gerontologist* 39:177–85.

Ory, M. G., Yee, J. L., Tennstedt, S. L., and Schulz, R. 2000. The extent and impact of dementia care: Unique challenges experienced by family caregivers. In R. Schulz (Ed.), *Handbook on dementia caregiving: Evidence-based interventions for family caregivers*. New York: Springer.

Pariante, C. M., Carpiniello, B., Orru, M. G., Sitzia, R., Piras, A., Farci, A. M. G., Del Giacco, G. S., Piludu, G., and Miller, A. H. 1997. Chronic caregiving stress alters peripheral blood immune parameters: The role of age and severity of stress. *Psychotherapy and Psychosomatics* 66:199–207.

Pearlin, L. I., Mullan, J. T., Semple, S. J., Skaff, M. M. 1990. Caregiving and the stress process: An overview of concepts and their measures. *Gerontologist* 30:583–94.

Pillemer, K., and Suitor, J. J. 1996. It takes one to help one: Status similarity and well-being of family caregivers to relatives with dementia. *Journal of Gerontology: Social Sciences* 51B: S250–57.

Pillemer, K., Suitor, J. J., and Wethington, E. 2003. Integrating theory, basic research, and intervention: Two case studies from caregiving research. *Gerontologist* 43(Special Issue):19–28.

Pruchno, R. A., and Resch, N. L. 1989. Husbands and wives as caregivers: Antecedents of depression and burden. *Gerontologist* 29:159–65.

Rice, D. P., Fox, P. J., Max, W., Webber, P. A., Lindeman, D. A., Hauck, W. W., and Segura, E. 1993. The economic burden of Alzheimer's disease care. *Health Affairs* 12:164–76.

Ryan, A. A., and Scullion, H. F. 2000. Nursing home placement: An exploration of the experiences of family carers. *Journal of Advanced Nursing* 32(5):1187–95.

Schulz, R., Biegel, D., Morycz, R., and Visintainer, P. 1990. Psychological paradigms for understanding caregiving. In E. Light and B. D. Lebowitz (Eds.), *Alzheimer's disease: Treatment and family stress* (pp. 106–21). New York: Hemisphere Publishing.

Schulz, R., O'Brien, A. T., Bookwala, J., and Fleissner, K. 1995. Psychiatric and physical morbidity effects of dementia caregiving: Prevalence, correlates, and causes. *Gerontologist* 35: 771–91.

Seeman, T. E., Kaplan, G. A., Knudsen, L., Cohen, R., and Guralnik, J. 1987. Social network ties and mortality among the elderly in the Alameda County Study. *American Journal of Epidemiology* 126(4):714–23.

Stephens, M. A. P., and Franks, M. M. 1999. Intergenerational relationships in late-life families: Adult daughters and sons as caregivers to aging parents. In J. Cavanaugh and S. K. Whitbourne (Eds.), *Gerontology: An interdisciplinary perspective* (pp. 329–54). New York: Oxford University Press.

Tarrier, N., Barrowclough, C., Ward, J., Donaldson, C., Burns, A., and Gregg, L. 2002. Expressed emotion and attribution in the cares of patients with Alzheimer's disease: The effect on carer burden. *Journal of Abnormal Psychology* 111(2):340–49.

Teri, L., Gibbons, L. E., McCurry, S. M., Logsdon, R., G., Buchner, D. M., Barlow, W. E., Kukull, W. A., LaCroix, A. Z., McCormick, W., and Larson, E. B. 2003. Exercise plus behavior management in patients with Alzheimer's disease: A randomized control trial. *JAMA* 290(15):2015–22.

Teri, L., Logsdon, R. G., and McCurry, S. M. 2002. Nonpharmacologic treatment of behavioral disturbance in dementia. *Medical Clinics of North America* 86(3):641–56.

Teri, L., Logsdon, R. G., Peskind, E., Raskind, M., Weiner, M. F., Tractenberg, R. E., Foster, N. L., Scneider, L. S., Sano, M., Whitehouse, P., Tariot, P., Mellow, A. M., Auchus, A. P., Grundman, M., Thomas, R. G., Schafer, K., and Thal, L. J., Alzheimer Disease Cooperative Study. 2000. Treatment of agitation in AD: A randomized, placebo-controlled clinical trial. *Neurology* 55(9):1271–78.

Tornatore, J. B., and Grant, L. A. 2002. Burden among family caregivers of persons with Alzheimer's disease in nursing homes. *Gerontologist* 42:497–506.

Vitaliano, P. P., Maiuro, R. D., Ochs, H., and Russo, J. 1990. A model of burden in caregivers in DAT patients. In E. Light and B. D. Lebowitz (Eds.), *Alzheimer's disease: Treatment and family stress* (pp. 267–91). New York: Hemisphere Publishing.

Vitaliano, P. P., Young, H. M., and Russo, J. 1991. Burden: A review of measures used among caregivers of individuals with dementia. *Gerontologist* 31:67–75.

Waldman, K. 1998. Benefits of caregiving. In-service presented to the Mental Health Care Line at the Veterans Affairs Medical Center, Houston, Texas.

Weiner, M. F., Tractenberg, R. E., Sano, M., Logsdon, R., Teri, L., Glasko, D., Gamst, A., Thomas, R., and Thal, L. J. 2002. No long-term effect of behavioral treatment on psychotropic drug use for agitation in Alzheimer's disease patients. *Journal of Geriatric Psychiatry and Neurology* 15(2):95–98.

Yaffe, K., Fox, P., Newcomer, R., Sands, L., Lindquist, K., Dane, K., and Covinsky, K. E. 2002. Patient and caregiver characteristics and nursing home placement in patients with dementia. *JAMA* 287(16):2090–97.

Yeh, S. H., Johnson, M. A., and Wang, S. T. 2002. The changes in caregiver burden following nursing home placement. *International Journal of Nursing Studies* 39(6):591–600.

Zarit, S. H., Reever, K. E., and Bach-Peterson, J. 1980. Relatives of the impaired elderly: Correlates of feelings of burden. *Gerontologist* 20:649–55.

Zarit, S. H., and Zarit, J. M. 1982. Families under stress: Interventions for caregivers of senile dementia patients. *Psychotherapy: Theory, Research, and Practice* 19(4):461–71.

PART 3

Interpersonal Aspects of Caregiving

Part III examines caregiving from an interpersonal context. In chapter 5, Sheila M. LoboPrabhu reviews the literature on attachment and its role in family caregiving. She then discusses the interpersonal affective bond between individuals and its role in caregiving. The chapter starts with a review of attachment theory, including the work of John Bowlby and Marie Ainsworth, and a description of the nine maturational tasks needed for a healthy marriage as described by Judith Wallerstein and Sandra Blakeslee. The role of the attachment bond in caregiving is discussed, as well as factors that promote continued caregiving in the face of adversity. Jerry Lewis's concept of rupture and repair of the bond between patient and family members in facilitating continued attachment is highlighted in the context of adult development. A healthy and positive bond will stand a caregiver in good stead during the difficult times. Of course, a damaged bond will place a caregiver and patient at risk for an unhealthy or abusive course of caregiving, with much pain experienced by patient, caregiver, and possibly the health care team. Practice implications for health care professionals based on an understanding of attachment theory are described and illustrated with the help of a clinical vignette.

In chapter 6, James W. Lomax offers a psychodynamic perspective on religion and spirituality. From this point of view, joy in caregiving results from creative illusion formation, which is an activity reinforced by participation in faith-based groups. In clinical encounters with patients and caregivers, Dr. Lomax urges appreciation of the positive and negative consequences of religious participation and recommends full use of community resources, including religious institutions and spiritual leaders, to guide treatment of mental health problems.

Naomi D. Nelson discusses in chapter 7 how intimacy and sexuality are affected by caregiving. Wright and Riegel's work on the principles of dialectical interaction suggests that the past, present, and future of marital relationships are intertwined and eventually become predictors of outcomes for a couple's relationship. It is the interaction of these three levels, rather than the illness severity, that determines the quality of the relationship when one member has dementia. This mutual dependency and interconnectedness of people explains why one spouse's behavior is so influenced by the behavior of the other spouse. Developmental dyssynchrony occurs when Alzheimer disease causes conflicts in various life dimensions. Dr. Nelson notes that such discord could have either positive or negative costs, depending on what actions are taken by the patient, caregiver, community, and health care team. Appropriate enactive skills learned by the caregiver, low levels of expressed emotion, interpretive caring by a caregiver, and a supportive health care team can all positively influence dialectical interaction and enhance quality of life.

Hana Osman addresses grief, bereavement, mourning, and death within the context of dementia in chapter 8. She first outlines the five stages of grief in anticipating one's own death as outlined by Elisabeth Kübler-Ross. She next discusses anticipatory grief on the part of both patient and caregiver, and how grief can add to stress in caregiving. She then describes how the loss of persona in dementia can cause anticipatory grief, and emphasizes the need for frequent monitoring, attention to the wishes of the patient, completion of advance directives, and end-of-life planning in an effort to honor the loved one's wishes. She concludes with a strong recommendation for involving both the care recipient and the caregiver in all aspects of treatment. Proper referrals to caregiver resources will ensure maximal support for the caregiver during and after the caregiving process.

CHAPTER FIVE

The Affective Interpersonal Bond in Caregiving

SHEILA M. LOBOPRABHU, M.D.

The concept of attachment styles is useful in examining adult caregiving relationships, in that throughout our lives attachment influences our basic interpersonal relationships and the way we interact with each other in familial, social, and environmental contexts. Attachment also plays an important role in normal aging. We would therefore expect attachment to be of great significance in how families cope with the onset of dementia in a family member. Dementia is devastating for both patient and family for many reasons: the loss of memory and independence of the afflicted person, the increasing reliance on family members initially for minor assistance, then with activities of daily living, and finally for total care. An extremely strong interpersonal bond between family members is needed to provide this extraordinary degree of care amidst the tremendous emotional, financial, and health burden to caregivers. This chapter explores attachment in the context of the interpersonal affective bond in caregiving relationships. It then reviews the psychodynamic and interpersonal aspects of the affective bond and discusses the role of disruption and repair of the interpersonal bond in facilitating healing and enabling ongoing caregiving in the context of dementia.

The three attachment styles beginning in early childhood can be identified in adult caregiving relationships as well. Secure attachment is characterized by positive feeling between caregiver and care recipient; insecure attachments are characterized by avoidance and ambivalence. Daily problems set the stage for empathic failures and misattunements between caregiver and care recipient. Successful repair of these misattunements strengthens the caregiving relationship, whereas repeated ruptures and withdrawals may result in a breach of the caregiver-recipient bond. Insecure attachment styles can lead to compulsive caregiving, defensive separation, and excessive dependency (Bowlby, 1969, 1973, 1980). These pathological styles of caregiving can lead to interpersonal conflict, which then initiates a cycle of negativity resulting in depression and guilt. Van Doorn et al. (1998) noted that "security increasing" marriages put spouses at risk for elevated grief symptoms on the death of one spouse. Security-increasing marriages are defined as those in which the marriage served a countervailing or compensatory function for the deficiencies of one or both spouses. Similarly, dementia in one spouse will change the dynamics of a stable relationship and increase the risk of depression and grief in the caregiving spouse.

AN OVERVIEW OF ATTACHMENT THEORY

Attachment is an enduring affective bond characterized by the tendency to seek and maintain proximity to a specific person, particularly when under stress (Ainsworth, 1973; Bowlby, 1969). Attachment is the deep and long-lasting connection between child and caregiver achieved during the first years of life. It profoundly influences every aspect of the human condition (i.e., mind, body, emotions, relationships, and values) (Levy and Thomas, 1999). Attachment to a loving caregiver is a basic human need. Children instinctively need the support and secure base that the parent provides within an ongoing reciprocal relationship.

Freud (1940) described the mother as the provider of basic satisfaction related to relief of hunger, cold, and other discomforts. Erikson (1963) described basic trust as one of eight stages of human development. Successful attainment of basic trust and positive experiences during the infant's early development will predispose the infant to secure attachment. Bowlby (1969) suggested that the infant develops an attachment to the mother not only because she is associated with gratification of physical needs but also because of basic behavioral patterns needed to promote infant survival. Bowlby (1969) and Ainsworth (1973) described the variable quality of the infant-mother attachment based on the dimension of security. Bowlby notes that if infants experience sensitive care consistently, they will develop a secure attachment to the caregiver. However, if infants experience sensitive care inconsistently or sporadically, or worse, if they do not experience sensitive care at all, they will develop insecure attachment. Ainsworth et al. (1978) described the Strange Situation procedure, in which infants are separated and then reunited with the mother, and then exposed to a stranger in the room in the presence and in the absence of mother. The infants are divided into three categories based on their behavior during the reunions with the mother after such exposures: secure attachment (in which the mother's return is greeted with unequivocal pleasure); insecure-avoidant attachment (in which the mother's return is greeted with conspicuous avoidance of mother by the infant); and insecure-resistant attachment (in which there is proximity-seeking behavior combined with angry, rejecting behavior at reunion with the mother).

Attachment persists into adulthood, with investment in adult loving relationships. Successful interpersonal bonding is essential to the capacity for sharing in the adult developmental stage of intimacy versus isolation (Erikson, 1963). Lewis (2000) suggested that a strong affective bond involves reciprocal gratification, which may be referred to as "quid pro quo." There is an ongoing dynamic in marriages and parent-child relationships in which each participant receives something important from the other. Harry Stack Sullivan (1953) first studied the importance of relationships and processes between people. In his interpersonal approach to therapy, the area of focus is the primary social group in a patient's life, defined as the immediate face-to-face involvement of the patient with one or more significant other. Humans of all ages are vulnerable to impairment in interpersonal relationships if there is failure or disruption in the development of strong early attachment bonds.

In his discussion of the role of relationships, Lewis (2000) stated that growth is facilitated when a strong affective bond is established with an important other, and when disruptions of this bond are repaired. Disruptions are inevitable, as it is impossible for perfect attunement to occur between two people all the time. Misattunements are common and can be thought of as failures in empathy. Healing occurs in the context of recognition of misattunement, acknowledgment of error, and exploration of the content or process which was not initially responded to. This healing of the relationship is the process of repair of the interpersonal affective bond.

A GOOD MARRIAGE

This section addresses what constitutes a good marriage and what makes a marital bond strong and helps sustain it through adversity (in this case, caregiving for a spouse with dementia). Caregiving and interpersonal bonding is examined from the context of the marital bond and how it is affected with the onset of dementia in one spouse. The next section discusses Jerry Lewis's work in rupture and repair of the interpersonal bond and its possible role in enabling spouses to continue caregiving in the face of enormous adversity.

The Elements of a Good Marriage

Marriage is defined as a "close union of husband and wife" or "joining together of husband and wife according to law or custom." Judith Wallerstein and Sandra Blakeslee (1996), in their book *The Good Marriage,* talk about the closeness between husbands and wives. They describe four types of marriage: romantic, rescue, companionate, and traditional. In the romantic marriage, couples keep alive within their marriage a sense of the original romantic love and intimacy that brought them together. Rescue marriages occur when one or both of the spouses enters the marriage to escape a difficult situation. The companionate marriage is noted for equally shared responsibilities between the spouses, when couples may both work outside the home and share child rearing and chores equally. The traditional marriage is characterized by the husband's being the breadwinner and the wife's staying home and caring for home and children. Wallerstein and Blakeslee also described the nine maturational tasks couples need to accomplish to build a healthy marriage:

1. to separate sufficiently emotionally from the family of origin, so that each spouse can fully invest in the marriage
2. to facilitate intimacy within the marriage, which will build togetherness while allowing each spouse sufficient autonomy
3. to embrace the daunting task of parenthood, while creating enough private time for the couple
4. to confront and master the inevitable crises of life, while maintaining the strength of the combined bond against adversity
5. to create a safe haven for the expression of differences, anger, and conflict
6. to establish a rich sexual relationship which is guarded against invasions from family and the outside
7. to use laughter and humor to keep things in perspective at all times
8. to nurture and comfort each other, while meeting each other's dependency needs and offering encouragement and support
9. to keep alive the early romantic idealized images of falling in love, while facing the sober realities of the changes wrought by time.

Wallerstein and Blakeslee (1996) noted in relation to task 4 that couples who stay together strive to overcome the inevitable crises of life while maintaining a strong combined bond against adversity. This bond is maximally tested when one or both spouses becomes seriously ill. This commonly occurs in old age, and especially when one spouse develops dementia.

Caregiving and Bonding

The caregiving situation is unique in that it involves change imposed by severe illness on a preexisting affective bond. Caregivers, as discussed above, are usually family members (the spouse being the most likely of all family members to provide care and adult children being the second most common). They have likely bonded with the afflicted individual over the course of a marriage or a lifetime. The bond formed during earlier experience with the patient when she was well is the basis for future caregiving. The more positive the bond, with its foundation of shared memories and interactions, the easier the caregiving. In the case of a conflicted prior relationship, it is harder for the caregiver to provide positive, nurturing care. Hodgson (1995), in her book *Alzheimer's—Finding the Words: A Communication Guide for Those Who Care*, describes her experience of caring for her mother with Alzheimer disease. She describes her love for her mother and her responses to the changes in her mother wrought by the illness: "Day by day, cell by cell, relatives are watching a loved one die and the emotional pain is unbearable" (p. 100). Hodgson describes caregivers' pain when the afflicted person fails to recall shared life events, and more so at the failure of facial recognition as the disease advances. She notes, "Moments of rare intelligence are like a gift. I'm gathering a mental bouquet of these moments and hope they will sustain me in the future. But I know these moments are becoming scarcer and will be gone soon. Therefore I cherish each one and clutch it to my heart" (p. 71). She poignantly describes the value of the interpersonal affective bond in human relationships and the joy brought by close attachments. However, disruption of the same bond can cause severe pain.

The Strength of the Marital Bond

One questions the particular strength and tenacity of the marital affective bond: is it because this is the most verbally expressed bond, with spoken words at the time of the wedding ceremony? Or is it because most religions consider this vow sacred? Many religions include the explicit promise of caregiving in the marital vow ("for richer or for poorer, in sickness and in health . . . till death do us part"). Most cultures recognize marriage as the predominant legal relationship, which supersedes the relationship between parent and adult children or between siblings. Spouses have special rights and responsibilities. Marriage is also a relationship of sexual intimacy and closeness, which sets it apart from other relationships. Disruption of the marital bond is often a devastating aspect of dementia. Caregiving spouses of persons with dementia need protection of their rights to enable them to fulfill their special responsibilities.

Marital Strain

The interpersonal affective bond is maximally tested when one spouse is seriously ill. Gladstone (1995) described four themes in marital perceptions when one of the spouses is afflicted with dementia: "marriage as a memory," the "illusory marriage," the "changed marriage," and the "unchanged or continuing marriage." In "marriage as a memory," spouses felt like their marriages were over, because of loss of companionship, or owing to the nonresponsiveness of the ill spouse due to cognitive impairment. In "illusory marriage," spouses described their situations as feeling not really married, but not really widowed either (i.e., an ambiguous marital status). In "changed marriage," spouses noted alterations in the nature of their marital relationships due to cognitive impairment in the afflicted spouse. They defined contacts with their spouses as that between friends, rather than that between marital partners. In the "unchanged or continuing marriage," spouses indicated that their marriages were unchanged or that their present circumstances were just another stage in their marriage. They referred to the ongoing love they felt for their spouses. The majority of spouses therefore indicated a difference in their marriage due to the cognitive deterioration of their partner. Clearly, the marital bond is tremendously at risk, and the challenge is how the spousal caregiver will cope. Spousal caregivers are at high risk for financial and health problems. Yet they provide the most extensive, comprehensive care to the most severely disabled. They are also the least likely to ask for help, and are therefore at greatest risk for caregiver strain and burden (Ade-Ridder and Kaplan, 1993). The marital bond can therefore be considered unique as compared to bonds with other family members and friends.

THE ROLE OF RUPTURE AND REPAIR IN PRESERVING
THE INTEGRITY OF A RELATIONSHIP
Rupture

Alzheimer disease is unique in its long-term course, the progressive nature of the illness, its severe financial burden (an estimated $172,000 per afflicted person), and its extreme cost to career, family, and health of the caregiver. Colarusso and Nemiroff (1987) described adult developmental tasks which include aging, increased awareness of time limitation and one's own death, illnesses or deaths of parents, family, and friends, altered relationships with family and a maturing spouse, planning for retirement and recognizing that not all personal goals will be reached in one's lifetime. Failure to successfully negotiate these developmental tasks results in a sense of failure and depression. This approach normalizes the caregiver's struggle with an expected developmental task, namely caring for an ill family member. There is inevitably conflict between the attainment of the caregiver's own personal goals while caring for a severely ill person. Caregivers often experience fatigue, anger, frustration, depression, role conflict, and guilt. These emotions may disrupt the relationship between caregiver and care recipient, often resulting in a sense of failure.

Grief and anticipatory mourning are common responses of the afflicted person and the family. Dementia can be seen as a moving target, characterized by a fluctuating but progressive course of the memory loss and cognitive changes of Alzheimer disease. The caregiver must cope with the repetitive questioning, derailment of thought processes, memory lapses, failure to recognize people and things, aphasia, apraxia (difficulty with executing learned movements or command), and dysarthria, which are common symptoms of dementia. Patients often deny that these things are happening. These could all be seen as ruptures in the affective bond between caregiver and patient.

What then is the process of repair which allows joy in caregiving and enables the caregiving relationship to continue despite great adversity?

Repair

Calvin Settlage (1988) proposed the concept of an adult developmental process. He suggests that disruption of a previously satisfactory and adaptive system is the stimulus for development, providing a challenge, which first leads to tension and then to conflict. Successful resolution leads to mastery and structural integration of the new function and attainment of a new level in the developmental process. Schore (1996) suggested that the infant's affect changes from despair to joy in the repair process. This is associated with the secretion of dopamine and endogenous opiates, which then prompt synaptic growth in the prefrontolimbic regions of the right brain. Internalization of a loved object is a factor in adult personality growth. Individuals are believed to incorporate into the self either admirable qualities of important others or characteristics of relationships with important others (Vaillant, 1977). Blatt and Behrends (1987) posited a model that centers on the formation of a gratifying relationship. Disruptions in this relationship may provoke internalization. When threatened by separation and loss in a relationship with an important other, the individual may attempt to retain the other by internalization of the other. Tronick and Gianino (1986) emphasized that successful repair turns despair into positive emotions, leading to a sense of mastery, development of effective coping mechanisms, and internalization of a relationship pattern which may prove valuable in later life. These authors provide different perspectives on the loss of the family role of the afflicted person and the struggle of the family to grieve that loss, cope with the challenge of letting go, and provide progressively increasing support.

There are other methods to repair the affective bond. One such method is through communication with loved ones, however fragmented their speech may be. Hodgson (1995) describes a story her mother with dementia loved to repeat. She comments, "My mother's pleasure in telling the story exceeds my displeasure at hearing it" (p. 42). Sensing the pleasure of the loved one may be a source of comfort to caregivers. Some caregivers attain pleasure in silence, in just sitting in the company of the loved one. Others communicate better with music even after speech is gone. Reality orientation is a way to cope by providing short, focused directions. That, accompanied by touch, is a method many caregivers describe as directing the person, while helping him or her feel safe and secure. Many caregivers describe this shared bonding through safety and security as rewarding. Validation therapy involves affirmation of the feeling behind an apparently disoriented interchange by the patient. In this form of therapy, caregivers look behind the words or behavior and examine the afflicted person's emotions leading to such behavior. This empathic effort aids in providing emotional support and strengthening the interpersonal bond. In summary, caregiving is an ongoing dance between caregiver and care recipient. In negotiating the complicated steps of this intricate dance, there is a sense of mastery and pleasure in a job well done.

Factors Modifying Successful Repair

Modifying factors in successful repair of the marital bond when it is ruptured by adverse circumstances can be listed as: (1) mastery, (2) boundary ambiguity, (3) perceived control, and (4) wishful thinking. Repair of the marital bond can be thought of in terms of "mastery" despite "boundary ambiguity," achieving greater "perceived control" over stressors, and minimizing "wishful thinking" coping behavior.

"Mastery" versus "helplessness" is a developmental challenge described in the cognitive therapy literature. Successful attainment of mastery indicates a successful outcome in the treatment of depression. There are mastery and pleasure scales which are used as subjective rating measures in the cognitive-behavioral approach to treatment of depression. One scale to measure mastery is the Pearlin Mastery Scale (Pearlin, Lieberman, Menaghan, and Mullan, 1981). Kaplan and Boss (1999) note that "boundary ambiguity" is the confusion experienced by a caregiver in caring for a person with dementia who is physically present but mentally and emotionally absent. The Boundary Ambiguity Scale for Dementia (Caron, Boss, and Mortimer, 1999) is a 21-item self-report instrument used to measure the degree to which the caregiver is preoccupied with the patient. It has two subscales measuring the two main factors representing boundary ambiguity: caregiver immobilization (which is the feeling of being trapped and overwhelmed in the caregiver role) and patient closeout (which is the extent to which the caregiver emotionally disengages from the care recipient). Obviously, caregivers of persons with dementia can rate high on both subscales, as the care recipient's cognitive difficulties place the caregiver in a very difficult situation. It is important that a caregiver retain a sense of mastery despite boundary ambiguity in order to cope well. Kaplan and Boss (1999) administered questionnaires to 84 community-dwelling spouses of persons with Alzheimer disease, in an attempt to identify factors that predict whether or not community-dwelling spouses experience depressive symptoms on institutionalization of a spouse with dementia. Boundary ambiguity alone accounted for 51 percent of the variability in the depressive symptoms score, whereas mastery alone was found to account for 32 percent. Mastery did not add significantly to the explanation of the depressive symptom score over and above boundary ambiguity. However, boundary ambiguity and mastery were linked together and were powerful in explaining caregiver symptoms of depression. Kaplan and Boss therefore infer that, in order to keep caregivers healthy, interventions and education about how to live with ambiguity and how to be masterful despite the ambiguous status of one's spouse seem necessary.

Wallhagen (1992) describes "perceived control" as the sense of control that a person experiences in a particular setting or situation. Perceived control has been implicated in the adaptation and well-being of older adults, and it may be especially relevant to older caregivers. Wallhagen notes that perceived control has a direct relationship with life satisfaction and depression and an indirect relationship with subjective symptoms of stress. Sistler and Blanchard-Fields (1993) studied 27 spouse caregivers of persons with dementia and 33 noncaregiving (healthy) spouses, aged 54 to 90, who described a stressful situation with their spouses. They completed measures of perceived control and subjective well-being. Both groups felt a similar perceived lack of control over the spouse's behavior, but they differed in how control influenced positive affect. Perceived control over the spouse was negatively related to positive affect for the healthy couples, but for caregivers it was positively related. Wishful thinking can be defined as wishing that things were different and that the spouse was not ill. Wishful thinking coping behavior had a negative relationship with all adaptation variables (Wallhagen, 1992/93).

Successful caregiver adaptation to the stress of caring for a person with dementia hinges on a variety of developmental outcomes. Spouses or family members who had a previously good marriage or relationship with the patient are better able to feel a sense of mastery in helping their now ill family member, and a positive relationship sets the stage for a better sense of perceived control. However, unhappy or abusive marriages or relationships are already characterized by a sense of anger and closeout. Such caregivers are therefore at higher risk for boundary ambiguity, wishful thinking that things were different, resentment at now having to care for the family member with dementia, and poor caregiver adaptation. Our role as health care professionals is early identification of at-risk marriages and relationships, maintaining sensitivity to patient and caregiver issues, validation of anger and hurt at past traumas or conflicts, and helping the caregiver and care recipient successfully adapt to the demands and stresses of caregiving.

JOY IN CAREGIVING

Gwyther (1990) suggests that values of commitment and family solidarity play a large role in caregiving. Older married couples have well-established values about commitment and family solidarity. Caregivers may feel pride and accomplishment in honoring their vows despite extreme sacrifice. Various comments from caregivers suggest that there is a core of strength that enables the relationship to survive and the caregiver to stay committed in the face of adversity.

An alternative suggestion is that dementia caregivers will tend to hold on to the familiar: to search for vestiges of familiarity in the loved one they once knew (Gwyther 1990). These vestiges, however minimal, bring great joy and enable the caregiver to go on. Gallagher-Thompson et al. (2001) videotaped caregiver and care recipient spouses with Alzheimer disease in their homes during nonstructured mealtime and structured planning activities when spouses planned for a future event such as a visit to a friend, a shopping trip, or a getaway. They measured three behavioral factors in the caregiving spouse: the supportive factor (assenting or paraphrasing behaviors such as expressing assent or approval), the facilitative factor (proposing a positive solution, clarifying statements, and inferring positive intentions in the spouse), and the rapport factor (includes smiling, laughing, using humor, and attending closely to the other person's speech). Caregiver spouses were noted to be most facilitative during the planning task, and care recipient spouses were highest on rapport-building interactions (e.g., smiling) during the same task. Caregiving wives increased their facilitative behavior from the mealtime to the planning task, probably reflecting the increased demand characteristics of the latter. These results may be used to conclude that smiling and expression of pleasure by the afflicted spouse has a positive feedback effect on the caregiver, thus providing the caregiver the necessary joy to continue caregiving.

Several authors suggest that mastery of the developmental task of separation-individuation brings a sense of accomplishment and satisfaction to the caregiver, which may strengthen the relationship (Colarusso and Nemiroff, 1987; Erikson, 1963). For spousal caregivers of persons with dementia, separation-individuation begins when they must make decisions without the guidance or support of the afflicted spouse, or when they are forced to seek outside help from family or formal sources. Caregivers must transition from their family role as spouse or adult child to caregiver, and ultimately from the caregiver stage to that of care manager, to cope with the progressive cognitive deterioration in the care recipient. This enables the caregiver to provide need-based care by attainment of separation-individuation along a moving continuum (Gwyther, 1990) where the caregiver needs to shoulder more responsibility while receiving less support from the impaired spouse. Separation-individuation conflicts may occur because of the need to share or relinquish part of the care of a spouse to family or other providers. Like any other stage in the developmental process, successful attainment of separation-individuation may provide a sense of mastery, which enables caregivers to generate feelings of success and pride.

Mr. A. is a 59-year-old male diagnosed with dementia after surgery for a ruptured cerebral aneurysm two years ago. He has severe memory and cognitive problems, is nearly aphasic with very little speech, and sometimes is incontinent of urine. He requires assistance to dress and groom himself. Mr. A. stopped driving two years ago. His wife wants to keep him at home as long as possible but fears that this will be hard to do because hallucinations and delusions sometimes keep him up at night. He wants his wife in the room at all times and in the same bed at night. Mr. A. has nightmares and often wakes his wife with his restless behavior. Mrs. A. is exhausted and feels that if she does not get some help, she will have to place him in a nursing home. She feels ashamed and frustrated at her perceived inability to cope with the situation. She also feels that she would be letting down her husband, who had been her best friend and a good husband and father.

Regarding caregiver burden, Mrs. A. says "Sometimes, I just want to run screaming through the house, and have at times done that. I have in the past gone into the backyard, dug holes, pulled weeds, and said everything out there I cannot say in the house, because it would not be fair. It is not his fault. The person I married is no longer there. I have learned that you do not ask God how much more of this you can take, because He will show you. We had planned to enjoy ourselves, go places and do things together. . . . I would see elderly wives taking their husbands in wheelchairs to their doctor's appointments. I never realized what these souls had to go through. The burden is unbelievable. You need a refuge for yourself, but you have to care for this person. You can't blame your partner and take it out on him; he didn't ask for this. I read the Bible and pray. I had too many problems when I was younger for me to be mad at God. I know that God does give you gifts. The only thing I can do is take one day at a time. There are so many people worse off than I. If I help others in greater need, I can remove myself from troubles. I am blessed with really good friends, who are empathic."

Yet this wife is able to feel joy in caregiving. "Oh, at times he is so loving with his friends and fun with the grandbabies and the kids. About joy in my private life . . . I love my gardening. I have friends who make me happy. They make me laugh, they call a lot and we just laugh. My husband brings me joy. We do have fun, if I can forget the things that we need done. I am not as compulsive now about the things that need doing around the house."

Mrs. A.'s comments suggest a strong bond between spouses. She clearly respects her spouse, who has been her best friend and confidant throughout their married life. Theirs is a romantic and traditional marriage, which has now become a "changed marriage" due to its irrevocable alteration by dementia. Mr. A.'s loss of functional ability, loss of memory, and cognitive problems are sources of pain for Mrs. A. She describes her perceived burden eloquently—she has a sense of losing the person she married, and instead having to care for a severely disabled spouse. At the same time, she describes the benefits of caregiving. In the case of this spouse, her strong spiritual convictions have enabled her to find joy. There is an uplifting sense of doing the right thing and fulfilling her part of the marital bargain. Her attempts to continue to find joy, even in this difficult situation, can be seen as her attempts to keep her marriage from becoming a "marriage as a memory." Her struggles can be seen as those of one attempting to hold on to the familiar, while gradually letting go. There are ruptures of the bond each time she has an empathic failure and an emotional outburst, which she so eloquently describes above. However, the consistent repair of this bond is what has brought her the most personal fulfillment and enabled continued caregiving. Treatment would focus on supporting this caregiver in fulfilling her personal obligations, while using appropriate pharmacotherapy to improve Mr. A.'s sleep, delusions, and hallucinations. Team involvement in helping this wife keep Mr. A. at home as long as possible will convey respect for the couple's wishes. The wife will also need support as the illness becomes too severe for her to adequately care for Mr. A. This is the time many caregivers need an exploratory discussion of their role as caregivers, involvement of adult children, and a reframed understanding of the spouse's responsibilities as a caregiver. Mrs. A.'s realistic appreciation of her caregiving role, along with an ability to examine her own thoughts and feelings, make this wife a good candidate for expressive-supportive psychotherapy, which can be incorporated into each clinic visit for Mr. A. We know that attainment of developmentally appropriate separation-individuation is associated with good caregiver coping. Constant empathic reframing of Mrs. A.'s struggles as a caregiver and providing support while she tries to master developmentally appropriate tasks will enable her to cope with her tremendous stress and grief.

SPECIAL BONDS

The section above discussed the special significance of the marital bond in dementia. In other chapters in this book, the role of spirituality in marriage and the role of intimacy in the sexual relationship are discussed in greater detail. This section addresses other important bonds in the care of persons with dementia, such as the bond between afflicted persons and their adult children and siblings and bonds with formal caregivers.

Adult Children

Adult children often have an important role to play in the care of persons with dementia. They form the second most common caregiving group, second only to spouses as caregivers of persons with dementia. Adult children may move in with an older family member or have the afflicted person live with them. They offer support such as cooked meals, homemaker services, driving, hands-on care, transportation to and from appointments, and help with treatment decisions. Areas of specific concern with adult children are issues of autonomy and loss. An example is when the parent afflicted with dementia has to relinquish driving to the son whom he first taught to drive. Parent-child relationships with prior conflicts predict problems with filial caregiving. Another special fear of a child of a person with dementia may be a fear that they too will develop dementia. Development of algorithms predictive of dementia based on family genetics and history may help alleviate some of the fears of adult children caring for parents with dementia.

Siblings as Caregivers

Many caregivers are siblings, especially in the case of the widowed or divorced elderly, or those without adult children or estranged from them. This is especially so in those cultures with large families (e.g., African American and Hispanic families). Faber and Mazlish (1998) suggested that there is typically positive bonding, sometimes accompanied by rivalry between siblings. Jewell and Stein (2002) stated that perceived sibling need, sibling affection, reciprocity with ill siblings, felt obligation toward parents, and parental requests for help with caregiving are associated with siblings caregiving for people with severe mental illness. Greenberg, Seltzer, Orsmond, and Krauss (1999) noted that the extent of current and future caregiving by siblings of disabled adults is a function of the demands and constraints of midlife, as well as the degree of closeness with family of origin. We need to know how such affective bonds differ from the marital bond and parent-child bonding, and the impact of sibling bonds in caregiving.

Bonds with Formal Caregivers

Clinical experience often suggests an attachment between a person with dementia and personal care or nursing home staff, especially in the context of long-term placement. Research is needed into the nature of such attachments, modifying factors, whether such attachments are with staff in general or with particular members of staff, and how this factor can be used to beneficially affect care in long-term facilities.

NEGOTIATING DEATH AND DYING: THE END OF THE RELATIONSHIP

As explained in more detail in chapter 8, whereas death most often represents the final opportunity to say good-bye to family members, for families in which the dying person has severe cognitive impairment, there is no possibility of saying good-bye. Death is a final disruption of the interpersonal bond. Yet, in death, as in caregiving, there is a chance for repair and healing. The important developmental task for the caregiver is that of final separation and letting go, along with internalization of the loved object. Elisabeth Kübler-Ross, in her book *On Death and Dying,* describes five stages of preparing for one's own death: denial, anger, bargaining, despair, and detachment. These stages are similar to anecdotal experiences of caregivers as they prepare for the death of a loved one with dementia. This process is often accompanied by anticipatory grief, when caregivers experience a process of decathexis in the loved one and they withdraw emotional attachment. This is a time of grief and intense emotional reaction for many caregivers and is further complicated by the complex medical care and decisions that accompany the dying process. Some such decisions are whether or not to implement tube feeds, whether to withdraw treatment and life support, and whether to proceed with end-of-life care. The caregiver may be responsible for surrogate decision making, a task made easier when there is an advance directive clearly expressing the afflicted person's wishes. Hospice and bereavement support groups have a valuable role in supporting families. Certain caregivers are at risk for traumatic grief (Shear et al., 2001) on the death of a spouse. Traumatic grief occurs in 10 to 20 percent of bereaved individuals and is characterized by traumatic stress and separation distress. Horowitz et al. (1997) first described the symptoms of traumatic grief as intrusive thoughts, strong pangs of severe emotions, strong yearnings, feelings of loneliness and emptiness, avoidance of people who serve as reminders of the loss, and loss of interest in personal activities. Traumatic grief is likely in the surviving spouse if the couple had a security enhancing marriage (as described earlier in this chapter), or if the caregiver-patient relationship was characterized by one of Bowlby's three insecure attachment styles: compulsive caregiving, excessive dependency, or a defensively separated attachment style. Preventive treatment for traumatic grief includes supportive psychotherapy, self-help groups, and widow-to-widow programs. These have shown moderate success in prevention of traumatic grief. Another treatment strategy is a three-phase approach outlined by Shear et al. (2001): (1) information gathering and rapport building, (2) addressing the core problems of traumatic stress and separation distress using re-experiencing exposure treatment and structured behavior therapy, and (3) flexible treatment with continued exposure therapy to reminders of the loss, or interpersonal therapy to assist reconnection of the bereaved spouse with others and to terminate the treatment.

IMPLICATIONS FOR CLINICAL PRACTICE

This review of the existing literature on the affective interpersonal bond in caregiving can help inform research-based practice guidelines in the management of caregiving in dementia. Caregiving in dementia can be viewed as an ongoing process, whose complex steps change constantly owing to the shifting needs of the person with dementia. Although it is important to be sensitive to the patient's needs, it is equally important to understand the role of the patient in the family and to maintain an adequate balance so that the needs of other family members may be met as well. Caregivers of persons with dementia are often struggling with other complex roles in the family in addition to caregiving, such as grandparenting and parenting, the caregiver's own medical problems, and financial troubles, which often accompany aging. Affirmation of the successes and joys of caregiving is essential in order for the caregiver to feel a sense of mastery. Validation and praise therefore are integral parts of visits to health care providers, providing the "refueling" needed for the caregiver to go on. I make the following six recommendations for the role of the health care team in assisting the caregiver:

1. *Identify the type of marriage or relationship that preceded the diagnosis of dementia.* In the case of couples, this would involve an assessment of the type of marriage and the degree of success in attaining the nine maturational tasks of a healthy marriage. In the case of all family caregivers, a thorough assessment of the attachment styles of patient and caregiver(s), both in their family of origin as well as in adult relationships, will help provide an informed approach to the nature of the adult caregiving relationship.

2. *Assess the changes in marital or relationship perceptions with the onset of dementia.* (i.e., whether the marriage is "unchanged," "changed," "illusory," or "marriage as a memory"). Obtaining a detailed marital history from both spouses will help the health care provider understand the nature of the prior relationship and the changes occurring in the marriage with the onset of dementia.

3. *Measure the degree of marital strain and burden imposed on the caregiver.* This will require assessment of the role of the caregiver and the nature of the caregiving relationship as well as identifying informal and formal social supports and the financial and emotional burdens of caregiving.

4. *Identify the joys of caregiving and what is particularly important to the caregiver in the creation of a sense of mastery or feelings of reward.* Praise and validation by the health care team are particularly helpful here, as the relationship is strengthened when the caregiver's struggles are acknowledged and when the caregiver is affirmed for the tremendously important role he or she plays in the care of the patient.

5. *Assess the areas of rupture and past/present/future repair of the affective interpersonal bond.* This will require a good understanding of the interpersonal relationship between the caregiver and care recipient and the role of the present caregiving relationship in bringing back past hurts, while providing an opportunity to heal and bring families closer.

6. *Assess and manage the factors affecting repair of the marital bond.* namely, "mastery," "boundary ambiguity," "perceived control," and "wishful thinking." The professional should attempt to maximize the caregiver's mastery and perceived control while minimizing boundary ambiguity and wishful thinking. This is the key to successful adaptation and a healthy caregiver–care recipient relationship.

CONCLUSION

Attachment is an enduring affective bond characterized by the tendency to seek and maintain proximity to a specific person, particularly when under stress. Dementia has been described as the "funeral that never ends," and it can strain even the strongest bonds of attachment. Caregiving for persons with dementia thus encompasses not only the usual demands of caregiving but is made worse by the progressive cognitive decline and loss of role in the family due to dementia. It is important for the health care team to treat, support, and provide vision and a sense of direction to the caregiver as he or she negotiates the difficult hurdles of caregiving. This can be done with a good understanding of attachment theory and the role it plays in caregiving.

Successful caregiving occurs in the context of repeated rupture and repair of the affective interpersonal bond between caregiver and care recipient. Repair brings joy to the caregiving relationship, providing a sense of satisfaction and reward, which is necessary for the caregiver to continue caregiving. Further research is necessary to better define the factors causing rupture and promoting repair of this bond. An explanation of the exact nature of separation and letting go in dementia will help clarify the developmental task faced by most caregivers. An appreciation of the type of marriage and the interpersonal aspects of the prior relationship provides an understanding of the specific conflicts for each caregiver-recipient dyad. This will help dementia care teams better understand the current caregiving situation within the context of the prior relationship and provide definitive guidelines for treatment to enhance the quality of life of both caregivers and care recipients.

REFERENCES

Ade-Ridder, L., and Kaplan, L. 1993. Marriage, spousal caregiving and a husband's move to a nursing home: A changing role for the wife? *Journal of Gerontological Nursing* 19:13–23.

Ainsworth, M. D. S. 1973. The development of infant-mother attachment. In *Review of child development research,* Vol. 3. Chicago: University of Chicago Press.

Ainsworth, M. D., Blehar, M. C., and Waters, E. 1978. *Patterns of attachment.* Hillsdale, N.J.: Lawrence Erlbaum Associated Press.

Blatt, S. J., and Behrends, R. S. 1987. Internalization, separation-individuation, and the nature of the therapeutic action. *International Journal of Psychoanalysis* 68:279–97.

Bowlby, J. 1969. *Attachment and loss: Attachment,* Vol. 1. New York: Basic Books.

Bowlby, J. 1973. *Attachment and loss: Separation-anxiety and anger,* Vol. 2. New York: Basic Books.

Bowlby, J. 1980. *Attachment and loss: Loss-sadness and depressive symptoms,* Vol. 3. New York: Basic Books.

Caron, W., Boss, P., and Mortimer, J. 1999. Family boundary ambiguity predicts Alzheimer's outcomes. *Psychiatry* 62(4):347–56.

Colarusso, C. A., and Nemiroff, R. A. 1987. Clinical Implications of adult developmental theory. *American Journal of Psychiatry* 144(10):1263–70.

Erikson, E. N. 1963. *Childhood and society.* New York: Norton.

Faber, A., and Mazlish, E. 1998. *Siblings without rivalry: How to help your children live together so that you can live too.* New York: Avon Press.

Freud, S. 1940. *An outline of psychoanalysis.* New York: Norton.

Gallagher-Thompson, D., Dal Canto, P., Jacob, T., and Thompson, L. 2001. A comparison of marital interaction patterns between couples in which the husband does or does not have Alzheimer's disease. *Journal of Gerontology* 56B(3):S140–50.

Gladstone, J. W. 1995. The marital perceptions of elderly persons living or having a spouse living in a long-term care institution in Canada. *Gerontologist* 35:52–60.

Greenberg, J. S., Seltzer, M. M., Orsmond, G. I., and Krauss, M. W. 1999. Siblings of adults with mental illness or mental retardation: Current involvement and expectation of future caregiving. *Psychiatric Services* 50:1214–19.

Gwyther, L. P. 1990. Letting go: Separation-individuation in the wife of an Alzheimer's patient. *Gerontologist* 30:698–702.

Hodgson, H. 1995. *Alzheimer's—Finding the words: A communication guide for those who care.* Minneapolis: Chronimed Publishing.

Horowitz, M. J., Siegel, B., Holen, A., Bonanno, G. A., Milbrath, C., and Stinson, C. H. 1997. Diagnostic criteria for complicated grief disorder. *American Journal of Psychiatry* 154:904–10.

Jewell, T. C., and Stein, C. H. 2002. Parental influence on sibling caregiving for people with severe mental illness. *Community Mental Health Journal* 38:17–33.

Kaplan, L., and Boss, P. 1999. Depressive symptoms among spousal caregivers of institutionalized mates with Alzheimer's: Boundary ambiguity and mastery as predictors. *Family Process* 38:85–103.

Levy, T., and Thomas, N. 1999. *Handbook of attachment interventions.* New York: Academic Press.

Lewis, J. M. 2000. Repairing the bond in important relationships: A dynamic for personality maturation. *American Journal of Psychiatry* 57:1375–78.

Pearlin, L. I., Lieberman, M. A., Menaghan, E. G., and Mullan, J. T. 1981. The stress process. *Journal of Health and Social Behavior* 22(4):337–56.

Schore, A. N. 1996. The experience-dependent maturation of a regulatory system in the orbital prefrontal cortex and the origin of developmental psychopathology. *Developmental Psychopathology* 8:59–87.

Settlage, C. F., Curtis, J., Lozoff, M., Lozoff, M., Silberschatz, G., and Simburg, E. J. 1988. Conceptualizing adult development. *Journal of the American Psychoanalytic Association* 36:347–69.

Shear, M. K., Zuckoff, M. A., and Frank, E. 2001. The syndrome of traumatic grief. *CNS Spectrums* 6(4):339–46.

Sistler, A. B., and Blanchard-Fields, F. 1993. Being in control: A note on differences between caregiving and noncaregiving spouses. *Journal of Psychology* 127(5):537–42.

Sullivan, H. S. 1953. *The interpersonal theory of psychiatry.* New York: Norton Press.

Tronick, E. Z., and Gianino, A. 1986. Zero to three. *Bulletin of the National Center for Clinical Infant Programs* 6(3):1–6.

Vaillant, G. E. 1977. *Adaptation to life.* Boston: Little, Brown.

Van Doorn, C., Kasl, S. V., Beery, L. C., Jacobs, S. C., and Prigerson, H. G. 1998. The influence of marital quality and attachment styles on traumatic grief and depressive symptoms. *Journal of Nervous and Mental Disease* 186:566–73.

Wallerstein, J., and Blakeslee, S. 1996. *The good marriage: How and why love lasts.* New York: Warner Books.

Wallhagen, M. I. 1992/93. Perceived control and adaptation in elder caregivers: Development of an explanatory model. *International Journal of Aging and Human Development* 36(3): 219–37.

CHAPTER SIX

Religious Participation and Caregiving

A Psychodynamic Perspective

JAMES W. LOMAX, M.D.

This chapter explores an important but often-neglected element in the care of persons with dementia: religious and spiritual participation on the part of the caregiver and patient. The chapter begins with a focused review of the health consequences of caregiving, emphasizing those that are relevant to the patient or caregiver's religious participation. These health consequences provide targets for therapeutic activity to attenuate the negative effects of caregiving by identifying and supporting the positive correlates of religious participation or by altering the type of religious participation that worsens health outcomes.

There is now a fairly robust and well-established literature on both the health consequences of caregiving in general (Schulz and Beach, 1999) and health consequences specific to caregiving in dementia (Schulz, O'Brien, Bookwala, and Fleissner, 1995). The synergy of loss, chronic distress, physical demands of caregiving, subjective sense of strain, and neglect of the caregiver's own health coalesce to produce negative health consequences for the caregiver (Schultz and Beach, 1999; Schulz et al., 2001). Such negative consequences include increased cardiovascular illness, depression, and diminished immune function and increased mortality. More specifically in caregiving for persons with Alzheimer disease, there is increased depression and anxiety (Martire and Hall, 2002) with the psychological and physical morbidities that are typical consequences of depression (Bruce, Seeman, Merrill, and Blazer, 1994; Hays et al., 1997). Those consequences range from alterations in immune function (Kiecolt-Glaser et al., 1991) to challenges in the marital relationship. Caring in Alzheimer disease often entails a significant modification of familiar marital coping patterns, the emergence of incongruent perceptions by the spousal pair, loss of companionship (particularly for the caregiver), and fears of abandonment, which may progress to the appearance or reemergence of delusional fears of spousal infidelity of the caregiver (Wright, 1991).

THE HISTORY OF RELIGIOUS PARTICIPATION
AS A PURSUIT OF HEALING

Before the mid-1990s, the great majority of health professionals and mental health professionals had very little exposure to religious participation as something that influenced health outcomes. Religious participation, if considered at all, had an association with punitive religiosity and guilt which might cause or exacerbate depression, or with the inconvenience of certain specific religious practices for medical interventions (e.g., Jehovah Witness's rejection of blood products which might cause ethical dilemmas).

However, in the mid-1990s, the confluence of several factors within medicine resulted in increased attention to religion and spirituality due to: (a) an irrational exuberance on the part of academic medicine for molecular medicine, (b) an emphasis on procedural expertise accompanied by increased distance of physicians from the personal experience of their patients, and (c) societal concerns about the spiraling cost of medical care, which has produced for-profit managed care with diminished emphasis on the best interests of the individual. At about this time, an increased number of epidemiological researchers conducted both their own studies and meta-analyses of other studies of religious participation and health outcomes. While there has been debate about the validity and specificity of some inferences from the studies (Sloan, Bagiella, and Powell, 1999), there is a growing consensus among medical practitioners (Puchalski and Larson, 1998), mental health researchers (Koenig, 1997), and nonmedical researchers (Levin, 2002) that there are reasonably strong correlates between religious participation and positive health outcomes.

Although a review of this extensive body of research is beyond the scope of this chapter, it is important to note some recurrent themes. The *causal* link between religious participation and health outcomes is fundamentally unclear, except that religious participation in general correlates with certain better health choices: diminished alcohol and tobacco use, and less inclination to participate in risky behaviors, such as reckless driving and reckless interpersonal intimacy (Oleckno and Blacconiere, 1991). The recurrent themes in this research are that a person's internal sense of religious involvement (usually termed religiosity), positive as opposed to negative religious coping strategy, healthy attachments, and generative community participation all seem correlated with better health outcomes (Ellison, Hummer, Cormier, and Rogers, 2000). Improved outcomes include quicker remissions from illnesses, diminished mortality and longer survival with chronic illnesses, and more positive self-rated perception of health (Coke, 1992).

It is important to emphasize the significant distinction between healing and curing. This distinction is pertinent from both religious and medical perspectives. On one hand, religious scholars inform us that Jesus viewed healing as restoration to community and considered such healing as a fundamental activity of the Christian faith (Johnson, 1999). Similarly, apart from some surgical problems and some infectious diseases, most physician activities seek to diminish morbidity and return patients to healthy developmental progress, as opposed to cure and complete remission of symptoms.

PUTATIVE MEDIATORS OF NEGATIVE HEALTH CONSEQUENCES OF CAREGIVING

Before describing the potential relationship between religious participation and caregiving, it is helpful to consider what might mediate (be the causal links for) the significant negative health outcomes for caregivers just described. The familiar biopsychosocial model for conceptualizing and intervening with behavioral disorders provides a synergistic framework to consider the different levels of mediating factors.

Biological

As is the case in many psychiatric disturbances related to stressors, there is data to suggest that altered hypothalamic-pituitary-adrenal axis function plays a role in mediating negative outcomes at the biological level. There is evidence for elevated cortisol levels and sympathetic tone, as well as altered immune function (Kiecolt-Glaser et al., 1991).

Psychological

Caregiving for a person with dementia produces a significant developmental interference with normal separation and individuation patterns of adult development (Gwyther, 1990; Vaillant, 2002). Incongruent perceptions of the current state of the marriage by the caregiving dyad are typically accompanied by repressed or suppressed (i.e., not well "metabolized") negative affects within both partners. The inability to manage negative affects intrapsychically or interpersonally commonly leads to the seeking of other supportive / accepting relationships outside of the marriage or the use of psychoactive substances, like alcohol, when such relationships are either unavailable or the caregiver is too depleted or exhausted to seek them out.

Social

At the social and community level, the loss of companionship for the caregiver, if not compensated for by appropriate community resources, intensifies loneliness for the caregiver. There are data to suggest both biological and psychological correlates of loneliness with resulting negative health outcomes (Cacioppo, Berntson, Sheridan, and McClintock, 2000; Cacioppo et al., 2000). Caregiver status is viewed positively in some religious communities, and in such circumstances caregiving may be seen as an opportunity for spiritual development.

The therapist trying to help a patient and a caregiver should assess and make interventions at each of these levels of the biopsychosocial spectrum. In the remainder of the chapter, I present a model for conceptualizing religious participation in a psychosocial framework, which allows mental health clinicians to use familiar professional skills to assess the health consequences of religious participation and to construct interventions that promote healing and positive health outcomes.

A PSYCHOSOCIAL PERSPECTIVE ON RELIGIOUS PARTICIPATION OF THE CAREGIVER AND CARE RECIPIENT

Dementia is a prototypical example of circumstances in which severe illness and / or the anticipation of the end of life challenges the healthy and progressive unfolding of life. Caregiving in dementia is a particularly desirable context for interdisciplinary study and collaboration. This desirability is not only due to the immense practical significance and the efforts to make the best of the "living-of-dying" experience, but also because of "the intermediate or transitional experience" between separation and attachment that such severe illness creates (Fricchione, 2000). It is precisely in this intermediate area that the relationship of spirituality, religion, and medicine can be examined and nurtured.

From a life span perspective, current religious experiences are influenced by and express consequences of earlier developmental progress. The psychiatrist and psychoanalyst Sigmund Freud was one of the first physicians to systematically attempt to consider religious experience in a health framework. Unfortunately, Freud saw religion only as a vehicle for the expression and maintenance of infantile and regressive needs and dependencies. For Freud, religious participation was either an obsessional neurosis (Freud, 1913) or a primitive oceanic merger (Freud, 1927; Parson, 1999), not a vehicle for the expression of adaptive creative attachments (in religious terms, a response to Grace).

Contemporary psychiatrists and psychoanalysts are more likely to contend that religious participation, like sexual behavior, is usually integrated within an individual's overall mode of personality function and development. Developmentally mature individuals tend to experience their religious and spiritual lives flexibly. In contrast, developmentally immature individuals express their religious and spiritual life in a rigid manner (Fowler, 1984).

One very important contribution of the Jesuit psychoanalyst William Meissner is his development of the concept of "transitional phenomena" (Meissner, 1984). Donald Winnicott had described the transitional object (the blanket or teddy bear to which the developing infant makes his first attachment outside of the mother) as a psychologically intermediate area of crucial developmental significance (Winnicott, 1971). Such transitional phenomena are neither totally subjective nor totally objective for the developing infant. They are best understood as an "illusion" in which the child plays out or practices "the drama of separation and attachment." Transitional objects are an enduring, significant dimension of human existence. They do not *disappear* with healthy development but are *transformed*. Growth-producing illusions have ties to reality but also measure the capacity of the person to transform reality into something *reflective* of inner significance and hope—the capacity for *creative illusion formation*. Humans do very poorly without illusion. Illusions give meaning and sustenance to the experience of self, other, and God. It is in this arena of illusion formation that Meissner and Winnicott positively, adaptively (and responsively to Grace for Meissner) place one important variety of religious experience.

From a psychological perspective, the spiritual dimension of religious participation can be viewed as an expression of attachment behavior. Of course the term *spiritual* means very different things, including beliefs (i.e., cognitions). However, in both the medical/scientific and religious/theological literature the term *spiritual* is used to refer to a type of seeking behavior satisfied by relationships of a particular quality. The experimental psychologist Jaak Panksepp suggests that there is also an "appetitive motivational/seeking system of the brain" which underlies many behaviors characterized by determined, active seeking (Panksepp, 1998). Spiritual pursuits involve seeking a connectedness with God, other people, or nature characterized by an interest in and valuation of the other as being intrinsically separate and important. Such attachment needs are part of normal human makeup. They promote human intimacy, facilitate procreation of the species, and influence the formation of groups and communities. Such products of attachment yearnings are of great evolutionary value.

Of course, there are also pathological expressions of attachment behavior. Individuals with schizoid or autistic disorders generally lack spiritual interests in the form of attachments to others that involve interest in the other as a separate, non-need-gratifying being. Other individuals have attachment needs that are desperate in nature, leading to preemptive, chaotic, and ill-advised connections. Such tendencies are often found in individuals with manic-depressive illness and cluster B personality disorders, particularly the borderline personality disorder. Such excessive and insecure attachment needs require therapeutic action that promotes the individual's capacity for modulation of those needs. Therapeutic action encouraging containment of the expression of such attachment needs is important in order to avoid chaos in all aspects of such individuals' lives, including the religious dimensions.

Formal religious organization and particularly religious rituals and religiously based moral or ethical reasoning can all be considered as expressions of the healthy human capacity to order experience and to seek meaning. Thus such cognitive expressions of religious experiences may represent a particular use of the "left brain interpreter" of cognitive psychotherapy (Wolford, Miller, and Gazzaniga, 2000). However, as with the attachment dimension, there are clinical excesses in the ordering of and attributing meaning to experience. Examples include individuals with obsessive-compulsive or paranoid spectrum disorders. Within a specifically religious framework, faith-based efforts to order experience can hypertrophy to the degree that rituals lose their spiritual base. Efforts to discern differences and prioritize experiences (Who is the best or most holy?) have led religious communities to make distinctions among themselves and outsiders leading to exclusions, discriminations, and religious wars. Therapeutic interventions with individuals who have paranoid or obsessive-compulsive disorders help them to express their needs to order experience with more creativity and flexibility. The therapist should encourage such individuals to seek personal meaning, while retaining as much tolerance toward others' ideas as a fundamentally rigid personality structure can manage. These individuals may benefit from empathic interventions to increase their own appreciation of other individuals with different answers to questions of what is meaningful and significant.

Finally, active religious participation is more likely to be health promoting than is passive religious participation (Burgener, 1994; Strawbridge, Cohen, Shema, and Kaplan, 1997). Activity that reflects the psychological capacity for "generativity" (Erikson, 1950) seems to be of particular value in this regard. Not only the being in community but also doing for others seems health promoting. Thus knowing what our patients do with their religious or spiritual experience is important in assessing the health care consequences of their religious participation.

IMPLICATIONS FOR CLINICAL PRACTICE

In clinical encounters with individual patient and caregiver pairs, an appreciation of the positive and negative consequences of religious participation can be translated into strategies for intervening with specific mental health problems and making full use of community resources, including religious institutions. In the clinical encounter it is most important to pay attention to the consequences and implications of the religious beliefs and practices of patient and caregiver while avoiding judgments about their validity. The therapist should consider the patient's religious and spiritual life as psychological and social elements of the biopsychosocial formulation to assess whether the patient and caregiver's manner of participation promotes healthy connectedness to self, to other individuals, and to his or her community.

From the psychological perspective, do the caregiver and patient's religious ideas or cognitions predict positive or negative religious coping with consequent implications for health outcomes? For example, does the patient or caregiver experience either the illness or the burden of the disease as a punishment for past sins and transgressions? When such negative religious coping is present, the therapist should challenge or redirect the negative cognitions either by appropriate psychotherapeutic interventions or in consultation with informed individuals acceptable to the patient's religious value system. Such consultation requires a familiarity with the religious leaders of one's community or the knowledge of how to gain such familiarity with new patient groups or faith traditions.

In contrast, does the person experience a feeling of being loved and accepted in spite of a stigmatizing illness? When positive religious coping is present, the therapist should actively inquire about the patient's religious belief system and express curiosity and interest in those beliefs. In explorations about religious communities a therapist often uncovers resources that are of immense practical value to caregiving, such as support groups and respite programs.

As information is gathered, the therapist needs to make decisions about whether to intervene in an empathic, interpretive, or redirecting manner (i.e., whether to facilitate or discourage further religious or spiritual self-reflection involvement on the part of the patient and caregiver and whether to support or discourage interpersonal and community religious activity on the part of the patient).

In this line of inquiry, which is similar to explorations of a patient's sexuality, there is a particular need to pay attention to one's own feelings and attitudes as such sensitive topics are discussed (i.e., countertransference). The therapist should pursue what might be considered a healing attitude in regard to religious participation. Such an attitude may promote the ability of patients to restore themselves to a community in which they can feel valued.

The therapist-patient relationship should become a sort of practice field in which patients feel connected to the therapist's interest in them as they talk about their religious lives. When the patient's religious traditions are quite at variance from the therapist's, it may be a challenge to focus on the consequences of the religious activities and to avoid becoming distracted by the content of religious beliefs that seem alien or even primitive. In more extreme examples, there is the potential for the therapist to intrude his or her religious values into a professional relationship, creating a significant ethical boundary violation (Lomax, Karff, and McKenny, 2002).

We should proffer an active curiosity about the subjective meaning and reality of the patient's religious participation. That curiosity will lead patients to elaborate on their spiritual lives, providing the information needed to guide therapeutic interventions. Such an atmosphere of respect in the therapist/patient relationship is an essential goal, even when religious and spiritual values of the patient/therapist dyad are quite different. Therapists who are deeply religious may find themselves needing to support a type of secular spirituality that may seem "deficient" in religious content, and agnostic or atheistic therapists may need to support an uncomfortable (to them) degree of religiosity because of the value that particular community experience has for that particular patient. In both instances, the spouse of a person with severe dementia may seek a community with a religious or secular spiritual quality as a compensation for the loss of the personal relationship with a spouse. It is the value of that *community* experience which the therapist should recognize and support separate from any religious bias of the therapist.

The health professional thus assesses whether the patient and caregiver's religious participation promotes a healthy connectedness to self, other individuals, and community. Three questions should be kept in mind. First, are the ordering and meaning-generating functions of the patient's religious participation likely to be health promoting? Second, is our patient (remembering that both the identified patient and the caregiver are our patients in this circumstance) involved in relationships in his or her religious life that lead to feeling accepted and involved? Finally, does the person's religious community provide opportunities for generative action and activity that can promote health and well-being?

Mr. A. is a 64-year-old laborer whose wife developed rapidly progressive Alzheimer disease a year before their long-anticipated retirement. As her memory and orientation difficulties escalated, he could feel the future they had planned slipping away. He was furious and depressed about the "unfairness" of these events. In an effort to find solace, he had changed from a conservative, nondenominational church to worship as a Jehovah's Witness. In this new religious participation, he "knew God's name as Jehovah for the first time." He found his solace in the "promised new order to come," in which good and decent people like him and his wife would be restored and rewarded and the wicked would be punished. He was also welcomed by a community that provided both a caring interest in his situation and practical support for his family.

Mr. A.'s religious participation is highly dependent on specific ideas and beliefs (i.e., very specific religious cognitions). His religious participation could be regarded as defensive, both psychologically (rationalization and reaction formation in his attitudes about God) and theologically (the creations of a wicked force and wicked people who would indirectly preserve the contrasting thought of a loving God). However, it was also adaptive. His religious faith produced hope, shared beliefs, and a community in which he both received help and had access to helping opportunities with other caregivers. The shared beliefs functioned as creative illusions that reflected the inner significance of a new, highly specific belief system shared by a socially active and involved community. There was a health-promoting synergy between Mr. A.'s beliefs and his faith community. When he was chosen to be an elder in the faith community, serving as a teacher and leader provided a significance to his current life which offset the loss of the long-treasured retirement years of travel and co-grandparenting he had planned with his wife. In an important way, his role in his faith community provided a much needed compensation for the unexpected loneliness and loss of the companionship he had anticipated sharing with his wife.

In stark contrast to what was meaningful to Mr. A. was the situation of Mrs. B. Mrs. B. was the caregiver for her husband, whose Alzheimer disease led to a marked change in his personality, with the emergence of aggressive outbursts and agitation, reflecting a significant change from the relational pattern in their more than 25 years of marriage. Her husband had become intermittently and unwarrantedly jealous of her relationship with a business associate. He loudly accused her of infidelity at a social gathering where he was feeling insecure because of his difficulty remembering names and roles of people he had met through her. A pivotal moment and spiritual encounter occurred when a neighbor of Mrs. B. came over to pray with her after this very disturbing event. Her neighbor, who had been present at the event, was somewhat older. She had gone through the experience of her husband's deterioration and death from Alzheimer disease. The course of the illness for the husbands of these two women was quite different. Her neighbor came to pray with Mrs. B., emphasizing religious content very little but offering a religiously based support like she had felt from her church community a decade earlier. Mrs. B. did not even remember much about what she and her neighbor prayed about. However, she remembered and treasured the connectedness her neighbor offered during a time of shame and confusion.

Mrs. B. described this encounter as "like meeting God" within her neighbor. For Mrs. B., her response was just as profound as what her neighbor experienced in her faith community. However, her response was expressed in a more "secular" spirituality. Mrs. B. became an active participant in the Alzheimer Association. There she began to give to others the type of encouragement and hope she had found in the generative giving of her neighbor. In my inquiries about Mrs. B.'s past religious participation, I learned that she had been traumatized as an adolescent when a youth minister had made inappropriate sexual advances to her. When she attempted to report this to the church hierarchy, she was accused of herself being sexually provocative. She therefore experienced further isolation and community censure instead of comfort. She could never "forgive" the church or its representatives for this "hypocrisy." Even the encounter with her religiously grounded neighbor could not lead her to any sort of organized religious activity, because of the betrayal she had experienced at a critical time in her life. It was important for the therapist to know why she was not making use of a formal religious community, and it would have been a mistake for a therapist to encourage her to reinvolve herself when she was not ready to do so. Readiness would have likely involved achievement of forgiveness, which was not on her agenda at the time of her therapeutic relationship.

Mr. A. and Mrs. B. had very different types of religious and spiritual participation. Mrs. B.'s was one of a more spiritual nature. It did not depend on specific religious beliefs, but on attachments in which she felt valued and understood. Her involvement in the caregiver support group provided a type of secular spirituality with health-promoting activities in the form of generative giving. Theologically, it could be debated whether her experience with her neighbor and subsequent giving in the support group was divinely inspired and whether her response was an act of grace. However, such coerced discussions with the patient may have been a possible boundary violation on the part of a therapist more concerned with convincing the patient than with listening to what was important and meaningful for her at this point in her life. What Mr. A. and Mrs. B. have in common is the opportunity to participate in generative giving, a spiritual and religious participation to be appreciated and supported by the therapist.

Neither the situation for Mr. A. nor that for Mrs. B. generated a need to contact or refer to a member of the clergy. There will often be times, however, that a therapist encounters a faith tradition with which he or she is unfamiliar. At such times, it may be helpful to read about other religious groups either in traditional books or Internet web sites. While reading may provide a good deal of factual or content information, discussions with religious officials or laity in different faith traditions often provides critically important exposure to the community dimension of religious participation that is hard to capture from written materials. There is also considerable difference in communities, even if the main denominational identifier is the same. Different Methodist, Baptist, or Presbyterian churches can have enormous differences in both religious beliefs and the spiritual attachments or engagements they offer. At times a patient or caregiver's interpretation of religious material can be highly idiosyncratic. Referral to a chaplain or other religious official can sometimes address personal rigidity and inflexibility. Of course, successful referrals require knowledge about the specific referral alternatives in terms of not only their theology but also their interpersonal/pastoral skills.

CONCLUSION

Caregiving in dementia typically represents an enormous challenge with serious health consequences. Being able to elicit and to understand the psychology of our patients' religious and/or spiritual participation may be quite useful at times in guiding the assessment of and intervention in the care of the caregiver. Using a traditional biopsychosocial formulation, the mental health counselor can combine knowledge and skills with a healing, accepting attitude to understand and intervene in a helpful way while maintaining appropriate therapeutic boundaries.

REFERENCES

Bruce, M. L., Seeman, T. E., Merrill, S. S., and Blazer, D. G. 1994. The impact of depressive symptomatology on physical disability: MacArthur studies of successful aging. *American Journal of Public Health* 84(11):1796–99.

Burgener, S. C. 1994. Caregiver religiosity and well-being in dealing with Alzheimer's dementia. *Journal of Religion and Health* 33(2):175–89.

Cacioppo, J. T., Berntson, G. G., Sheridan, J. F., and McClintock, M. K. 2002. Multilevel integrative analyses of human behavior: Social neuroscience and the complementing nature of social and biological approaches. *Psychological Bulletin* 126(6):829–43.

Cacioppo, J. T., Ernst, J. M., Burleson, M. H., McClintock, M. K., Malarkey, W. B., Hawkley, L. C., Kowalewski, R. B., Paulsen, A., Hobson, J. A., Hugdahl, K., Spiegel, D., and Berntson, G. G. 2000. Lonely traits and concomitant physiological processes: The MacArthur social neuroscience studies. *International Journal of Psychophysiology* 35(2–3): 143–54.

Coke, M. M. 1992. Correlates of life satisfaction among elderly African Americans. *Journal of Gerontology* 47(5):316–20.

Ellison, C. G., Hummer, R. A., Cormier, S., and Rogers, R. G. 2000. Religious involvement and mortality risk among African American adults. *Research on Aging* 22(6):630–67.

Erikson, E. H. 1950. *Childhood and society.* New York: W. W. Norton.

Fowler, J. W. 1984. *Becoming adult, becoming Christian.* San Francisco: Harper.

Freud, S. 1913. Totem and taboo. In J. Strachey (Ed.), *The standard edition of the complete psychological works of Sigmund Freud,* Vol. 13 (pp. 1–164). London: Hogarth Press.

Freud, S. 1927. The future of an illusion. In J. Strachey (Ed.), *The standard edition of the complete psychological works of Sigmund Freud,* Vol. 21 (pp. 3–56). London: Hogarth Press.

Fricchione, G. L. 2000. Religious issues in the context of medical illness. In A. Stoudemire, B. S. Fogel, and D. B. Greenberg (Eds.), *Psychiatric care of the medical patient* (2nd ed.) (pp. 91–101). New York: Oxford University Press.

Gwyther, L. P. 1990. Letting go: Separation-individuation in a wife of an Alzheimer's patient. *Gerontologist* 30:698–702.

Hays, J. C., Krishnan, K. R., George, L. K., Pieper, C. F., Flint, E. P., and Blazer, D. G. 1997. Psychosocial and physical correlates of chronic depression. *Psychiatry Research* 72(3): 149–59.

Johnson, L. 1999. *Living Jesus: Learning the heart of the Gospel.* San Francisco: Harper.

Kiecolt-Glaser, J. K., Dura, J. R., Speicher, C. E., Trask, O. J., and Glaser, R. 1991. Spousal caregivers of dementia victims: Longitudinal changes in immunity and health. *Psychosomatic Medicine* 53(4):345–62.

Koenig, H. G. 1997. *Is religion good for your health?* New York: Haworth Press.

Levin, J. 2002. *God, faith, and health: Exploring the spirituality-healing connection.* New York: John Wiley & Sons.

Lomax, J. W., Karff, R. S., and McKenny, G. P. 2002. Ethical considerations in the integration of religion and psychotherapy: Three Perspectives. *Psychiatric Clinics of North America* 25:547–59.

Martire, L. M., and Hall, M. 2002. Dementia caregiving: Recent research on negative health effects and the efficacy of caregiver interventions. *CNS Spectrums* 7(11):791–96.

Meissner, W. W. 1984. Religion in psychoanalytic perspective. In *Psychoanalysis and religious experience* (pp. 135–60). New Haven: Yale University Press.

Oleckno, W. A., and Blacconiere, M. J. 1991. Relationship of religiosity to wellness and other health-related behaviors and outcomes. *Psychological Reports* 68:819–26.

Panksepp, J. 1998. Seeking systems and anticipatory states of the nervous system. In *Affective Neuroscience* (pp. 9–23). Oxford: Oxford University Press.

Parson, W. B. 1999. The oceanic feeling revisited. In *The enigma of the oceanic feeling* (pp. 89–169). Oxford: Oxford University Press.

Puchalski, C. M., and Larson, D. B. 1998. Developing curricula in spirituality and medicine. *Academic Medicine* 73(9):970–74.

Schulz, R., and Beach, S. R. 1999. Caregiving as a risk factor for mortality: The Caregiver Health Effects Study. *Journal American Medical Association* 282(23):2215–19.

Schulz, R., Beach, S. R., Lind, B., Martire, L. M., Zdaniuk, B., Hirsch, C., Jackson, S., and Burton, L. 2001. Involvement in caregiving and adjustment to death of a spouse: Findings from the Caregiver Health Effects Study. *Journal American Medical Association* 285(24): 3123–29.

Schulz, R., O'Brien, A. T., Bookwala, J., and Fleissner, K. 1995. Psychiatric and physical morbidity effects of dementia caregiving: Prevalence, correlates, and causes. *Gerontologist* 35:771–91.

Sloan, R. P., Bagiella, E., and Powell, T. 1999. Religion, spirituality, and medicine. *Lancet* 353: 664–67.

Strawbridge, W. J., Cohen, R. D., Shema, S. J., and Kaplan, G. A. 1997. Frequent attendance at religious services and mortality over twenty-eight years. *American Journal of Public Health* 87(6):957–61.

Vaillant, G. E. 2002. *Aging well.* Boston: Little Brown.

Winnicott, D. W. 1971. *Playing and reality.* New York: Basic Books.

Wolford, G., Miller, M. B., and Gazzaniga, M. S. 2000. The left hemisphere's role in hypothesis formation. *Journal of Neuroscience* 15;20(6):RC64, 1–4.

Wright, L. K. 1991. The impact of Alzheimer's disease on the marital relationship. *Gerontologist* 31:224–37.

CHAPTER SEVEN

Caregiving and the Sexual Relationship in Dementia

NAOMI D. NELSON, PH.D.

Sexuality and intimacy are important at every stage of life and assume a central position in many diverse forms of human interaction. Sexual difficulties may occur with older couples even when dementia is absent—most notably, depression, physical illness, side effects of medication, and inhibited sexual desire (Cohen and Eisdorfer, 1986). These more natural challenges of sexuality become more complicated, however, when a partner experiences dementia and when behavioral or cognitive changes create unpredictable difficulties in a sexual relationship. Socially inappropriate behavior such as intermittent incontinence, physically aggressive behavior, and verbal agitation can become problematic for partners who live with dementia (Cohen-Mansfield, 1996), and the presence of these behaviors can negatively affect the desire for sexual contact. Additionally, sexual functioning may become stressful when the person with dementia forgets the sequence of the sexual act, is unable to perform due to impotency, and/or makes inappropriate sexual demands (Davies, Zeiss, and Tinklenberg, 1992).

In the classic book on dementia, *The 36-Hour Day,* Mace and Rabins (1999) suggest that lifetime habits of modesty and attitudes toward sexuality and intimacy remain fairly consistent throughout life. Accidental behaviors and memory lapses may complicate sexuality and intimacy but are less likely to cause stress for the well spouse than other more disruptive actions such as inappropriate sexual behavior (Mace and Rabins, 1999). Personality changes may also impact the affectional bond for couples living with dementia (Garner, 1997); these personality changes may include passivity, diminished emotional responsiveness, and decreased initiative (Askin-Edgar, White, and Cummings, 2002).

SEXUALITY

Sexuality can be defined in many ways but is usually understood as the behavior directly associated with having sexual relations or being sexually aroused, involving both biological and psychological components (Sinnott and Shifren, 2001, p. 457). Sexuality is also understood as an intimate physical act occurring between two people who are expressing feelings for each other during a superficial encounter or who are committed to a long-term relationship. For most couples, the sex act is as natural to body functioning as other activities such as eating and exercising (Ornstein and Sobel, 1989). Sexuality combines many needs, the needs for being touched, caressed, and feeling close to others. Although some persons are able to live without sex, for most individuals the sex act is a necessary function that contributes to warm feelings of affection and understanding.

Intimacy, an important aspect of sexuality, is expressed among couples in a myriad of ways—by being physically close to another, by sharing deepest secrets and dreams, by creating friendships, by communicating privately, and by developing an intimate sexual relationship with a partner. The essence of intimacy does not necessarily change when a partner is afflicted with dementia, but the needs for affection and the manner of sexual expression may change and disrupt the familiar pattern of the couple's sexual relationship. For some individuals who live with dementia, expressions of intimacy without actual sexual intercourse may be just as critical for meeting their needs of being loved and being accepted.

I begin this chapter by presenting three vignettes and discussions. Following this, several constructs useful in understanding couple interactions are presented along with a brief review of selected research studies. The chapter concludes with a discussion of implications for clinical practice. All information in the vignettes has been changed to protect the privacy of the individuals and couples.

Mr. W. is 65 years old and has been married to his second wife for 10 years. Two years ago, when his wife was 64 years old, she was diagnosed with Alzheimer disease (AD) and since that time her memory and her ability to perform activities of daily living (ADLs) have progressively worsened. Mr. W. reported a very active sex life until recently, when Mrs. W. began to doubt that they had ever been married. When questioned by his wife, Mr. W. would patiently respond with the facts even to the point of showing her their marriage certificate; nothing was convincing to her. Her delusion about not being married progressed to her refusal to have sex with him because as she stated: "We're not married and I don't believe in sex before marriage." She would permit them to share the same bed if they slept on opposite sides. One evening, Mrs. W. told her husband that he would need to move out because it was sinful to live together without marriage. He was devastated and came to the clinician asking for help in understanding this behavior.

Initially, Mr. W. needs an opportunity to express his feelings of loss and confusion, while at the same time, to learn more about AD, paranoia, and delusions. Together with the clinician, Mr. W. can discuss aspects of delusional thinking and can learn about the intense anxiety his wife is experiencing. Mr. W. should be referred to relevant AD literature, videotapes, and a caregiver support group. Second, Mr. W. needs assistance in developing behavioral interventions that are based less on reasoning (i.e., less on "proving" their marriage) and more on physical expressions of comfort and security. For example, Mr. W. benefited from discussions about behavioral diversions that were initiated at times when his wife became suspicious and insecure. Mr. and Mrs. W. began taking pleasure outings that didn't require elaborate explanations but provided physical activities—trips to the zoo, neighborhood parks, and community gardens. As time progressed, Mrs. W. appeared to be calmed during these outings, and as some of her former laughter returned, she even permitted the holding of hands. Because his wife got upset when he prepared himself for bed, the clinician suggested that he transfer his clothes to a different bedroom closet and then both of them could undress in private but still share the same bed. As he began to share her care with paid companions, Mr. W. resumed regular tennis matches and the refinishing of antiques. He also began to regularly attend an AD support group. Over time, Mrs. W. expressed less paranoia and he was able to occasionally kiss her and physically provide comfort for her. They continued to act as if they were dating but they no longer had sexual intercourse or intimate physical touching.

Mrs. L., age 59, had been married for thirty-two years to her husband when he developed frontotemporal dementia (FTD) at age 63 and was no longer able to work. Mr. L. had always been flirtatious with other women but he had never demonstrated much affection to his wife other than perfunctory sex twice a month. In the months before the diagnosis of FTD, Mrs. L. began to realize that his behavior had changed; he was now overly affectionate with her and he nightly requested sex with her. He became quite irritable when Mrs. L. rebuffed him or continued with other tasks when he wanted sex. Mrs. L. made an appointment with the clinician hoping that they could receive some help with this change in behavior and in order to plan some strategies that would reduce her husband's desire for sex.

Mr. L. readily agreed to meet with the clinician because "I know that you can help my wife to better understand her sexual responsibilities." His impulsiveness and disinhibition were quite apparent by his flirtatiousness with the clinician, his lack of insight into his disorder, his frank talk of desiring to have an affair with a woman at his church, and his complete disregard for the feelings of his wife concerning their sexual activity.

The clinician began working with Mr. and Mrs. L. by helping both of them understand FTD and specifically the idiosyncratic nature of the behavioral changes associated with the illness. Although Mr. L. would participate in the discussion and appeared to cognitively understand the changes in his behavior, he was not able to transfer this insight into behavioral changes when they returned home. The clinician also spent time with the couple assessing the quality of their relationship before FTD and, together with them, examining factors that influenced the quality of that relationship.

When discussing his need for more physical activities, Mr. L. suggested that he could volunteer in senior programs at his church. With her husband's permission, Mrs. L. communicated with the church staff and offered to them a brief explanation about his condition and his need for supervision. Mr. L. thoroughly enjoyed his volunteer activities, and his friendly and gregarious style, together with his limited attention span, were well accepted by the group. As a result of these volunteer activities, his sense of self-worth and meaningful purpose improved and alleviated some, but not all, of his demands for more sex with his wife. Mrs. L. began attending a support group for those caring for demented family members and he enrolled in a community-sponsored early-stage peer support group. As supportive therapy progressed, Mrs. L. became more motivated for her work, community activities, and hobbies. As an adjunct to the support group, the clinician continued to see them twice monthly for six months and they both participated in their support groups for one year.

Mrs. V., age 70, requested a counseling session because of her distress about a recent sexual activity with her husband. Mr. V., age 72, had been diagnosed with AD 14 months previously; although his memory difficulties were mild, he did experience apraxia while performing ADLs. Mrs. V. reported that they had had a satisfactory sex life during their 50 years of marriage, although she admitted that her husband's libido was much greater than hers. One night as she and her husband were preparing for bed, Mr. V. indicated that he would like to have sex. She readily agreed because she knew that being affectionate had great meaning for him and she was in need of physical closeness also. When it came time for sequencing the steps of the sex act, Mr. V. promptly forgot and he became very flustered and said "I just give up." When his wife tried to help him, he was unable to reach an erection and became very anxious, was unable to perform, and left the bed in frustration. She also was distressed and knew that they needed help.

Mrs. V. had many questions and frustrations to share with the clinician. "Can you imagine what it's like to have to explain all the steps of sex to your husband of fifty years? I just can't do it. What should I do to make him feel that I still love him? What if we did sometime have sex, and then he immediately forgot that we had shared the intimacy? How would we interact the next day?"

Mrs. V.'s perceptive questions were very disturbing to her. She needed encouragement and support to talk about her feelings and the situation with her husband. She expressed feelings of embarrassment when she had to touch her husband and show him the steps about an act that had been so automatic in their intimate relationship. Mrs. V. needed reassurance that this type of forgetting is not that unusual for someone who has AD and that the physical comfort and affection shared with each other in bed, even without the sex act, may be one way that her husband can still express his fond feelings for her. The V.'s benefited from discussing the incident with a clinician, and were encouraged to talk about it further if the anxiety level of Mr. V. would be respected and minimized. Mrs. V. did choose an appropriate setting at home to discuss with her husband their sexual preferences and they were able to be physically close to each other without the expectations for perfect performance each time.

THEORETICAL CONSTRUCTS

These vignettes illustrate some of the sexual concerns that spousal caregivers have difficulty dealing with. The following section introduces five constructs that may help to explain the complex interactions of the couples described. These assumptions provide a theoretical base for understanding elements of human connectedness, conflicted growth, problem solving, emotional expression, and meaningful caring inherent in the caregiving relationship. The social scientists describe these concepts by the terms *dialectic interaction, dyssnchrony, enactive skills, expressed emotion,* and *interpretive caring.*

Dialectic Interaction Theory

Dialectic interaction theory, as postulated by Riegel (1973), is a systematic group of assumptions that examines the connection between the person and the environment (sociocultural and historical) and suggests that human survival depends on this interconnectedness. Rosenwald (1975), like Riegel, also emphasized the social nature of individuals and the necessity of forming human interrelationships as a precursor for growth and development. This belief in the mutual dependency or interconnectedness of people assists in understanding that the outcome of one spouse's behavior is dependent on and influenced by the behavior of the other spouse (Wright, 1994). Together these interrelations and intimate connections between the individual and the social structures (environment) contribute to developmental progression and growth (Ryff, Kwan, and Singer, 2001). All caregivers cited in the vignettes craved the social exchange and interconnectedness with their partners as described by Riegel. Persons with dementia and their caregivers are influenced by the behavior of each other and by the physical environment in which their interactions occur.

Dyssnchrony

These dialectic interactions or interconnections are not always in synchrony, or harmony, with one another. According to Riegel (1976), the process of dyssnchrony occurs when various life dimensions (biological, sociocultural, and/or psychological) conflict with one another. When individuals are faced with difficult life situations, such as Alzheimer disease, a developmental crisis, or dyssnchrony, may occur. As a result of the crises arising from these opposing and conflicted life dimensions, something new emerges from the dyssnchrony (Wright et al., 1999), and these new changes are described as dialectical leaps or developmental jumps (Riegel, 1976). The outcomes resulting from these leaps become positive or negative, depending on what actions are taken by the individual to ease the difficulties. This developmental trend toward movement and change requires the formulation of special skills so that qualitative transformations can occur.

Following professional assistance, opportunities for developmental leaps emerged. The three caregivers described in the vignettes demonstrated positive leaps, but for some caregivers not illustrated here, the changes from dyssnchrony become more negative and often take the form of anger, resentment, helplessness, and prolonged bitterness that continue even after the caregiving role is terminated.

Enactive Skills

The term *enactive skills* (Goulet, 1973) refers to those skills that are positively cor-related with task mastery and problem solving. Enactive skills are a major theme in learning theory as discussed by Bornstein and Bruner (1989) and by Riegel (1973), who suggest that learning is a social process involving the environment and an in-dividual. In the development of enactive skills, the learner constructs new ideas or concepts based on current or past knowledge or direct manipulation of objects and spatial awareness. Riegel (1973) assumed that the development and use of enactive skills increased through adulthood and accounted for changes in learning over the life span.

Most caregivers living with dementia have implemented enactive skills, acquired through the use of problem-solving skills and a knowledge base, for coping with changes in spousal behavior. Caregivers in the vignettes sought professional assis-tance with sexuality concerns and actively participated in professionally led support groups and/or individual counseling sessions. This supports the idea that learning about a new challenge, albeit a relationship challenge in the midst of caregiving tasks, may often be enhanced within a social context. Not all caregivers seek socially directed formal "learning opportunities," but previous task-mastery in related areas of problem solving may influence their ability to cope with sexuality concerns.

Expressed Emotion

Expressed emotion refers to negative attitudes of criticism (dislike, annoyance, resentment) and/or emotional overinvolvement (overprotectiveness, overconcern, self-sacrifice) that parents, spouses, or siblings sometimes communicate toward significant others in their families, particularly those with mental health problems and/or dementia. With certain types of mental health problems, high levels of ex-pressed emotion can be a negative force for certain patients, and a barrier to close-ness and intimacy between dementia caregivers and patients (Fearon, Donaldson, Burns, and Tarrier, 1998).

Fearon et al. (1998) examined the significance of expressed emotion among cou-ples when one was affected with dementia. They suggested that high levels of ex-pressed emotion can become a deterrent in the intimacy patterns between the well partner and the one with dementia and may be influenced by a past history of resentment and unresolved interpersonal problems. The work of Fearon et al. (1998) also confirmed the findings of Morris, Morris, and Britton (1988) when they discovered that intimacy declined as the dementia progressed.

Without professional intervention, the caregivers in the vignettes would predictably experience more expressed emotion. Feelings of resentment and relationship discord are best expressed within the context of a confidential support group setting or counseling session, where interpersonal problems may be safely confronted.

Interpretive Caring

Interpretive caring is a complex cognitive, emotional, and behavioral process through which well partners in a relationship put into action their knowledge and understanding of their partners with dementia, the disease process, and themselves in order to overcome their experience of vulnerability (Perry, 2002). The interpretive caring concept encourages the caregiver to make changes based on the knowledge gained from new perceptions and observations about their relationship and the meanings inferred from new roles and responsibilities. This focus on the cognitive dimension in dementia caregiving, in addition to the emotional dimension, brings to both partners a more "couple-oriented or family-unit" relationship than the more traditional dependent-independent roles of the couple.

In Perry's study of 20 wives providing care, interpretive caring was described as a process of finding some meaning or coherence to the role of a caregiver. The changes for these wives involved constructing a new daily life that would sustain both partners. One could argue that this emergence of a new daily life could be understood within the context of Riegel's (1973) theories of dialectical interaction, dyssnchrony, and the development of enactive skills.

All caregivers in the vignettes demonstrated some level of interpretive caring, particularly in their determination to learn more about specific sexual behaviors and reactions within the context of dementia. By explicitly seeking new ways of handling behavioral changes, they were indirectly bringing new meaning and coherence to their roles as caregivers.

APPLICATIONS OF DIALECTIC INTERACTION

Wright (1991, 1994, 1995, 1999) explored the multidimensional process of the dialectic as postulated by Riegel (1973, 1976) and applied it to the social phenomena of the marital relationship, aging, and chronic illness. The basic premise underlying Wright's relationship studies is the dialectical assumption that the outcome of one spouse is intrinsically linked to the outcome of the other spouse. Wright was intrigued by Riegel's belief that the outcomes of these interactions could be positive (control, concordance, and adaptation) or negative (disorder, discordance, or distortion). These outcomes do not simply happen; they are influenced by actions or coping behaviors which in turn may change individuals, their relationships, and their environment (Wright, 1991, p. 225). Riegel would likely call these coping behaviors learned or enactive skills (Riegel, 1973).

One of the major contributions of Wright's marital interaction studies is the finding that the past, the present, and the future of marital relationships are intertwined and eventually become predictors of outcomes for the couples' relationship (Wright, 1991). She believes that when one member has dementia, it is in the interaction on these three levels, rather than the illness severity, that determines the outcome and quality of the relationship.

In one of Wright's seminal studies (1991), she compared caregiver and AD affected spouses with healthy married couples (n = 47) and examined the impact of AD from a human developmental perspective as contrasted with a caregiver burden approach. By using several standardized tools and an interview questionnaire assessing marital quality and coping techniques, Wright identified a variety of coping outcomes and four marital dimensions.

Representative coping strategies used by well partners, in a dyad with a spouse who had AD, were self-control, limit setting, low levels of expressed emotion, escape into other activities, and outright rejection of their spouses. Less is reported about well couples' coping skills other than their experience of more shared meaning and mutual discussions. The marital dimensions that Wright (1991) identified were the consensus/instrumental dimension, the tension dimension, the companionship/confidant dimension, and the affectional/sexual dimension.

The consensus/instrumental dimension is defined as the sharing or lack of sharing between couples on matters of money and financial resources. Wright (1991) learned that for AD couples, in contrast to well couples, the responsibility for handling the money was a major role change for the AD caregiver and produced more incompetent feelings and worries about financial resources.

When considering the tension dimension of marriage, the most frequent source of tension for the AD caregiver was repetitive questioning, clinging behavior, and restless walking on the part of the person with dementia. The persons with AD minimized tension and described it as being nonproblematic (Wright, 1991, p. 231). In contrast, the well spouses described less behavioral tension but cited differences of opinions and attitudes about travel, relatives, church attendance, grown children, and household tasks.

The third dimension of marriage, the companionship/confidant dimension, also indicated differences between the two groups. The caregivers expressed lack of companionship with their spouses and frustration with clinging behavior; in contrast, the well couples expressed enjoyment and pleasure of being with each other even to the point of being "too close" at times.

The last dimension of marriage, affectional/sexual, was viewed by the AD caregiver as being abnormal and was accompanied by feelings of resentment and exploitation when sexual demands were made. For the well couples, they seemed more aware of their own beliefs and their partner's feelings about sexual activity and they were more likely to mutually decide issues of sexual frequency and expressions of intimacy.

The findings of this study have many implications for understanding sexuality and the marital relationship within the context of dementia. One of the most revealing outcomes affirms that even in early to middle stages of AD, much of the shared meaning between spouses in all aspects of the marital dimensions is lost. This finding is in contrast to the healthy couples, for whom shared meaning was present in all aspects of the marital dimensions.

RELATED STUDIES

One of the first studies to address marital intimacy and spousal reactions of persons with dementia was conducted by Morris et al. (1988). In this article, the authors assessed the quality of the relationship before the onset of dementia and again at the time of the study. Although the sample was small (n = 20 dyads) and the instruments were not standardized, the findings indicated that the degree of change in the level of intimacy presumably contributed more to caregiver depression and less to caregiver stress. A decline in intimacy was estimated from the difference reported between the past and present intimacy patterns. Those caregivers who were presently experiencing less intimacy than before the onset of dementia were more likely to be depressed but not necessarily more stressed or strained. The authors suggest that this loss of intimacy and a poor premorbid relationship may be vulnerability factors for those partners caring for persons with dementia.

Ballard et al. (1997) conducted an interesting study on couples when one of the partners experienced mild to moderate changes in AD. Of the 40 couples that completed the questionnaires, 22.5 percent continued to have a satisfactory sexual relationship and were satisfied with the situation. Of those couples who were no longer sexually active, the majority (61%), were satisfied with the situation, whereas 38 percent were dissatisfied. The study revealed a trend for male partners to be more sexually active and that satisfaction with sexual activity had an inverse relationship with age, hallucinations, and vascular dementia.

IMPLICATIONS FOR CLINICAL PRACTICE

The aforementioned theories and research approaches offer the clinician a substantive conceptual framework for understanding couples living with dementia and for providing resourceful interventions. Underlying these interventions is the belief in the uniqueness of each individual and of each couple, an understanding of their intimate relationship with each other, and an appreciation for their relationship within the social context of family, friends, and community. These basic principles inherent in couples' counseling require that the clinician practice with an authentic and other-directed presence. The recommendations of unconventional interventions that are too outlandish for the couple's cultural context or value system and the suggestions of rigidly traditional relationship encounters may have destructive effects for the couple seeking to share intimacy under the difficult situation. An approach that encourages the clinician to combine a solid scientific foundation and clinical wisdom about gerontology, sexuality, and relationships will be more constructive and helpful for these couples.

The clinician confronts a myriad of issues when working with couples when one of them is impaired by dementia. The issues surrounding sexuality and dementia are complex and the clinician may feel personal discomfort in addressing such concerns and may benefit from professional consultation or referral at the outset. Before working with these couples, it is essential that the clinician become an expert in understanding the intricacies of dementia and become knowledgeable about specific brain disorders and the resultant changes in cognition, language, behavior, and insight. It is also important for the clinician to be proficient in dealing with sexual problems among couples of all ages, and to examine personal views about sexual practices in general, about sexuality in the older adult, and about sexuality in couples when one has a dementia.

Additional concerns for the clinician may include insecurity about professional competence in dealing with these issues, the uncertainty of mutual sexual consent for both individuals, and the priority of the sex act itself in a relationship where the impaired person may be lacking insight and the well spouse may be already overwhelmed with caregiving responsibilities.

A good assessment precedes any interventions. The use of the dialectic theory focuses on the past, present, and future of the relationship and the way these factors interact (Wright, 1991). To strengthen this assessment, the clinician begins to form assumptions about these interactions by observing behavior and by asking questions about the developmental phase of the individuals and of their relationship as a couple, the past and present commitment of the couple to each other, the length of time they have been together, the manner in which conflict and stress have been handled, the past and present history and frequency of intimacy and sexuality practices, the characteristics and preferences for communication, the nature and quality of their relationships with family members and friends, their involvement in the community, and the nature of support for them individually and for them as a couple. Additionally, a prior history of physical and emotional illnesses and how they have been handled would be helpful when examining the interaction of all these factors.

For the clinician, the clinical milieu needs to be relaxed, professional in nature, and safe for persons to talk about sexuality and dementia. Many older adults are open in talking about sexual issues with a trusted professional when respectful questions are posed and a confidential environment is ensured. However, for some couples living with dementia, the sexual behavior/attitudes may be embarrassing for the caregivers to discuss and they may show reticence in discussing topics that at one time were socially taboo (Litz, Zeiss, and Davies, 1990). The clinician should avoid stereotypic views of older adults, their behaviors, and their responses to illness and aging. Categorizing people by age, gender, and perception of life events should be avoided.

A clinician who approaches the couple using an interaction theory of person and environment is interested in the perspective of many—the person with dementia, the partner, the family, and society—and is attentive to the meaning of illness and the experience of illness for each of these entities (McDaniel, Hepworth, and Doherty, 1992). This interaction theory may also be strengthened by the application of brief psychotherapy models, object-relations theory, adult development theory, and cognitive/behavioral suggestions.

When possible, I prefer to explore sexual and intimacy concerns within the context of individual and/or couples counseling that is conducted in a relatively short period of time over several weeks. During these first sessions, I also introduce the couple to the resources of the Alzheimer's Association, the day activity centers, if appropriate, and ask them to bring members of their family to at least one session. I introduce the caregiver to an appropriate support group, facilitated by a professional or an experienced community leader, and I refer the person with dementia to an early-stage peer group if available in the community. I provide information and educational materials about dementia based on the learning needs and preferences of the individual/couple/family.

Early on in the process of counseling, I encourage the application of enactive, problem-solving strategies that are familiar to the caregiver and/or the couple and that can be useful when discussing challenging intimacy and sexuality issues. I introduce specific coping skills that usually involve diversional tactics, time management skills, stress reduction, self-care, respite care, enlisting help, and the ABCs of behavioral management strategies (antecedent, behavior, and consequence).

The most difficult issues for the caregiver and the person with advanced dementia include the uncertainty of mutual consent, the decline in insight, the lack of partner recognition, the fading memory of the nature of the relationship, and the forgetting of the required steps for the sexual act. Thorough discussions of these issues are essential.

CONCLUSION

The clinical vignettes presented here and the description of five constructs of the unique interactive processes that occur in couples who live with dementia underscore how the behavior of one spouse becomes very dependent on the behavior of another, how growth and change are made possible through dialectical leaps, and how the use of enactive skills, the application of interpretive caring, and the presence of low expressed emotion may benefit the interconnectedness of the couple.

From a clinical perspective, no expert has all the answers, and dealing with the uncertainty of the dementia situation is one of the greatest challenges for the caregiver, the person with the dementia, and the clinician. The needs for connections, friendship, love, sex, affection, and a close relationship remain for most individuals throughout the life span and are deserving of respect and compassion. It is possible that when these basic needs of the individuals and the couple are confronted, the sexual desires will be more comfortably addressed.

There is a need to develop improved methods for assessing sexuality within the context of caregiving and dementia and to create relevant intervention strategies within the context of rigorous research and practical application to the clinical setting. The clinicians working with these issues of intimacy experience professional opportunities that are filled with learning and challenges. But more importantly, these clinical experiences have the potential to offer unique and compelling concrete encounters for couples who value even the elusive nature of intimate relationships.

REFERENCES

Askin-Edgar, S., White, K. E., and Cummings, J. L. 2002. Neuropsychiatric aspects of Alzheimer's disease and other dementing illnesses. In S. C. Yudofsky and R. E. Hales (Eds.), *Neuropsychiatry and clinical neurosciences* (4th ed.) (pp. 954–56). Washington, D.C.: American Psychiatric Publishing.

Ballard, C. G., Solis, M., Gahir, M., Cullen, P., George, S., Oyebode, G. F., et al. 1997. Sexual relationships in married dementia sufferers. *International Journal of Geriatric Psychiatry* 12:447–51.

Bornstein, M. C., and Bruner, J. S. 1989. *Interaction in human development*. Hillsdale, N.J.: Lawrence Erlbaum Associates.

Cohen, D., and Eisdorfer, C. 1986. *The loss of self: A family resource for the care of Alzheimer's disease and related disorders*. New York: New American Library.

Cohen-Mansfield, J. 1996. Inappropriate behavior. In Z. S. Khachaturian and T. S. Radebaugh (Eds.), *Alzheimer's disease: Cause(s), diagnosis, treatment, and care*. Boca Raton, Fla.: CRC Press.

Davies, H. D., Zeiss, A., and Tinklenberg, J. R. 1992. Til death us do part: Intimacy and sexuality in the marriages of Alzheimer's patients. *Journal of Psychosocial Nursing* 30(11):5–10.

Fearon, M., Donaldson, C., Burns, A., and Tarrier, N. 1998. Intimacy as a determinant of expressed emotion of carers of people with Alzheimer's disease. *Psychological Medicine* 28:1085–90.

Garner, J. 1997. Dementia: An intimate death. *British Journal of Medical Psychology* 70:177–84.

Goulet, L. R. 1973. The interfaces of acquisition: Models and methods for studying the active, developing organism. In J. R. Nesselroade and H. W. Reese (Eds.), *Life-span Developmental Psychology* (pp. 281–98). New York: Academic Press.

Litz, B. T., Zeiss, A. M., and Davies, H. D. 1990. Sexual concerns of male spouses of female Alzheimer's disease patients. *Gerontologist* 30:113–16.

Mace, N. L., and Rabins, P. V. 1999. *The 36-Hour Day: A family guide to caring for persons with Alzheimer's disease, related dementing illness and memory loss in later life* (3rd ed.). Baltimore: Johns Hopkins University Press.

McDaniel, S. H., Hepworth, J., and Doherty, W. J. 1992. *Medical family therapy: A biopsychosocial approach*. New York: Basic Books.

Morris, L. W., Morris, R. G., and Britton, P. G. 1988. The relationship between marital intimacy, perceived strain and depression in spouse caregivers of dementia sufferers. *British Journal of Medical Psychology* 61:231–36.

Ornstein, R., and Sobel, D. 1989. *Healthy pleasures*. Reading, Mass.: Perseus.

Perry, J. 2002. Wives giving care to husbands with Alzheimer's disease: A process of interpretive caring. *Research in Nursing and Health* 25:307–16.

Riegel, K. F. 1973. Developmental psychology and society: Some historical and ethical considerations. In J. R. Nesselroade and H. W. Reese (Eds.), *Life-span developmental psychology* (pp. 1–23). New York: Academic Press.

Riegel, K. F. 1976. The dialectics of human development. *American Psychologist* 31:689–700.

Rosenwald, G. C. 1975. Epilogue: Reflections on the universalism of structure. In K. F. Riegel and G. C. Rosenwald (Eds.), *Structure and transformation: Development and historical aspects* (pp. 215–19). New York: John Wiley.

Ryff, C. D., Kwan, C. M. L., and Singer, B. H. 2001. Personality and aging: Flourishing agendas and future challenges. In J. E. Birren and K. W. Schaie (Eds.), *Handbook of the Psychology of Aging* (5th ed.) (pp. 477–99). San Diego: Academic Press.

Sinnott, J. D., and Shifren, K. 2001. Gender and aging: Gender differences and gender roles. In J. E. Birren and K. W. Schaie (Eds.), *Handbook of the psychology of aging.* (5th ed.) (pp. 454–76). San Diego: Academic Press.

Wright, L. K. 1991. The impact of Alzheimer's disease on the marital relationship. *Gerontologist* 31:224–37.

Wright, L. K. 1994. Alzheimer's disease afflicted spouses who remain at home: Can human dialectics explain the findings? *Social Science and Medicine* 38:1037–46.

Wright, L. K., Hickey, J. V., Buckwalter, K. C., and Clipp, E. C. 1995. Human development in the context of aging and chronic illness: The role of attachment in Alzheimer's disease and stroke. *International Journal of Aging and Human Development* 41:133–50.

Wright, L. K., Hickey, J. V., Buckwalter, K. C., Hendrix, S. A., and Kelechi, T. 1999. Emotional and physical health of spouse caregivers of persons with Alzheimer's disease and stroke. *Journal of Advanced Nursing* 30:552–63.

CHAPTER EIGHT

Grief and Loss in Dementia

HANA OSMAN, PH.D., M.S.S.W.

Throughout our lives, we experience losses, and in response we feel a variety of emotions, such as sadness, remorse, sorrow, fear, anger, and sometimes even relief. In early childhood, the feelings can be exaggerated, such as when a child sobs uncontrollably after breaking a toy or misplacing a favorite possession. As we grow older, we learn to accept loss as a natural occurrence in life. Three terms are frequently used interchangeably in discussing our reaction to loss: bereavement, grief, and mourning. Although related, each term describes a specific aspect of the reaction to the loss, as we process the event and live to accept it. DeSpelder and Strickland (2000) define the terms in the following manner:

Bereavement refers to the "objective event of loss" (p. 224). It is the state of being when we are suddenly and forcibly deprived of something meaningful in our lives.

Grief is a set of complex physical, emotional, and/or behavioral reactions to the loss that can include disturbances in one's ability to eat or sleep, or feelings of a heavy weight on the chest. Emotional reactions range in severity, depending on a variety of factors such as life experiences, the circumstances leading to the loss, or the individual person's emotional health before the event. People can react to grief with sadness, depression, or anger—and in times of intense grief with visual and/or auditory hallucinations. Behavioral expressions of grief may vary among cultural groups, from stoicism to overt forms of crying, hitting one's chest, and wailing.

Finally, *mourning* is the process through which a grieving person can integrate the loss in everyday life. Cultural influences frequently define mourning rituals, and they may serve to identify the grieving individual through outward appearances. People in mourning are distinguished from others by wearing either all white or all black clothing, by not wearing makeup or jewelry, by wearing a black armband, or by altering their physical appearance as by cutting off their long hair, a native American tradition. Mourning the death of a loved one serves as a transitional period between experiencing the loss and the resumption of a new routine. Although the experience of loss is universal, our reactions may vary by culture, tradition, and individual preferences. Actions viewed by some as helpful in the process of accepting the loss of a loved one due to a sudden death may be perceived by others as being inappropriate or disrespectful. It is important to accept these variations because they represent the individuality of the mourner and the circumstances surrounding the loss or the death.

This chapter focuses on grief as persons with dementia and their caregivers experience it and offers suggestions for dealing with it.

THE STAGES OF GRIEF

In a dramatization of what happens to the minds of persons with dementia, such as persons who are diagnosed with Alzheimer disease, Doka and Aber (2002) liken the feelings experienced by patients and families to the horror described in the film *Invasion of the Body Snatchers*. The process is described as "the bodies are invaded by what seem to be mind snatchers" (p. 218). In response to the situation of a healthy body being attacked by an invader that destroys the mind, those affected "suffer a profound sense of loss" (p. 219). Although generally persons with dementia do not die until years after the initial diagnosis is made, caregivers may feel that the patient has experienced a type of psychosocial death. Doka and Aber (2002) define psychosocial death as "those cases in which the psychological essence, individual personality, or self is perceived as dead though the person remains alive" (p. 219). When patients lose the memory of who they are and what their lives have been, the personality of the person who occupies the physical body essentially dies. Caregivers feel depression, grief, and loss as the person with dementia loses emotional, physical, and social abilities and interactions.

Family members, as well as patients, learn to adjust to feelings of loss incrementally. In an attempt to help us understand how people who experience loss in their lives cope, several models have been developed. Sadock and Sadock (2001) describe two models of grief and bereavement as outlined by John Bowlby and C. M. Parkes. Bowlby's stages are summarized as numbness or protest; yearning and searching for the lost figure; disorganization and despair; and finally reorganization.

Parkes's stages focus on alarm; numbness; pining or searching; depression; and recovery and reorganization.

In spite of the emergence of many stage theories of grief, the early work and contributions of Elisabeth Kübler-Ross (1969) to the field of thanatology remain the gold standard. She describes five stages of adjustment that people go through when facing their own deaths. Although her theory was formulated to apply primarily to individuals who are themselves dying, some of these stages are applicable to the process of adjustment to any life change, and may apply to degrees to persons with dementia. The process of adjustment can also be applied to patients' family members who are also grieving over the progressive loss of their loved ones. Kübler-Ross studied patients who were diagnosed with cancer, and she summarized their experiences in five stages: denial, anger, bargaining, depression, and acceptance. These stages were later given the acronym DABDA.

Denial is reportedly "used by almost all patients" (Kübler-Ross, 1969, p. 35) at different times during the course of terminal illness, but particularly at the beginning of the illness. Denial can be considered healthy because it allows patients to distance themselves from the reality of their illness and it helps them deal with the painful realization of their impending death. Kübler-Ross asserted that patients are likely to use denial as a defense mechanism, particularly when they are not comfortable discussing death. This stage is characterized by statements such as: "No, not me, it cannot be true" (p. 34); "the doctor is wrong"; "the lab made an error"; or "this can't possibly happen to me because . . ." Persons who are newly diagnosed with dementia may not be prepared to accept interventions by service agencies because they are not acknowledging the presence of the memory problems that may now require intervention. Although denial can be a protective defense mechanism that allows patients the time to cope with their losses, it may also hinder their ability to seek help with activities that they are no longer capable of performing. Continuing to drive an automobile after it is established that cognitive functioning is impaired is one example of how denial can pose a threat to the person with Alzheimer disease, as well as to the general public. When it is clear that the patient's denial puts him or her in peril, families and other caregivers have an obligation to break through the denial and intervene to protect the patient from self-injury.

Family members in denial may "doctor shop" and misinterpret explanations to support their hope that the individual does not have a progressive cognitive impairment. In the example above, family members may also want the patient to continue to drive because of convenience or because of their own need to maintain peace in the family, as when the patient resists relinquishing the driver's license or the car keys. Patients vacillate between Kübler-Ross's stages of adjustment, but denial is frequently the first stage because it is a way of allowing the information about the inevitability of one's own death to be processed and to "sink in." After patients have been forced to face the reality of their illness, either when the symptoms become too obvious to ignore or when the diagnosis is confirmed and the treatment process makes it impossible to continue in their denial, the patient's reaction can turn to anger.

Anger is the stage that is most easily recognized by questions such as: "Why me?" and "I've been a good person, why couldn't this have happened to . . . instead of me?" Patients at this stage may be the most difficult for family members and caregivers to deal with, because they themselves may become the focus of the patient's anger. Cognitively impaired persons become increasingly demanding, with frequent complaining, and they are generally difficult to please.

As persons with dementia become more difficult to care for, caregivers experience anger, and the focus of their anger may become the patients themselves for becoming increasingly dependent and for not meeting their companionship or sexual needs. Guilt over feeling angry with the care recipient frequently develops, and it may contribute to the caregivers' depression. Caregivers also focus their anger on relatives who are considered neither helpful nor realistic, or on society or God for the circumstances in which they find themselves (Doka and Aber, 2002). When anger becomes counterproductive, and as the patient progresses through the process of adjusting, anger subsides, and the person may try bargaining to be a better person.

Bargaining is the stage of trying to postpone the inevitable, and is characterized by statements such as: "I'll quit smoking, if only I can live until I see my daughter graduate from college." It symbolizes negotiating with a higher power to extend life, in an attempt to regain control over seemingly uncontrollable events. Bargaining frequently includes a promise of "a life dedicated to God" (Kübler-Ross, 1969, p. 74) or to the church. When bargaining fails to achieve the intended reprieve, the person moves to the next stage.

Depression is the next stage, when there is no hope for reversal of the diagnosis or the prognosis and the person realizes that there is no escape from death. Depression and feelings of despair can affect patients and their caregivers alike. This is the stage in which patients grieve the loss of their health and of the future they anticipated and planned for themselves. This stage may start with sadness at the realization that the course of the illness is irreversible. Feelings of sadness should be accepted by those who witness it, and should in fact be expected. The presence of social support, assuring the patient that he or she will not be abandoned, is crucial during this stage. Assessing depression in older adults can be challenging because it is frequently difficult to separate symptoms of clinical depression from manifestations of the "normal aging processes" (Scogin, 1994, p. 76). It is important to distinguish between the sadness that people experience when their life situations change, and clinical depression that should be treated. Persons with dementia who are depressed, and depressed caregivers, can benefit from assessment and treatment of their depression. It is important to note that older males have an elevated risk of self-destructive behavior, and suicide assessment is an integral part of the management of depression in all older patients. Traditional treatment of depression by the use of psychotropic medications and/or by various psychotherapeutic interventions varies in outcome depending on the cause of the depression and the mental health history of the depressed individual. Families can help the depressed individual by acknowledging the person's feelings and seeking help through support groups, counseling, and eventually hospice programs. The clinical approach to treating depression experienced by a person with dementia is different from the approach used for the caregiver who is grieving over the loss of a loved one to dementia or to death. Whereas psychotropic medications may be appropriate for the patient, caregiver support groups, respite from caregiving, and social support may be more appropriate for the caregiver.

Many depression assessment tools are available to clinicians who specialize in the care of older adults. Among these are the Beck Depression Inventory (Beck et al., 1961), the Zung Self-Rating Depression Scale (Zung, 1965), the Geriatric Depression Scale (Yesavage et al., 1983), the Inventory for Diagnosing Depression (Zimmerman and Coryell, 1988), and the Cornell Scale for Depression in Dementia (Alexopoulos, Abrams, Young, and Shamoian, 1988), an assessment scale which is specifically designed to assess depression in older adults with dementia.

Acceptance is the final stage in the Kübler-Ross (1969) stage theory of adjusting to a life-altering event, such as being diagnosed with cancer. Some patients experience acceptance when they are closest to death, or just before death occurs. In fact, they are often described as "void of feelings" (Kübler-Ross, 1969, p. 100) and as not being angry, hopeless, or depressed. In this stage, patients doze off frequently and gradually increase their sleeping hours. Some patients do not reach this stage because of their attempt to continue to fight. When exhausted, this group of patients may make comments such as "I just cannot make it anymore" (Kübler-Ross, 1969, p. 101), and after uttering such words, they die without ever reaching acceptance.

Acceptance is particularly relevant to individuals whose cognitive abilities are intact when they are close to death, such as patients dying of cancer, the population that Kübler-Ross worked with and described. Experiencing acceptance for this population may be demonstrated by making final health care plans, saying goodbye to loved ones, and preparing for one's funeral.

Although they can occur sequentially for some, for others the different stages identified by Kübler-Ross may recur as the illness progresses. Many patients die in denial of their illness, angry or depressed. Persons in the advanced stages of dementia may not experience acceptance in the manner described by Kübler-Ross because of their progressive cognitive impairment. Caregivers, however, can reach the stage of acceptance as they become accustomed to the caregiving role by becoming skilled in providing care. This stage may also provide the caregiver with the opportunity to make future health, end-of-life care, and funeral plans for the person with dementia.

Critics of Kübler-Ross's stage theory point out the inaccuracy in implying that everyone experiences death in the same way and that the stages occur in a particular sequence. In fact, Kübler-Ross disavowed an "invariant sequence" interpretation of her work. It is best to view Kübler-Ross's stage theory as descriptive of the feelings that people can experience as they face their own death, or as they adjust to caring for a person with dementia. Every model of grief has its unique taxonomy. What all models have in common is their assertion that adjustment to grief is incremental and that it slowly occurs in stages that are unique to each person.

ANTICIPATORY GRIEF

Everyone involved in the care of the person with dementia experiences grief at some point. As patients realize that their memory is becoming increasingly impaired, and as they struggle to cope with the impairment, they grieve the loss of their past as well as their present and future (LaBarge and Trtanj, 1995; Rando, 1986). Family members grieve for the patient before death (Kasl-Godley, 2003), and this continuum of grief continues after the person dies (Bass, Bowman, and Noelker, 1991). Grief that occurs before death is commonly referred to as "anticipatory grief" (Kasl-Godley, 2003). Dementia can develop over a long period of time, during which the afflicted person is aware of the gradual increase in impairment. The slow progression of dementia allows patients and caregivers alike to adjust to the changes that are occurring and prepares the caregivers for the inevitable death of their loved ones (Mullan, 1992). Anticipatory grief can also facilitate the bereavement process after the person dies, by allowing caregivers to address unresolved conflicts and prepare for the transition into new relationships (Fulton and Gottesman, 1980) before death occurs. In studies reported by Farran et al. (1991), Kasl-Godley (2003), Bull (1998), and Loos and Bowd (1997), the focus of the grief was on losing the relationship the caregivers had with the care recipient. They mourned the change in their communication patterns, grieved the loss of their own freedom, and processed their distress over observing the cognitive, psychological, social, and physical decline of their care recipient.

Grief of the caregiver before the death of the person with dementia can be characterized by the isolation of the grieving caregiver from social support and from the recognition of the grief by others (Doka, 2000). In her book *Caring for People with Alzheimer's Disease,* Anderson (1995) lists symptoms of stress experienced by caregivers:

1. *Anger:* The unpleasant tasks associated with caring for a person with dementia, such as cleaning up after incontinence or feeling that the care recipient is not sufficiently appreciative, can lead to feelings of anger. This may represent a change in attitude toward the person with dementia and a change in their relationship. This change may be accompanied by grief over the loss of the prior relationship with the loved one.

2. *Helplessness:* Not being able to understand the person's behavior, or if the caregiver's best efforts to alleviate the person's discomfort are not successful.

3. *Embarrassment:* Some of the actions of the care recipient that are socially unacceptable, such as masturbation or incontinence, can cause embarrassment.

4. *Guilt:* This is a complex emotion that can result from needing to move the care recipient to a facility that can provide a more advanced level of care, or can result from feeling angry that the care recipient is not getting better.

5. *Grief:* As the condition of the care recipient continues to deteriorate, the caregiver grieves the loss of the person that was once a life partner and the relationship that was once intimate.

6. *Depression:* The caregiver can experience different levels of depression as the care recipient moves into a different stage of the condition or as placement to a long-term facility becomes inevitable.

7. *Isolation:* Family caregivers can become isolated as their social support dwindles, the initially acute condition becomes a long-term way of life, and the caregiver feels the absence of resources.

8. *Concern:* As the care receiver shows diminishing emotional reaction, the caregiver may feel concern over not doing enough to help.

These significant stressors may necessitate forming a new relationship with the care recipient based on hands-on caring rather than reciprocal emotional attachment, but also incorporating some of the elements of the prior interpersonal relationship.

Doka and Aber (1989) described caregivers' grief over the continuous deterioration of persons with Alzheimer disease as grief over the social death rather than the physical death of the care recipient. Social death occurs gradually, as the person who is afflicted with any progressive dementia slowly withdraws from societal roles and is "treated like a corpse" (Doka and Aber, 1989) while still alive. Mourning the social death of a person is complicated, and it causes role ambiguity because, although the spouse is essentially socially widowed, he or she is still legally married. Societal pressures do not allow spouses to grieve, as in response to a physical death, and therefore they cannot progress through the entire process of grief (Lezak, 1978), a process that eventually leads to accepting the inevitable and moving on with one's life. In a study of caregivers of persons with dementia, Meuser and Marwit (2001) reported that anticipatory grief is as "real" and can be as intense as grief that is experienced after death. However, as these authors note, studies of anticipatory grief in cases of progressive dementia have not been thoroughly reported in the literature.

CHRONIC GRIEF

"Chronic grief" (Rabins, 1984, p. 374) is a label used to describe grief that is experienced by caregivers of persons with progressive dementia as the condition develops, possibly over many years, and it continues after the person dies. But, when, then, should grief be considered pathological? There are frequent reports in the literature of healthy individuals experiencing auditory and visual hallucinations for extended periods of time during the grief period after the death of their loved ones (Rees, 1971; Olson et al., 1985; Byrne and Raphael, 1994; Grimby and Berg, 1995). In healthy older individuals, these hallucinations eventually resolve as the mourning process progresses. However, pathological grief may be an early manifestation of cognitive decline in the grieving individual, when it persists without resolution or when it takes unusual forms. For example, Venneri, Shanks, Staff, and Della Salla (2000) reported on a case of a 78-year-old widow who appeared to be physically and mentally healthy before the death of her husband, on whom she was very dependent. After his death, she had delusions of her husband visiting her in their home, and she insisted that he was still alive and that he married their 20-year-old neighbor. Her delusions persisted, and her cognitive functioning continued to deteriorate until she was hospitalized and eventually placed in a residential facility for persons with dementia.

One vehicle to address anticipatory and chronic grief may be hospice care, in which all efforts are made to provide a psychologically nuanced context for death. As Robert Kastenbaum (2004) noted, before hospice care, death was shrouded in secrecy. The death awareness movement opened communication on death between patients, families, physicians, and society in general. In a sense, patient and family members could now use their emotional energy and attachment to pave the way for a "good death" that was individualized and perhaps free of recrimination and bitterness. For example, if patient and family members can accept the fact that Alzheimer disease (AD) is a terminal illness and the patient is going to die soon, perhaps direct and open communication (in whatever form it might take in an individual with dementia) between patient and family members can begin a healing process that will carry over after the patient dies. Even with the limited cognitive capacities of one in the terminal stages of AD, such family acceptance, attempts at comfort care, and expressions of love may be optimal preventive medicine which may expedite a healthy grief process.

THE LOSS OF PERSONA IN DEMENTIA

The stress caused by caregiving has been reported to lead to depression, as well as to introspection, self-evaluation, and doubt in one's abilities to successfully perform assigned duties (Lewinsohn, Hoberman, Teri, and Hautzinger, 1985). Contributing to the stress felt by caregivers is the constriction of their own lives, as they devote more time and energy to the care of the progressively ill care recipient. As care recipients' needs and dependence increase, the caregivers gradually give up their own interests and outside activities to devote their time to their caregiving duties. Caregivers frequently are forced to give up outside employment, their social contacts diminish, and their personal identities are gradually lost to their roles as caregivers (Skaff and Pearlin, 1992).

Alzheimer disease causes loss of self of the patient in a different manner. Although some authors recognize that those with dementia may remain open to pastoral interventions (Kimble, McFadden, and Park 2003), and a few others believe that AD can even be viewed as a transcendent state that allows individuals to obtain a form of higher consciousness, most emphasize that it robs them of their identity and their sense of who they are (Cohen and Eisdorfer, 1986). Until Alois Alzheimer medicalized the concept of dementia in 1907, the symptoms that we now recognize as the syndrome of Alzheimer disease were considered a normal decline associated with the process of aging (Herskovits, 1995), and some of its effects were expected. The causes of dementia may vary, but memory loss is common to all causes of dementia (Silverstein, Flaherty and Tobin, 2002). Losing one's memory, including the ability to remember one's identity, may be one of the most devastating effects. Regardless of what caused the memory loss, its effects are the same, namely the loss of a sense of identity, which is the essence of being human. It is evident that the early signs of the disease, such as inability to perform one's job, being disoriented and not being able to relate to family, friends, and acquaintances affect the core of what it means to be an individual. This is the reason that a main therapeutic approach for individuals with dementia involves supplying external sources of self-validation (Feil, 1993). We should never forget that these individuals must be accorded the profound respect accorded to all human beings. Such affirmation serves an immediate goal of buttressing a demented person's flagging self-identity, reflecting an interpersonal stance honoring his or her long developmental history. It also serves an overarching beneficent social goal (i.e., the individual should not be treated "just" as one with Alzheimer disease, and reduced self-awareness does not rob a person of identity).

PLANNING FOR THE FUTURE

The time between diagnosis of early dementia and the point at which cognitive functioning is severely impaired can be used to make future health care plans and to consult financial and legal advisors for estate planning. Persons in the early stages of dementia are legally competent and can make most of their own decisions. To spare the family and other caregivers the burden of making difficult end-of-life health care decisions for the patient, the patient can make such decisions in advance. A study by Gessert, Forbes, and Bern-Klug (2001) concludes that caregivers are largely unprepared to make these decisions for persons with dementia and are emotionally burdened by anticipatory grief and guilt. They strongly recommend that persons in the early stages of dementia engage their family members in discussions about clinical end-of-life care, while they still possess decisional capacity and before such decisions need to be made. In this study, families were clear on their desire to "do the right thing" but did not know how to "operationalize their intentions" (p. 279). Patients and family members may be in the throes of one of the early grief stages and not fully accepting of the illness. Clinician-led discussions about patient wishes in anticipation of treatment decisions may be necessary on an ongoing basis. As caregivers and family members of persons with dementia may not be aware of the type of decisions they could be asked to make, discussions between patients, family members, and health care providers about the use of mechanical ventilation, feeding tubes, dialysis, cardiopulmonary resuscitation, and antibiotics can be very useful. Based on these discussions, persons in the early stages of dementia can then complete legal documents such as a living will, the appointment of a health care decision maker, and selecting a guardian-in-need (designating one person to become guardian when and if guardianship becomes necessary); they can articulate their wishes about end-of-life care and can relieve their family members of the burden that making end-of-life decisions can be. However, it is important that the patient be screened for depression to make sure that his "true" wishes are being expressed. These documents can be particularly useful to the care-givers because they provide assurance that the decisions made on the patient's be-half are in fact in congruence with the patient's wishes.

To ensure that financial concerns are also addressed, the patient can (1) avoid costly and time-consuming court procedures to appoint a legal guardian by ap-pointing a trusted family member or friend as a durable power of attorney to han-dle financial transactions, (2) establish a living trust, and (3) execute a will to dis-tribute property at the time of death. Some patients and their caregivers may choose to consult an attorney to assist in the completion of these documents. How-ever, many states require only that the documents are signed, dated, and appropri-ately witnessed. A more thorough discussion of these documents is addressed in the chapter on the ethics of dementia caregiving.

Mr. A. is a 79-year-old man who lives with his wife of 45 years. At age 75, he completed a living will and designated his son Robert as his surrogate de-cision maker. Mr. A. felt that he prepared the necessary papers to ensure that his end-of-life wishes would be followed when he was no longer able to make his own health care decisions. At age 77, Mr. A. was diagnosed with dementia, and he again reiterated to his wife and son his concerns about liv-ing in a state of dependency on mechanical interventions to prolong his life.

One year after his diagnosis, Mr. A. tripped and fell in his house and sus-tained a head injury. He was hospitalized, and during the hospital stay he had a stroke that left him with severe physical and cognitive deficits. Mr. A. then developed pneumonia, and his kidneys failed. The medical team re-quested consent for dialysis and for the insertion of a feeding tube to pro-vide him with nutrition and hydration.

Robert refused to give consent for further invasive intervention. He re-quested that his father be discharged from the hospital to his home, with services from the local hospice for palliative care, in accordance with Mr. A.'s living will.

The medical team felt that Mr. A.'s medical condition was not terminal and that he could improve with the use of antibiotics, dialysis, and a feed-ing tube. The physicians refused to allow Robert to dictate limiting medical intervention on behalf of his father, because Mr. A.'s living will was specific to interventions related to the progression of dementia. Mrs. A. visited her husband daily, and she was clearly distraught over the prospect of his death. She was reluctant to limit medical care for her husband, and the medical team felt that because there appeared to be lack of consensus within the family, they needed to continue treatment. The case was referred to the hospital ethics committee to determine if limiting care under these circumstances would be considered ethical, and whether the conditions of the living will were met.

The consultation team of the ethics committee met with Mrs. A., Robert, and the attending physician. Mrs. A. was tearful throughout the meeting, and she deferred the decisions to her son. Robert explained that he had discussed the living will thoroughly and repeatedly with his father. Although Mrs. A. was present during many of these discussions, she was mostly an observer rather than an active participant. Robert described his parents as being emotionally close and his mother as having been particularly dependent on her husband. He related discussions about his father's wish to designate him rather than his wife as his surrogate decision maker because he (Mr. A.) felt that his wife would not be emotionally capable of making end-of-life decisions for him. The attending physician described Mr. A.'s medical condition, stating that although medical intervention could conceivably resolve Mr. A.'s pneumonia and the feeding tube would provide him with the nutrition and hydration that he needed to survive, there was little chance for recovery from the cognitive deficits, and he would continue to need dialysis treatments. He also commented on Mrs. A.'s frail physical condition and recommended placement in a nursing home for Mr. A. The physician gave the family no hope for complete recovery or for a return to his pre-stroke condition. Mrs. A. and Robert then agreed that Mr. A. had repeatedly made them promise that they would never place him in a nursing home.

The threat of a discharge from the hospital to a nursing home, coupled with understanding the irreversible complications of the stroke, were sufficient to convince Mrs. A. that her husband was indeed now in the clinical situation that he so strongly opposed. The ethics committee concurred with the family's conclusion that applying Mr. A.'s living will would be the ethical approach to dealing with his current condition.

The feeding tube was not inserted, the dialysis was not initiated, and the antibiotics were withheld. Mr. A. was discharged from the hospital to his home, with a referral to hospice, and he died four days after discharge, attended by his loving wife and son. Such ethics committee family meetings may serve a "therapeutic" function. Given such prior planning, it is to be expected that the normal family mourning process will be expedited and that pathological grief patterns will be less likely to occur.

How caregivers deal with their own stress may affect the level of care they are able to provide the person with the dementia and the length of time that they are able to provide the care before placement in an alternative living arrangement becomes necessary. Relieving the stress experienced by caregivers can take different forms. Caregivers need to learn about and become very familiar with the natural progression of the condition of dementia because this knowledge can be very helpful in anticipating the next stage of the dementia and preparing to deal with it. In addition to taking care of themselves by staying healthy, exercising, visiting their own physicians on a regular basis, getting sufficient sleep and rest, and using respite care that is provided in the community for families of patients with dementia, caregivers can start making the appropriate financial and medical planning for the patient.

IMPLICATIONS FOR CLINICAL PRACTICE

As the process of dealing with dementia progresses, clinicians can prepare the care recipient, as well as the caregiver, to deal with the inevitable need for making difficult decisions, including medical decisions concerning end-of-life care. Such planning will facilitate the management of grief and loss in dementia for both caregiver and care recipient. Steps that can be taken to assure a systematic and relatively smooth transition between optimal health and the eventual death of the care recipient include developing a partnership between the clinician and the patient/caregiver dyad (Schulz and Martire, 2004). This partnership needs to address typically difficult topics that relate to mental health as well as medical interventions. The following is a suggested approach for clinicians:

1. Monitoring of care recipient and caregiver mental health needs and referral to mental health professionals for the assessment and treatment of anxiety and depression
2. Referral to caregiver support groups
3. Recommendation for professional estate planning
4. Discussion of care recipient medical and end-of-life wishes for the use of technological advances such as cardiopulmonary resuscitation and ventilator support, feeding tubes, dialysis, and antibiotics
5. Completion of health care advance directives including a living will, designation of a health care surrogate, and a physician's do-not-resuscitate order

6. Conversation about the care recipient's wishes regarding admission to health care facilities for acute and / or long-term care when there is little or no hope for recovery

7. Initiate discourse about the use of available resources including hospice care.

Involving the care receiver and the caregiver in all aspects of the care of the person with dementia can assure the clinician that the needs of both members of the dyad are assessed and addressed. Relieving some of the caregiver burden of grief and loss may be achieved when there is knowledge that all available resources and alternatives are considered and that all that needs to be done for the care of the care recipient is in fact done.

REFERENCES

Alexopoulos, G. S., Abrams, R. C., Young, R. C., and Shamoian, C. A. 1988. Cornell Scale for depression in dementia. *Biological Psychiatry* 23:271–28.

Anderson, G. 1995. *Caring for people with Alzheimer's disease: A training manual for direct care providers.* Baltimore: Health Professions Press.

Bass, D. M., Bowman, K., and Noelker, L. S. 1991. The influence of caregiving and bereavement support on adjusting to an older relative's death. *Gerontologist* 30:32–42.

Beck, A. T., Ward, C. H., Mendelson, M., Mock, J., and Erbaugh, J. 1961. An inventory for measuring depression. *Archives of General Psychiatry* 4:561–71.

Bull, M. A. 1998. Losses in families affected by dementia: Coping strategies and service issues. *Journal of Family Studies* 4:187–99.

Byrne, G., and Raphael, B. 1994. A longitudinal study of bereavement phenomena in recently widowed elderly men. *Psychological Medicine* 24:411–21.

Cohen, D., and Eisdorfer, C. 1986. *The loss of self: A family resource for the care of Alzheimer's disease and related disorders.* New York: W. W. Norton.

DeSpelder, L. A., and Strickland, A. L. 2002. *The last dance: Encountering death and dying.* Boston: McGraw Hill.

Doka, K. J. 2000. Mourning psychosocial loss: Anticipatory mourning in Alzheimer's, ALS, and irreversible coma. In T. A. Rando (Ed.), *Clinical dimensions of anticipatory mourning: Theory and practice in working with the dying, their loved ones, and the caregivers.* Champaign, Ill.: Research Press.

Doka, K. J., and Aber, R. A. 1989. Psychosocial loss and grief. In K. J. Doka (Ed.), *Disenfranchised grief: Recognizing hidden sorrow.* Lexington, Mass.: Lexington Books.

Doka, K. J., and Aber, R. A. 2002. Psychosocial loss and grief. In K. J. Doka (Ed.), *Disenfranchised grief.* Champaign, Ill.: Research Press.

Farran, C. J., Keane-Hagerty, E., Salloway, S., Kupferer, S., and Wilken, C. S. 1991. Finding meaning: An alternative paradigm for Alzheimer's disease family caregivers. *Gerontologist* 31:483–89.

Feil, N. 1993. *The validation breakthrough: Simple techniques for communicating with people with "Alzheimer's-type dementia."* Baltimore: P. Brooks Pub.

Fulton, R., and Gottesman, D. J. 1980. Anticipatory grief: A psychosocial concept reconsidered. *British Journal of Psychiatry* 137:45–54.

Gessert, C. E., Forbes, S., and Bern-Klug, M. 2000–2001. Planning end-of-life care for patients with dementia: Roles of families and health professionals. *Omega* 42(4):273–91.

Grimby, A., and Berg, S. 1995. Stressful life events and cognitive functioning in late life. *Aging Clinical and Experimental Research* 7:35–39.

Herskovits, E. 1995. Struggling over subjectivity: Debates about the "self" and Alzheimer's disease. *Medical Anthropology Quarterly* 9(2):146–64.

Kasl-Godley, J. 2003. Anticipatory grief and loss: Implications for intervention. In D. W. Coon, D. Gallagher-Thompson, and L. W. Thompson (Eds.), *Innovative interventions to reduce dementia caregiver distress: A clinical guide.* New York: Springer Publishing.

Kastenbaum, R. 2004. *On our way: The final passage through life and death.* Los Angeles: University of California Press.

Kimble, M. A., and McFadden, S. H., and Park, M. 2003. *Aging, spirituality, and religion: A handbook,* Vol. 2. Minneapolis, Minn.: Augsburg Fortress Press.

Kübler-Ross, E. 1969. *On death and dying.* New York: Macmillan.

LaBarge, E., and Trtanj, F. 1995. A support group for people in the early stages of dementia of the Alzheimer's type. *Journal of Applied Gerontology* 14:289–301.

Lewinsohn, P. M., Hoberman, H., Teri, L., and Hautzinger, M. 1985. An integrative theory of depression. In S. Reiss and R. Bootzin (Eds.), *Theoretical issues in behavioral therapy.* New York: Academic.

Lezak, M. 1978. Living with the characterologically altered brain injured patient. *Journal of Clinical Psychiatry* 34:592–98.

Loos, C., and Bowd, A. 1997. Caregivers of persons with Alzheimer's disease: Some neglected implications of the experience of personal loss and grief. *Death Studies* 21:501–14.

Meuser, T. M., and Marwit, S. J. 2001. A comprehensive, stage-sensitive model of grief in dementia caregiving. *Gerontologist* 41:658–70.

Mullan, J. 1992. The bereaved caregiver: A prospective study of changes in well-being. *Gerontologist* 32:673–83.

Olson, P., Syddeth, J., Peterson, M., Peterson, P., and Egelhoff, C. 1985. Hallucinations of widowhood. *Journal of the American Geriatrics Society* 33:543–47.

Rabins, P. V. 1984. Management of dementia in the family context. *Psychosomatics* 25:369–71, 374–75.

Rando, T. A. 1986. *Loss and anticipatory grief.* Lexington, Mass.: Lexington Books.

Rees, W. D. 1971. The hallucinations of widowhood. *British Medical Journal* 4:37–41.

Sadock, B. J., and Sadock, V. A. 2001. *Kaplan and Sadock's pocket handbook of clinical psychiatry* (3rd ed.). Philadelphia: Lippincott Williams & Wilkins.

Schulz, R., and Martire, L. M. 2004. Family caregiving of persons with dementia. *American Journal of Geriatric Psychiatry* 12(3):240–49.

Scogin, F. R. 1994. Assessment of depression in older adults: A guide for practitioners. In M. Storandt and G. R. VandenBos (Eds.), *Neuropsychological assessment of dementia and depression in older adults: A clinician's guide.* Washington, D.C.: American Psychological Association.

Silverstein, N., Flaherty, G., and Tobin, T. S. (Eds.). 2002. *Dementia and wandering behavior: Concern for the lost elder.* New York: Springer.

Skaff, M. M., and Pearlin, L. I. 1992. Caregiving: Role engulfment and the loss of self. *Gerontologist* 32:656–64.

Venneri, A., Shanks, M. F., Staff, R. T., and Della Salla, S. 2000. Nurturing syndrome: A form of pathological bereavement with delusions in Alzheimer's disease. *Neuropsychologia* 38:213–24.

Yesavage, J. A., Brink, T. L., Rose, T. L., Lum, O., Huang, V., Adey, M., and Leirer, V. O. 1983. Development and validation of a geriatric depression screening scale: A preliminary report. *Journal of Psychiatric Research* 17:37–49.

Zimmerman, M., and Coryell, W. 1988. The validity of a self-report questionnaire for diagnosing major depressive disorder. *Archives of General Psychiatry* 45:738–40.

Zung, W. W. K. 1965. A self-rating depression scale. *Archives of General Psychiatry* 12:63–70.

PART 4

Implications for Treatment
The Multidisciplinary Approach

Part IV uses a biopsychosocial model to draw clinical implications from research on the individual and interpersonal aspects of caregiving. In chapter 9, Melissa Martinez and Mark E. Kunik explore pharmacological options for the care of patients with behavioral disturbance. They discuss the pharmacological management of disruptive behaviors such as insomnia, agitation, and aggression, which limit patients' positive interaction with others and consume large amounts of caregivers' time and resources. They emphasize, however, that nonpharmacological behavior management should be attempted first. A multidimensional assessment of the patient, caregiver, and environmental determinants affecting such disruptive behavior will guide combined nonpharmacological and pharmacological treatments to achieve state-of-the-art care.

In chapter 10, Silvia Sörensen, Deborah King, and Martin Pinquart discuss individual and family therapies as they apply to dementia care in clinical and home settings. These include individual interventions aimed at reducing stress; providing psychoeducation, support, psychotherapy, and multicomponent interventions; and family interventions such as family education, family consultation, and family therapy. The authors outline the role of "mutuality" and "filial maturity" in the context of successful family caregiving relationships. They discuss caregiving and the various types of family systems, such as "securely attached" families, "overwhelmed" families, "closed/fixed" families, and "wounded" families. To best address the needs of the patient and family, they recommend combining various therapeutic modalities into a multimodal approach within the context of the prior relationship.

David A. Chiriboga discusses the role of social supports in caregiving in chapter 11. He notes that the amount of available positive social support is inversely correlated with distress in caregiving. He categorizes supports into informal supports (i.e., unpaid assistance by families and friends) and formal supports (i.e., paid assistance provided by professionals and semiprofessionals such as social workers, nurses, visiting homemakers, and the clergy). He also tackles the less well studied subject of invisible supports. For example, he creatively challenges our thinking regarding care recipients as not just sources of distress but as potential sources of support as well.

As suggested by all the chapters in this section, a multidisciplinary team is optimal in the care of patient and caregiver. Such a team should include a primary care physician or geriatrician, a psychiatrist with some expertise in geriatrics, a psychologist, a social worker, a nurse, and a chaplain. However, in real life it is hard to obtain a team comprising all the above disciplines in every setting. While such a team may be available in the hospital, it is hard to have a full team in nursing homes, smaller health care centers, or in private practice. In such settings, it is up to the individual clinician to attempt to apply a biopsychosociospiritual model, even when other disciplines are not readily available. This would involve using all the resources at hand, while spending sufficient time with the patient and caregiver to pay attention to the multidimensional needs of the patient. The chapters in this section provide a multidisciplinary framework for thinking, which may be adapted by individual clinicians to their various practice settings. Clinicians may need to network to form relationships with providers from various disciplines in the community, who can be called on in a reciprocal manner to assist in the care of the patient with dementia. The clinician's prior relationship with the local hospital and emergency room staff can be helpful when trying to assist the patient and caregiver in a time of crisis. Use of community supports such as the Alzheimer's Association, pastoral care, the religious community, and various charities may further enhance treatment. The clinician should feel free to assist the caregiver and patient in reaching out to every available support to enhance care.

CHAPTER NINE

The Role of Pharmacotherapy for Dementia Patients with Behavioral Disturbances

MELISSA MARTINEZ, M.D.
MARK E. KUNIK, M.D., M.P.H.

Behavioral disturbances occur in up to 90 percent of persons with dementia (Tariot and Blazina, 1994), and these disturbances affect many of those involved in the patients' care. Unfortunately, these behaviors not only are distressing but can be dangerous as well. More than 24,000 incidents of assaultive behavior were reported by 166 VA facilities over a one-year period, with psychosis and dementia cited as two of the conditions most commonly associated with these assaults (Lehman, McCormick, and Kizer, 1999). The psychological, occupational, and emotional consequences of these incidents are substantial, as these incidents have been observed to contribute to stress, caregiver burnout, and decreased quality of care (Kunik et al., 2003a). Disruptive behaviors, such as insomnia, agitation, and aggression, severely limit patients' potential for positive interactions with others and force caregivers to devote considerable time and resources to patient management. In the health care setting, this can detract from the care of other patients. In the home setting, this can severely disrupt the personal and professional lives of family members. Thus, establishing effective preventive measures and treatment strategies for behavioral dyscontrol is necessary for maintaining safety, preserving quality of care, maximizing the patient's quality of life, and protecting the caregiver's quality of life. Evidence-based reviews provide guidelines for the evaluation, management, and treatment of behavioral disturbances in persons with dementia (AGS and AAGP, 2003; APA, 1997; Doody et al., 2001).

Although physicians categorize dementia according to different etiologies, most types have similar consequences. All dementias involve damage or death of brain cells. Depending on the location of the damage, patients can develop different symptoms. These symptoms often include loss of memory, personality changes, language impairment, and behavioral changes. The unique pattern of damage and neurochemical balance in each person complicates treatment strategies. Certain treatments that may be helpful for some patients may not be helpful for others. Assuring the provision of appropriate and effective treatment for behavioral disturbances in these patients presents a major challenge to caregivers. Developing a systematic, rational, and pragmatic approach for assessing and addressing these behaviors can improve quality of life for patients and caregivers alike.

A MULTIDIMENSIONAL MODEL

In the past, the conceptualization of the causes of behavioral symptoms in persons with dementia neglected environmental, caregiver, and patient influences. Instead, it focused on the disease itself as the primary determinant of disruptive behaviors. This led to the possible overuse of stereotyped treatment interventions, such as physical restraints and nonspecific sedative medications. While there is a role for these treatments in the care of persons with dementia, considering a broader, more explicit conceptual model that includes multiple causes of behavioral symptoms expands caregivers' treatment options.

The multidimensional model considered in this chapter categorizes the causes of behavioral problems in persons with dementia into those derived from the patient, the caregiver, and the environment, with each group divided further into untreatable and treatable determinants (see table 9.1). By highlighting potentially treatable causes, while placing them in context with those causes unlikely to change, this model provides a systematic, rational, and pragmatic approach to the treatment of these symptoms (Kunik et al., 2003b).

Treatable causes of behavioral symptoms are those conditions that can be improved through the efforts of clinicians, family, and/or staff. These causes include comorbid medical conditions, caregiver knowledge and caregiving skills, and the physical aspects of the setting, such as lighting and noise level. Through addressing these issues, distressing behaviors may be decreased or even prevented. Untreatable causes include the patient's pre-illness personality or temperament, the gender of the caregiver, and caregiver turnover or staff mix; they define the context in which interventions occur. Thus untreatable determinants place a baseline constraint on the amount of improvement attainable through the modification of other causes (Kunik et al., 2003b).

TABLE 9.1
The Multidimensional Model

Factors Related to Individuals with Dementia		Caregiver Factors		Environmental Factors	
Fixed	Treatable	Fixed	Treatable	Fixed	Treatable
Dementia and related disease characteristics	Psychological or emotional needs	Gender	Psychological factors and emotional needs	Staffing issues	Physical aspects of facility
Pre-illness personality or temperament	Pain and other medical conditions	Quality of past relationship with family caregiver	Education	Setting	Social interaction and stimulation
Socioeconomic status	Physiological needs		Quality of the current relationship and caregiving skills		Change
					Use of restraints
Gender and patient preferences	Existential issues				Traffic flow
	Medications				

SOURCE: Kunik et al., 2003a.

DISTRESSING BEHAVIORS:
INSOMNIA, AGITATION, AGGRESSION
Patient Determinants

Whether verbal or physical, distressing behaviors exhaust both the patient and the caregiver. As a person's dementia progresses, his or her ability to communicate clearly decreases. This can lead to patient agitation and aggression, which can stimulate feelings of frustration and helplessness in the caregiver. In the more advanced stages of the illness, a patient can lose insight regarding his or her inability to communicate. The agitation and aggression, which initially resulted from frustration, can become the patient's primary, and possibly only, means of communicating unmet physical, physiological, emotional, and existential needs (Algase et al., 1996; Magliocco, 1996). For example, screaming may express pain, hunger, or anxiety, while hitting may express fear or discomfort with the caregiver. Furthermore, lack of participation in meaningful activities may lead to agitation, persistent vocalizations, or apathy (Magliocco, 1996). The tasks of the caregiver include learning to interpret these behaviors and addressing the patient's unmet needs appropriately, without neglecting his or her own emotional health.

With elderly patients, one of the most common causes of altered mental status, or delirium, is a change in medical condition. When a caregiver notes a sudden change in a patient's behavior or mental status, he or she must consider the possibility of an infection, such as pneumonia or a urinary tract infection. Other medical conditions that cause changes in mental status and subsequent changes in behavior include electrolyte imbalances, strokes, and cerebral hemorrhages. The management of delirium superimposed on a dementia is a complicated matter that often needs to be conducted in a hospital setting. This will help to assure that all factors are addressed and to optimize chances that the individual will return to premorbid levels of cognitive functioning without excess disability.

New medications and changes in medication dosage can also alter a patient's sensorium and behavior. The complicated nature of brain damage in persons with dementia leads to unpredictable responses to medication. For example, while benzodiazepines or anticholinergic medications cause relaxation and sedation in most patients, persons with dementia can experience a paradoxical agitation. Caregivers often respond to this increased agitation, insomnia, and possible aggression by giving more of these medications, usually to no avail, leading to a vicious cycle in which the distressing behaviors continue or worsen.

Caregiver Determinants

Caregivers' knowledge of dementia and their caregiving skill also have an impact on patient care (Kunik et al., 2003a). In addition, caring for persons with dementia requires understanding, flexibility, and endurance—qualities that typically erode with fatigue in the absence of appropriate supports. Feelings of anger or depression can develop and affect the caregiver-patient interaction. Although comprehension is lost as the disease progresses, patients remain sensitive to the tone of communications, which can promote or inhibit disruptive behaviors (Rabins, Mace, and Lucas 1982). Through the efforts of the health care team and the family, conditions such as caregiver burnout and depression can be minimized or avoided. Combining these efforts with increased caregiver education can help maintain or improve the quality of the caregiver-patient relationship.

Environmental Determinants

Characteristics of the environment, including physical design, ambient noise, social interactions, and level of care provided, can modify behavioral symptoms. Lighting, wall patterns, floor patterns, and temperature can influence behavior, depending on the amount of stimulation and comfort, or overstimulation and discomfort they provide. Sensory modulation activities, such as listening to music,

also decrease agitation, especially if the music is individualized to the patient's preferences (Gerdner, 2000). Level of social interaction plays a role as well, as isolation
is associated with wandering and screaming (Cohen-Mansfield, Werner, and Marx
1990; Synder et al., 1978), while increased social activity may worsen agitation. If the
level of care provided is not appropriate to the patient's needs, then behavioral
dyscontrol may increase. Thus awareness and modification of these conditions according to the needs of each patient can significantly alter the presence of the distressing behaviors.

Mrs. L. is a 68-year-old African American woman with a history of vascular dementia, hypertension, and diabetes mellitus who lives in a nursing
home, as her family is unable to provide the intensive care she requires. At
the time of her placement, she was unable to perform any of her activities of
daily living. Over the past few days, the staff noted that the patient was beginning to behave differently. Whereas she usually isolates herself from others
and spends most of her time watching television, Mrs. L. recently started
screaming uncontrollably at times and walking aimlessly around the unit.

In responding to this abrupt change in the patient's behavior, the staff's
primary concern was to ensure that no new medical problem was contributing to her symptoms. The staff measured her blood pressure, pulse,
temperature, respiratory rate, oxygenation, and blood glucose—everything
was stable and within normal limits. No one noted a recent cough, fever, or
changes in the patient's urinary or bowel habits. She was taking all her medications, and no medications had been changed within the past few
months. She was eating and sleeping well. As far as the staff could tell, she
was not in any pain. None of the patient's usual caregivers at the nursing
home had changed, and her physical environment had been stable as well.
On further exploration, one of the nurses noted that the patient's daughter,
who usually visits her every day, had not visited her in the prior few days.
The next morning, one of the staff called the patient's daughter, who stated
that she had been very busy but planned to come to the nursing home later
that day. Throughout the day, the patient remained agitated; however, after
her daughter visited, the patient's behavior returned to normal.

The above vignette describes a systematic approach for addressing this patient's
behavior. Initially, the staff evaluated for treatable patient determinants of behavioral
dyscontrol, such as a medical problem, changes in medications, or unmet needs.
After determining that the patient's medical and physiological needs had been met
and that no changes to the patient's care regimen had been made, the staff was able

to evaluate caregiver determinants. As stated above, the caregivers involved in this patient's care were trained professionals who had a history of providing good care. However, environmental determinants of the patient's behavior had changed. Although no recent staff changes had occurred, the patient's daughter had stopped visiting her. Soon after, the patient's level of social interaction had decreased and she had become more agitated. Once the patient's environment returned to "normal," her agitation resolved.

PHARMACOTHERAPEUTIC OPTIONS

Although assessing and addressing treatable patient, caregiver, and environmental determinants will minimize behavioral problems, at times these efforts are not sufficient, and medications become necessary. Adding medications to a patient's care regimen involves careful consideration of the patient's medical condition and the degree to which his or her behavior is disruptive or dangerous (American Psychiatric Association, 1997). The degree to which the safety and the quality of life of the patient and those around him or her are affected helps determine the need for medications. If the patient's behavior is not significantly distressing or potentially harmful, then no changes to the medication regimen may be necessary, and distraction or redirection may suffice (American Psychiatric Association, 1997). For example, if a patient occasionally wanders aimlessly around the house or nursing unit, then treatment with medication is unnecessary, as this behavior is neither harmful nor very disruptive. If, however, the quality of life or well-being of the patient or those in his or her environment is compromised, then pharmacological therapy may be called for. For example, if a patient starts hitting the caregiver while he or she is trying to bathe or dress the patient, then giving a small amount of medication to help control this aggression is helpful. By treating disruptive and dangerous behaviors, the caregiver is able to maintain his or her own safety while appropriately caring for the patient. When used judiciously, medication helps protect the caregiver's quality of life by making it safer and easier to provide care. Some caregivers are reluctant to use medications because they view them as stigmatizing or selfish (i.e., "the easy way out"). Another perspective is to view the use of medications as either an augmentation strategy or the next step in treatment. It may be helpful to counsel the caregiver that dementia and its consequences are similar to other chronic medical illnesses, such as diabetes, which often require medication for better control of symptoms (see figure 9.1).

Persons with dementia often have comorbid medical conditions, such as liver failure or renal impairment, which can alter the metabolism and excretion of sub-

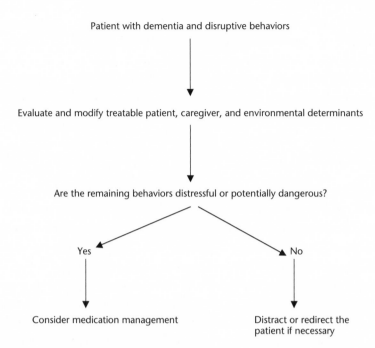

Patient with dementia and disruptive behaviors

Evaluate and modify treatable patient, caregiver, and environmental determinants

Are the remaining behaviors distressful or potentially dangerous?

Yes

No

Consider medication management

Distract or redirect the patient if necessary

Figure 9.1 Decision Tree.

stances present. As polypharmacy is common in elderly persons with dementia, the addition of a medication to a patient's regimen requires considerable thoughtfulness regarding dosages used and potential interactions with other medications. Depending on the medication added and the patient's medical condition, higher or lower doses may be necessary to produce the desired effect without causing significant side effects or toxicity. Similarly, the addition of a medication may alter blood levels of other medications, rendering those medications ineffective or potentially lethal. Therefore, medication is often considered a treatment of "last resort." Prescribing smaller starting doses and increasing dosages at smaller increments over longer intervals help to minimize problems and potential harm.

Medications prescribed for the treatment of disruptive, impulsive, and/or dangerous behaviors in persons with dementia are often chosen from three general classes of medications: antipsychotics, antidepressants, and anticonvulsants. When choosing the appropriate medication for a patient, the clinician must take into account multiple factors. As stated earlier, the patient's medical condition and medication regimen significantly influence this choice. The medication's side effect profile and the type of behavior requiring treatment also guide this decision (American Psychiatric Association, 1997). For example, if a patient has auditory or visual hallucinations and his or her agitation is due to these hallucinations, then starting an antipsychotic medication would be appropriate. If, however, the patient's agitation stems from an underlying depression, then starting an antidepressant medication would be more reasonable. There is no standard medication that is recommended for all patients; rather, the choice hinges on the specific needs of the individual receiving treatment (see table 9.2).

Antipsychotics

Antipsychotic medications are well documented as modestly effective treatments for disturbing behaviors in persons with dementia (Lawlor, 2002; Lee et al., 2004; Snowden, Sato, and Roy-Burne, 2003). Approximately 20 percent of patients have delusions and 15 percent of patients have hallucinations (Lyketsos et al., 2000). By affecting dopamine and serotonin receptors in the brain, antipsychotic medications reduce or eliminate these symptoms. Not uncommonly, persons with dementia develop the paranoid delusion that their caregivers are trying to hurt them. As a result, patients act aggressively toward the caregivers, possibly causing injury to themselves and/or the caregivers. In addition, patients' perceptions of reality can be altered significantly by auditory or visual hallucinations. These hallucinations distress the patient as well as the caregiver and may contribute to patient agitation, aggression, and insomnia. Persons with dementia often become suspicious of others in their environment and accuse them of stealing personal belongings. Both the patients and those accused can become agitated or aggressive. By treating these symptoms, antipsychotics minimize disruptive behaviors in persons with dementia and help maintain safety for all.

As with any medication, the risks and benefits associated with antipsychotic use must be weighed before initiating treatment. Persons with dementia are particularly sensitive to medication side effects. In addition to causing sedation, antipsychotic medications can lower a patient's seizure threshold, cause a decrease in blood pres-

TABLE 9.2
Medications

Antipsychotics	Antidepressants	Anticonvulsants	Acetylcholinesterase Inhibitors
Quetiapine	SSRIs	Gabapentin	Galantamine
Aripiprazole	Mirtazapine	Carbamazepine	Donepezil
Ziprasidone	Trazodone	Valproic acid	Tacrine
Olanzapine	Venlafaxine		Rivastigmine
Risperidone	Buproprion		
Haloperidol	Duloxetine		

sure when rising from a seated or lying position, and produce potentially dangerous changes in heart rhythms. Seizures can cause falls, and changes in heart rhythm and blood pressure can contribute to dizziness and confusion. Not surprisingly, an increased risk of hip fractures, often caused by falls, is associated with antipsychotic use (Ray et al., 1987). The use of antipsychotic medications in the elderly can result in changes in the lipid, blood glucose, and weight profile of these patients, setting them up to be at risk for what is popularly know as the "metabolic syndrome." These medications should therefore be used with care because of the increased cardiovascular and cerebrovascular risks. Lastly, older adults on typical antipsychotics are at increased risk for tardive dyskinesia—abnormal face, trunk, and extremity movements—which may be irreversible. The newer antipsychotic medications, such as risperidone, olanzapine, quetiapine, ziprasidone, and aripiprazole, appear to be at least as effective as older antipsychotics such as haloperidol and thorazine and appear to be less likely to cause side effects (Kindermann et al., 2002). Although studies support the effectiveness of risperidone (Katz et al., 1999) and olanzapine (Clark et al., 2001; Street et al., 2000) in decreasing disruptive behaviors in persons with dementia, randomized controlled trials testing the use of quetiapine and ziprasidone in this population are currently lacking.

Antidepressants

Depression and anxiety (Lyketsos et al., 2000) each affect approximately 20 percent of persons with dementia and can contribute to or cause considerable agitation, aggression, and insomnia. While insomnia is a common symptom of depression and anxiety (regardless of age or health), agitation and aggression may be more common in persons with dementia who have depression than in other populations. As dementia progresses and patients' abilities to communicate verbally decrease, they begin expressing their anxiety and depression through behaviors, such as agitation and aggression. The most appropriate course of action in these situations is to treat the underlying anxiety and/or depression.

The medications often chosen to treat persons with depression and/or anxiety are selective serotonin reuptake inhibitors (SSRIs). This class of antidepressants includes the following medications: fluoxetine, paroxetine, citalopram, and sertraline. These medications work by altering serotonin levels in the brain and receptor responses. Although all appear to have equal efficacy for treating depression in the general population (Kaplan and Sadock, 1998), their side effect profiles and potential interactions with other medications vary. For example, fluoxetine often activates patients, whereas paroxetine frequently causes sedation. Citalopram carries the advantage of interacting least with other medications compared to the other SSRIs, while fluoxetine and paroxetine can inhibit the metabolism of acetylcholinesterase inhibitors.

Although SSRIs are considered a first-line treatment for anxiety and depression in the general population, few studies have evaluated their efficacy in persons with dementia, and they have yielded mixed results (Bains, Birks, and Dening, 2004; Lyketsos and Lee, 2004; Magai et al., 2000; Trappler and Cohen 1998; Oslin et al., 2000; Rosen et al., 2000). This is possibly because of their relatively recent introduction to the market, the variability in study criteria and the course of depressive symptoms, concomitant treatments provided during the study, and placebo response (Lyketsos and Lee, 2004). Nortriptyline, an older antidepressant which belongs to the tricyclic antidepressant category, has been shown to significantly decrease depressive symptoms in persons with dementia (Katz et al., 1990; Streim et al., 2000). Tricyclic antidepressants work by affecting the levels of multiple neurochemicals thought to be involved in depression, such as dopamine, norepinephrine, and serotonin. Their use, however, is limited, due to their side effect profiles and potential to be lethal in overdose. Side effects of tricyclic antidepressants include blurred vision, dry mouth, constipation, urinary retention, irregular heart rhythms, and at times, confusion (Marangell et al., 2002). Therefore, SSRIs are chosen more frequently, as their side effect profile is generally less problematic in these patients and they are not lethal in overdose. Side effects associated with SSRI use include headache, nausea, weight loss, insomnia, diarrhea, sexual dysfunction, and increased sweating (Marangell et al., 2002; Schatzberg and Nemeroff, 2001). Although most of these side effects abate with time, patients may initially feel worse and become more agitated before they feel better. Occasionally, patients develop low serum sodium (hyponatremia), which can cause changes in mental status and behavior.

If the patient remains agitated or worsens despite weeks of treatment, then switching to a different antidepressant within the same class or to an antidepressant in a different class, such as venlafaxine, duloxetine, or buproprion, might be warranted, after ruling out or addressing the possible medical causes that may be contributing to increased agitation. Venlafaxine works by affecting serotonin and norepinephrine but carries a risk of causing high blood pressure, and it is less well tolerated in frail elderly patients (Oslin et al., 2003). Buproprion can cause seizures (Marangell et al., 2002; Schatzberg and Nemeroff, 2001). Since duloxetine was approved for treatment of depression in the general population in 2004, clinical experience with this medication is extremely limited. Treatment with any medication carries some risk. These risks must be weighed carefully against the benefits before initiating treatment.

For some patients, doctors may choose to take advantage of a medication's side effect profile to tailor treatment to the specific needs of that patient. Mirtazapine, an antidepressant that affects serotonergic and noradrenergic receptors, causes sedation and increased appetite at low doses, rendering it a good medication for persons with dementia who are not eating or sleeping well. It can be used either alone or in combination with other antidepressants to enhance treatment. Another benefit of using mirtazapine is that it has relatively few drug interactions; one disadvantage is that a few patients may develop low white blood cell counts, which will decrease their ability to fight infection (Marangell et al., 2002; Schatzberg and Nemeroff, 2001).

Another antidepressant that is helpful for persons with dementia is trazodone. Trazodone functions as a weak SSRI and directly affects serotonergic receptors. This medication is rarely used alone, as effective antidepressant doses are too sedating; instead, it is often used as an adjunct to other antidepressants. In addition to enhancing treatment, it causes sedation and is therefore helpful for insomnia (Marangell et al., 2002; Schatzberg and Nemeroff, 2001). Avoiding benzodiazepines in the treatment of anxiety and insomnia is wise, as these medications are addictive, may cause a paradoxical agitation in persons with dementia, and have depressive effects.

Anticonvulsants

Although their mechanisms of action are not well understood, anticonvulsants, such as carbamazepine and valproic acid, have been used as treatments for agitation, aggression, and disinhibition in persons with dementia. However, studies measuring the efficacy of these agents have yielded conflicting results (Trehan 1998). Potential side effects of both medications include liver toxicity and changes in blood cell counts. More specifically, the potential side effects of carbamazepine include nausea, dizziness, difficulty with walking, bone marrow suppression, hyponatremia, and a life-threatening rash (Marangell et al., 2002; Schatzberg and Nemeroff 2001). The potential side effects of valproic acid include difficulty with blood clotting, hair loss, nausea, weight gain, tremor, sedation, and rarely, inflammation of the pancreas (Marangell et al., 2002; Schatzberg and Nemeroff 2001). These medications also have multiple interactions with other medications. Whereas carbamazepine increases the metabolism of other medications, valproic acid decreases their metabolism (Schatzberg and Nemeroff, 2001). Therefore, extreme caution is necessary when using these medications. Medication levels, liver function studies, and complete blood counts should be monitored throughout treatment.

Interestingly, another anticonvulsant, gabapentin, has recently been reported as a possible alternative treatment for behavioral and psychological disturbances in persons with dementia (Miller, 2001). Compared to valproic acid and carbamazepine, its side effect profile is more favorable, and no laboratory monitoring is necessary. Additional studies are needed, however, to evaluate this medication's efficacy for treatment of behavioral disturbances in persons with dementia.

Acetylcholinesterase Inhibitors

In addition to improving cognitive function and delaying cognitive decline in persons with mild to moderate dementia, acetylcholinesterase inhibitors may also help improve behavioral disturbances (Kindermann et al., 2002). The most well-known acetylcholinesterase inhibitors are tacrine, donepezil, rivastigmine, and galantamine. Increasing evidence suggests that these agents have modest and clinically important effects on behavior, with a concomitant decrease in reported caregiver distress (Cummings et al., 2004). However, there have been no large randomized controlled trials, which randomize patients based on the presence of behavioral disturbances. Therefore, there is inconclusive evidence on the effects of these medications on psychiatric symptoms (Warner, Butler, and Arya, 2004).

Mr. Q. is a 74-year-old Caucasian man with a history of Alzheimer dementia, hypertension, and benign prostatic hypertrophy who is living at home with his 65-year-old wife, his primary caregiver. The patient has a history of becoming agitated occasionally in the evenings but is calmed easily with redirection. Last evening, when the patient's wife returned home from her support group, her son informed her that the patient had become more agitated than usual. Whereas his usual episodes of agitation consisted of pacing around the house, the patient had started yelling and was becoming physically aggressive. His wife and son, who are well educated and trained to care for the patient, were unable to calm him with redirection. Eventually, they had to restrain him for his safety as well as their own.

The next morning, Mr. Q. was calmer. His wife and son took him to his family physician. The wife explained to the doctor that no changes in the patient's care routine, physical environment, or medications had been made. She noted, however, that over the past few weeks the patient had begun eating less, sleeping less, and interacting less. His energy had been low as well. After a thorough medical work-up was completed, including a physical exam, laboratory studies, and imaging studies, the doctor concluded that the patient was well medically. On reviewing his record more closely, the physician noted that the patient had experienced a depressive episode in his twenties that had been treated with medication. She discussed with the family the possibility that the patient's increased agitation and aggression were due to depression. They decided to start an antidepressant and to give a low dose of an antipsychotic as needed for periods of increased agitation or aggression. The wife was advised to note behavior patterns before these episodes so she could try to give the antipsychotic before the behavior became severe or dangerous. Within weeks, the patient's increased agitation and aggression resolved. The antipsychotic was discontinued, but the antidepressant was maintained.

This vignette highlights the importance of a systematic, pragmatic approach to patient management whereby caregiver skill is maximized. The wife had been educated about dementia and was actively involved in support groups to preserve her own mental health. Although neither the patient's caregivers nor the environment had changed, the patient's medical condition had. The diagnosis of depression was made only after the completion of a thorough medical work-up assessing whether other conditions such as infections or electrolyte imbalances were contributing to his behavior. Other determinants to consider include medication changes and unmet physiological needs. Once the diagnosis of depression was made, the appropriate treatment was started and the patient's disruptive and dangerous behaviors resolved.

The above vignette underscores the importance of looking beyond presenting symptoms in order to identify and treat the patient's underlying condition. If the patient's symptoms had been treated with an antipsychotic only, then although his agitation and aggression might have resolved, his depression would have continued. By considering multiple patient, caregiver, and environmental determinants, his caregivers were able to identify the primary cause of his symptoms and provide appropriate care.

IMPLICATIONS FOR CLINICAL PRACTICE

If a person with dementia starts exhibiting dangerous or disruptive behaviors, the clinician should complete a thorough evaluation of the potentially treatable patient, caregiver, and environmental determinants that could be contributing to these behaviors.

If potentially treatable determinants are identified, they should be addressed.

If the behaviors pose a threat to the patient or others, then medication may be necessary.

The medications chosen are determined by the source and nature of the behavior. If the patient is hallucinating or having delusions, then an antipsychotic might be helpful. If the patient is agitated due to depression or anxiety, then starting an antidepressant should be considered. If antipsychotics or antidepressants are contraindicated in the patient, other medications, such as mood stabilizers, acetylcholinesterase inhibitors, or anxiolytics such as buspirone, may be helpful for controlling disruptive or dangerous behaviors.

CONCLUSION

A multidimensional approach is crucial for assessing and addressing behavioral problems in persons with dementia. By considering patient, caregiver, and environmental contributions to a patient's behavior, the caregiver is more likely to identify and treat the cause of the disruptive behaviors and less likely to focus only on the symptoms. The caregiver is also able to tailor treatment to an individual patient's needs and thereby improve the quality of care provided. With time, the caregiver will become familiar with the meanings of a patient's behavioral patterns and will likely be able to address the causes of certain behaviors before these behaviors become disruptive or dangerous. If modifying patient, caregiver, and environmental determinants is not sufficient to maintain safety and quality of life for the patient and those around him or her, then medications may become necessary. Adding even small doses of medication to a patient's treatment regimen can significantly improve the quality of life of both the patient and the caregiver by making it easier for the caretaker to provide care in a safe environment. The patient's medical condition, the medication side effect profile, and the type of behavior needing treatment will help determine which medication is chosen. Although these medications can be helpful, they can also be harmful. As dementia is a progressive illness, the level of care and types of treatment necessary will most likely change with time. Intermittent reevaluations of the patient's condition are necessary in order for caregivers to continue to provide the most appropriate treatment and best quality of care possible.

REFERENCES

Algase, D. L., Beck, C., Kolanowski, A., Whall, A., Berent, S., Richards, K., and Beattie, E. 1996. Need-driven dementia-compromised behavior: An alternative view of disruptive behavior. *American Journal of Alzheimer's Disease* 11(6):10–19.

American Geriatric Society (AGS) and American Association for Geriatric Psychiatry (AAGP). 2003. The American Geriatric Society and American Association for Geriatric Psychiatry recommendations for policies in support of quality mental health care in U.S. nursing homes. *Journal of the American Geriatric Society* 51(9):1299–1304.

American Psychiatric Association (APA). 1997. Practice guidelines for the treatment of patients with Alzheimer's disease and other dementias of late life. www.psych.org/psych_pract/treatg/pg/pg_dementia_32701.cfm. Accessed 1/4/2003.

Bains, J., Birks, J. S., and Dening T. R. 2004. Antidepressants for treating depression in dementia (Cochrane Review). *The Cochrane Library,* Issue 4. UK: John Wiley & Sons (online abstract only).

Clark, W. S., Street, J. S., Feldman, P. D., and Breier, A. 2001. The effects of olanzapine in reducing the emergence of psychosis among nursing home patients with Alzheimer's disease. *Journal of Clinical Psychiatry* 62:34–40.

Cohen-Mansfield, J., Werner, P., and Marx, M. S. 1990. Screaming in nursing home residents. *Journal of the American Geriatrics Society* 38:785–92.

Cummings, J. L., Schneider, L., Tariot, P. N., Kershaw, P. R., and Yuan, W. 2004. Reduction of behavioral disturbances and caregiver distress by galantamine in patients with Alzheimer's disease. *American Journal of Psychiatry* 161(3):532–38.

Doody, R. S., Stevens, J. C., Beck, C., Dubinsky R. M., Kaye, J. A., Gwyther, L., Mohs, R. C., Thal, L. J., Whitehouse, P. J, DeKosky, S. T., and Cummings, J. L. 2001. Practice parameter: Management of dementia (an evidence-based review). Report of the quality standards subcommittee of the American Academy of Neurology. *Neurology* 56(9):1154–66.

Gerdner, L. A. 2000. Effects of individualized versus classical "relaxation" music on the frequency of agitation in elderly persons with Alzheimer's disease and related disorders. Abstract. *International Psychogeriatrics* 12:49–65.

Kaplan, H. I., and Sadock, B. J. 1998. Delirium, dementia, amnestic and other cognitive disorders and mental disorders due to general medical condition. In *Kaplan and Sadock's synopsis of psychiatry: Behavioral sciences/clinical psychiatry,* ed. R. Cancro (chap. 10). Baltimore: Lippincott Williams & Wilkins.

Katz, I. R., Jeste, D. V., Mintzer, J. E., Clyde, C., Napolitano, J., and Brecher, M. 1999. Comparison of risperidone and placebo for psychosis and behavioral disturbances associated with dementia: A randomized, double blind trial. *Journal of Clinical Psychiatry* 60:107–15.

Katz, I. R., Simpson, G. M., Curlik, S. M., Parmelee, P. A., and Muhly, C. 1990. Pharmacologic treatment of major depression for elderly patients in residential settings. *Journal of Clinical Psychiatry* 51(Suppl.):41–47.

Kindermann, S. S., Dolder, C. R., Bailey, A., Katz, I. R., and Jeste, D. V. 2002. Pharmacological treatment of psychosis and agitation in elderly patients with dementia. *Drugs and Aging* 19(4):257–76.

Kunik, M. E., Lees, E., Snow, A. L., Cody, M., Rapp, C. J., Molinari, V. A., and Beck, C. K. 2003a. Disruptive behavior in dementia: A qualitative study to promote understanding and improve treatment. *Alzheimer's Care Quarterly* 4(2):129–40.

Kunik, M. E., Martinez, M., Snow, A. L., Beck, C. K., Cody, M., Rapp, C. G., Molinari, V. A., Orengo, C. A., and Hamilton, J. D. 2003b. Determinants of behavioral symptoms in dementia patients. *Clinical Gerontologist* 26 (3/4):83–89.

Lawlor, B. 2002. Managing behavioural and psychological symptoms in dementia. *British Journal of Psychiatry* 181:463–65.

Lee, P. E., Gill, S. S., Freedman, M., Bronskill, S. E., Hillmer, M. P., and Rochon, P. A. 2004. Atypical antipsychotic drugs in the treatment of behavioral and psychological symptoms of dementia: Systematic review. *British Medical Journal* 329:75–78.

Lehman, L. S., McCormick, R. A., and Kizer, K. W. 1999. A survey of assaultive behavior in Veterans Health Administration facilities. *Psychiatric Services* 50(3):384–89.

Lyketsos, C. G., and Lee, H. B. 2004. Diagnosis and treatment of depression in Alzheimer's disease. *Dementia and Geriatric Cognitive Disorders* 17:55–64.

Lyketsos, C. G., Stenberg, M., Tschanz, J. T., Norton, M. C., Steffens, D. C., and Breitner, J. C. S. 2000. Mental and behavioral disturbances in dementia: Findings from the Cache County Study on memory in aging. *American Journal of Psychiatry* 157:708–14.

Magai, C., Kennedy, G., Cohen, C. L., and Gomberg, D. 2000. A controlled clinical trial of sertraline in the treatment of depression in nursing home patients with late-stage Alzheimer's disease. *American Journal of Geriatric Psychiatry* 8:66–74.

Magliocco, J. S. 1996. Therapeutic activities for low-functioning older adults with dementia. In C. R. Kovach (Ed.), *Late stage dementia care: A basic guide.* Washington, D.C.: Taylor & Francis.

Marangell, L. B., Martinez, J. M. Silver, J. M., and Yudofsky, S. C. (Eds.). 2002. *Concise guide to psychopharmacology.* Washington, D.C.: American Psychiatric Publishing.

Miller, L. J. 2001. Gabapentin for treatment of behavioral and psychological symptoms of dementia. *Annals of Pharmacotherapy* 35(4):427–31.

Oslin, D. W., Streim, J. E., Katz, I. R., Smith, B. D., DiFilippo, S. D., Ten Have, T. R., and Cooper, T. 2000. Heuristic comparison of sertraline with nortriptyline for the treatment of depression in frail elderly patients. *American Journal of Geriatric Psychiatry* 8:141–49.

Oslin, D. W., Ten Have, T. R., Streim, J. E., Datto, C. J., Weintraub, D., DiFilippo, S., and Katz, I. R. 2003. Probing the safety of medications in the frail elderly: Evidence from randomized controlled trial of sertraline and venlafaxine in depressed nursing home patients. *Journal of Clinical Psychiatry* 64(8):875–82.

Rabins, P. V., Mace, N. L., and Lucas, M. J. 1982. The impact of dementia on the family. *JAMA* 248(3):333–35.

Ray, W. A., Griffin, M. R., Schaffner, W., Baugh, D. K., and Melton, L. J. 1987. Psychotropic drug use and the risk of hip fracture. *New England Journal of Medicine* 316(7):363–69.

Rosen, J., Mulsant, B. H., and Pollock, B. G. 2000. Sertraline in the treatment of minor depression in nursing home residents: A pilot study. *International Journal of Geriatric Psychiatry* 15:177–80.

Schatzberg, A. F., and Nemeroff, C. B. (Eds). 2001. *Essentials of clinical psychopharmacology.* Washington, D.C.: American Psychiatric Publishing.

Snowden, M., Sato, K., and Roy-Burne, P. 2003. Assessment and treatment of nursing home residents with depression and behavioral symptoms associated with dementia: A review of the literature. *Journal of the American Geriatrics Society* 51:1305–17.

Street, J. S., Clark, W. S., Gannon, K. S., Cummings, J. L., Bymaster, F. P., Tamura, R. N., Mitan, S. J., Kadam, D. L., Sanger, T. M., Feldman, P. D., Tollefson, G. D., and Breier, A. 2000. Olanzapine treatment of psychotic and behavioral symptoms in patients with Alzheimer disease in nursing care facilities: A double-blind, randomized, placebo-controlled trial. *Archives of General Psychiatry* 57:968–76.

Streim, J. E., Oslin, D. W., Katz, I. R., Smith, B. D., DiFilippo, S., Cooper, T. B., and Ten Have, T. 2000. Drug treatment of depression in frail elderly nursing home residents. *American Journal of Geriatric Psychiatry* 8:150–59.

Synder, L. H., Rupprecht, P., Pyreck, J., Brekhus, S., and Moss, T. 1978. Wandering. *Gerontologist* 18:272–80.

Tariot, P. N., and Blazina, L. 1994. The psychopathology of dementia. In *Handbook of dementing illnesses.* New York: Marcel Dekker.

Trappler, B., and Cohen, C. I. 1998. Use of SSRIs in "very old" depressed nursing home residents. *American Journal of Geriatric Psychiatry* 6:83–89.

Trehan, R. 1998. Pharmacological treatment of dementia and behavior disorders in dementia. In M. Kaplan and S. B. Hoffman (Eds.), *Behaviors in dementia: Best practices for successful management,* chap. 12. Baltimore: Health Professions Press.

Warner, J., Butler, R., and Arya, P. 2004. Dementia. In F. Godlee (Ed.), *Clinical evidence mental health.* London: British Medical Journal Publishing Group.

CHAPTER TEN

Care of the Caregiver

Individual and Family Interventions

SILVIA SÖRENSEN, PH.D.

DEBORAH KING, PH.D.

MARTIN PINQUART, DR.PHIL.HABIL.

Caregiving for older adults with physical ailments and/or dementia has important consequences for the psychological health and the general well-being of caregivers. Results from many studies on the effectiveness of interventions for caregivers (Knight, Lutzky, and Macofsky-Urban, 1993) suggest that interventions provide some relief for caregivers but that existing programs still require substantial refinement to enhance their effectiveness. One such refinement may be to include the caregiver's family members in the intervention, for education, consultation, or even therapy.

This chapter first summarizes aspects of caregiving that are most often associated with caregiver stress, with a focus on relational aspects of the caregiving situation. Subsequently we describe six types of intervention, including both individual and family-based interventions. Family-based approaches to caregiver intervention have been gaining popularity but have not been systematically evaluated. We discuss the effectiveness of both individual and family approaches and suggest situations in which each would be most effective.

THE EFFECTS OF CAREGIVING

The effect of the physical, psychological, social, and financial demands of providing care has been termed *caregiver stress* (Vitaliano et al., 1991) or *caregiver burden* (Zarit, Zarit, and Reever, 1982), which can be further differentiated into objective and subjective burden. Objective burden involves primary stressors, including having to manage the caregiver's physical, cognitive, and behavioral changes. It also includes secondary stressors, such as having less time for family, friends, work, vacations, hobbies, or leisure activities, and experiencing financial hardship (National Alliance for Caregiving and AARP, 1997). Subjective burden involves negative emotional reactions of the caregiver, such as worry, anxiety, anger, frustration, and fatigue, as well as grief and loss.

Four aspects of caregiving are most often associated with negative effects on caregivers: (1) characteristics of the care recipient, (2) characteristics of the care situation, (3) characteristics of the caregiver, and (4) relational effects of the care situation, such as changes in closeness between caregiver and care recipient, and family conflicts. Among *care recipient characteristics,* behavior problems cause the most stress and burden for the caregiver, followed by the care recipient's cognitive deficits and physical impairments. Also, people caring for elders with dementia are often more burdened than those caring for individuals with other illnesses (Pinquart and Sörensen, 2003a, 2003b). The *aspect of the care situation* that is most related to burden and depression is the amount of care provided. Caregivers who live with the care recipient are at higher risk for stress and burden than those who do not co-reside with the care recipient, because they tend to spend more hours providing care and take on more caregiving tasks. *Characteristics of the caregiver* also affect the stressfulness of caregiving: spousal caregivers are at greater risk for depression than adult child caregivers (Pinquart and Sörensen, 2003b), and minority caregivers may be less likely to experience burden and depression than majority culture caregivers (Roth et al., 2001; Lawton, Rajagopal, Brody, and Kleban, 1992). Finally, the *effect of caregiving on family relationships* may directly affect caregiver stress. For example, Kaplan and Boss (1999) demonstrate that "boundary ambiguity" (i.e., the confusion caused by the experience of caring for a family member with dementia who is physically present but mentally and emotionally absent) often emerges for dementia caregivers and is strongly related to depressive symptoms. Spousal caregivers often experience decreased companionship and changes in sexual intimacy (Wright, 1993), resulting in a sense of loss. Patterns of interaction in the larger family context may change in response to caregiving and may therefore also influence caregiver well-being. For example, Shields and colleagues (Shields, 1992; Speice, Shields, and Blieszner, 1998) suggest that disagreements about the focus of caregiving conversations may increase depressive symptoms in the caregiver.

Increased attention has been focused on caregiving as a source of positive affect. In addition to being stressed, caregivers also report feeling useful, appreciating closeness to the care recipient, and experiencing pride in their ability to handle crises (Farran et al., 1999; Kinney, Stephens, Franks, and Norris, 1995; Kramer, 1997).

INTERVENTIONS

Caregiver interventions can be divided into five major groups of individual intervention and three types of family intervention.

Individual Intervention

1. *Interventions Aimed at Reducing Objective Stress.* Interventions in this category are aimed at reducing the objective amount of care provided by caregivers. They include respite care and programs to enhance the competence of the care recipient. Respite care entails either in-home or site-specific supervision, assistance with activities of daily living, or skilled nursing care designed to give the caregiver time off. It does not imply that activities or programs are offered to the care recipient (e.g., Burdz, Easton, and Bond, 1988). Adult day care programs provide a combination of respite and activity programs. These interventions often engage the care recipient away from home and offer stimulating programs tailored toward the patient population's specific needs (e.g., Burdz et al., 1988; Zarit, Stephens, Townsend, and Greene, 1998). Interventions to improve care recipient competence include memory clinics for persons with dementia and activity therapy programs designed to improve affect and everyday competence (LoGiudice et al., 1999; Zarit et al., 1982).

2. *Psychoeducational Interventions.* These interventions are aimed at decreasing the caregiver's subjective and objective burden by providing education and skills training. They involve structured programs geared toward providing information about the care recipient's disease process and information about resources and services, as well as training caregivers to respond effectively to disease-related problems, such as memory and behavior problems in persons with dementia or depression and anger in persons with cancer (e.g., Gallagher-Thompson et al., 2000; Ostwald et al., 1999; Teri, Logsdon, Uomoto, and McCurry, 1997). Intervention formats usually include lectures, group discussions, and written materials and are always led by a trained leader. Support may be part of a psychoeducational group but is secondary to the educational content.

3. *Supportive Interventions.* These are aimed at reducing subjective burden by providing social support and helping caregivers create their own social support networks, for example through self-help groups. Professionals or peers may lead these interventions. They are typically unstructured, focused on building rapport among

participants, and aimed at creating a space in which to discuss problems, successes, and feelings regarding caregiving (e.g., Toseland, Rossiter, and Labrecque, 1989). Rather than using the principles of group therapy to explore deeper psychological conflicts or confront participants with problematic behaviors, support groups rely strongly on group members to provide mutual emotional support and to share concrete information on the nature of the care recipient's needs, how to manage problem behaviors, and where to obtain services. In contrast to psychoeducational programs, these interventions are rarely standardized or manualized. Education is not their primary focus, and descriptions typically provide little detail on the exact content or procedure (e.g., Gonyea and Silverstein, 1991).

4. *Psychotherapeutic Interventions.* Aimed at reducing personal response patterns and mental health problems that increase stress and reduce effective responses to care recipient's needs, this type of intervention involves a therapeutic relationship between the caregiver and a trained professional. Many psychotherapeutic interventions with caregivers follow a cognitive-behavioral approach, in which therapists may teach self-monitoring, challenge negative thoughts and assumptions that maintain the caregiver's problematic behavior, and help caregivers develop problem solving abilities by focusing on time management, overload, and management of emotional reactivity. Psychotherapeutic interventions also may help the caregiver reengage in pleasant activities and positive experiences (e.g., Goldberg and Wool, 1985; Lovett and Gallagher, 1988). Others focus on grief and mourning, as caregivers adjust to the gradual loss of a loved one due to cognitive or physical decline. Such interventions typically involve the facilitation of grief processes that have been blocked by the "ambiguous" nature of loss when a care recipient has a cognitive disorder that leaves him or her physically present but psychologically absent (Boss and Couden, 2002).

5. *Multiple-component Interventions.* These include various combinations of educational interventions, support, psychotherapy, and respite (e.g., Drummond et al., 1991; Hinchliffe et al., 1995; Montgomery and Borgatta, 1989). Some interventions also combine the traditional methods with family consultation or therapy (as described below). For example, Mittelman et al. (1995) combined individual family counseling sessions with weekly support group participation, and Montgomery and Borgatta (1989) offered a combination of educational services and respite care. Eisdorfer et al. (2003) also described an intervention in which both brief strategic family therapy intervention adapted from Szapocznik and Kurtines (1989) and a computer-telephone integrated communication system are used with family caregivers. Combining several methods of intervention is a promising approach, particularly if those methods are tailored to the needs of the caregiver.

Charlotte, a 46-year-old mother of three children, worked part time outside the home as a librarian and writing instructor at a local college. She sought help for recurrent headaches and feelings of depression in the context of numerous family stressors, including her father's death six months previously from lung cancer and her mother's insidious decline due to Alzheimer disease. It emerged during the first interview that Charlotte and her younger sister Susan had always had conflictual relationships with their mother, Mrs. P., whom Charlotte perceived as being "critical and selfish all her life." Before his death, her father had served as Mrs. P.'s emotional ally and caregiver, as well as being the buffer and conduit for communication between mother and daughters. His death triggered an exacerbation of Mrs. P's comorbid depression and put Charlotte in the position of being the primary source of support and caregiving for her mother, especially because Susan lived far away in another state.

The first three sessions of therapy with Charlotte involved grief work focused on the loss of her father. The therapist facilitated the mourning process by encouraging her to talk and write about her memories of her father, encouraging her to visit his gravesite, and suggesting she write some of her memories and feelings in a journal, which she would share from time to time with the therapist.

Charlotte had already contacted a local Alzheimer disease support group but found it difficult to attend because she was already overextended in terms of child rearing and caregiving responsibilities. Thus the next stage of therapy involved an examination of Charlotte's constant feelings of guilt and self-reproach and the fact that she was still waiting for her mother's approval. Recognizing that her mother's dementia and personality features precluded such approval, she began to mourn the fact that she would never get the warmth and support from her mother that she had longed for all her life. Although deeply painful, this process allowed her to set more realistic expectations for herself as a caregiver. She decided to hire someone to provide in-home assistance to her mother. She also negotiated that her sister would make quarterly visits so that Charlotte would have predictable periods of respite from caregiving responsibilities. Once these changes were made, Charlotte's headaches and depressed feelings decreased. After twelve sessions the therapy was terminated, with the understanding that Charlotte could "check back in" at any time she needed more assistance.

Family Intervention

Family intervention is the process of bringing two or more family members to-gether to address problems encountered in the caregiving process. We include un-der family interventions (1) *family psychoeducational approaches* aimed at more than one caregiver, (2) *family consultation* in crisis situations when family problem-solving that is normally intact has been stymied temporarily, as well as (3) *family therapy,* which focuses on modifying long-standing family interaction patterns.

1. *Family Psychoeducation.* The focus of family psychoeducation is on management of the illness per se, rather than on family relational patterns. It involves increasing family members' knowledge of the disease, including possible treatments and likely prognosis, as well as engaging family members in a skill-building process that teaches unique methods for managing illness-related behaviors and personal coping. Essen-tially, existing individual psychoeducational approaches are modified to enhance mas-tery and self-efficacy of more than one family caregiver. Family members are encour-aged to avoid generating additional stress for the caregiver, but rather to be available as a resource (Hepburn, Caron, and Mach, 1991; Mittelman et al., 1995).

2. *Family Consultation.* This form of intervention is applied when, despite solid, positive bonds of attachment and a history of effective problem solving, the family is overwhelmed by an unfamiliar care-related problem and thus is unable to cope (Shields, King, and Wynne, 1995). In these cases, families may need assistance in reor-ganizing roles and responsibilities (Hepburn et al., 1991). Family consultation may also subsume the family mediation approach, which is often indicated when there is dis-agreement between family members as to how to proceed with a caregiving plan (Beck and Sales, 2001) and when disagreement is not part of a long-standing pattern of conflictual family relationships. Conflict among family members about caregiving is-sues has been associated with caregiver depression (Semple, 1992). Thus consultation is highly indicated in families where conflict has arisen in the context of caregiving.

3. *Family Therapy.* In contrast to family psychoeducation and family consultation, family therapy brings two or more family members together to alter the nature of relational dynamics. It is conducted after family members explicitly agree to engage in a more rigorous process of change. Although caregiving itself may constitute a serious stressor and threat to family members' well-being, in some families the dif-ficulties experienced by family caregivers may be due to long-standing problematic family interaction patterns. For example, when the family has a history of negative, conflict-ridden communication, or is unable to communicate at all, a family therapist

who actively intervenes in negative interactions and models positive communication can contribute substantially to the well-being of the caregiver and care recipient. Family therapy is often helpful to caregivers because the degree of burden experienced by adult-child caregivers is related to the early quality of the "attachment" or affectional bond between parent and child (Cicirelli, 1993; Carpenter, 2001), as well as to later feelings of closeness and conflict in the adult intergenerational relationship (Townsend and Franks, 1995). Although many adult-child caregivers maintain positive affectional bonds with ill aging parents, some work suggests that it is hard to maintain strong bonds of attachment as parents become too frail to offer emotional closeness and security (Cicirelli, 1991). Whitbeck and colleagues show that the quality of the early parent-child relationship is often related to later development of filial concern and the likelihood that adult offspring will provide instrumental and emotional support to their ill parents (Whitbeck, Hoyt, and Huck; 1994). This research suggests a need for family interventions that support, strengthen, or rekindle bonds of attachment between adult offspring and aging parents.

Other family dynamics that may affect caregiving relationships have been suggested in the clinical literature. Two concepts, "mutuality" and "filial maturity," convey the adaptive, dynamic nature of successful relationships in the second half of life. Wynne (1984) defined *mutuality* as the ability to maintain long-term commitment to family relationships and to adjust them over time in the face of life cycle transitions. Mutuality is attained only when prior basic relational functions—positive bonds of attachment, clear and effective modes of communication, and shared problem solving—have developed as a relational foundation. Filial maturity is attained when adult offspring increase their caring support for aging parents, and aging parents become more able and willing to accept input and help from their children (Blenkner, 1965; King, Bonacci, and Wynne, 1991). Such transformation rests on the family's ability to renegotiate intergenerational power hierarchies and attain "adult-to-adult" relationships between parents and grown children (Qualls, 1999; Williamson, 1981).

Several models of family therapy with older adults have been developed (Hargrave and Hanna, 1997; Knight and McCallum, 1998; Mitrani and Czaja, 2000; Qualls, 2000), although few if any have been evaluated empirically. Shields, King, and Wynne (1995) suggested that family therapists must develop clinical interventions that are congruent with the family's stage of relational and life cycle development. Consistent with this approach, we propose several levels of intervention that reflect work at successively deeper strata of family relational functioning.

At the level of least complexity, families who exhibit solid attachment bonds, open communication, and good problem-solving skills do not require therapy but instead benefit from brief education and consultation, as noted above. Many caregiving families fall in this category.

At the next level are "overwhelmed" families, who have good relational abilities but are temporarily stymied by the complexity and emotional intensity of the caregiving process. These families need minimal help to fully accept the reality of the patient's prognosis, grieve this reality and "jump start" their natural abilities to communicate and collaboratively make decisions. Family consultation and mediation is often appropriate in this context, but in certain cases brief therapeutic interventions aimed at improving communication may also be necessary.

At more challenging levels of relational competence are the "closed" and/or "fixed" families, who struggle with long-standing relational difficulties. These families have the greatest need for a more intensive approach to treatment. "Closed" families characteristically avoid discussion of complex, emotionally charged issues; "fixed" families have rigid roles of authority (e.g., highly matriarchal or patriarchal families) and limited ability to collaboratively solve problems or make decisions. "Closed" families need help opening communication and expressing feelings in adaptive ways, whereas "fixed" families need help with role transitions and finding new patterns of decision making.

At the deepest level of relational difficulty are "wounded" families, who lack basic bonds of affection between family members, typically because of past or current substance abuse or mental illness. They have great difficulty coming together as a family and they exhibit a critical communication style, a pattern associated with increased risk of depressive relapse in older adults (Hinrichsen and Pollack, 1997). Practitioners set limits on their negative interactions and quickly establish guidelines for more positive forms of communication. Often this level of relational difficulty requires more intensive therapy to help family members engage in a process of reparation, forgiveness, and healing (Hargrave and Anderson, 1992; King, 2001).

In a family consultation model, during the first one or two sessions the therapist establishes which level of intervention the family needs and then proceeds to develop an intervention plan. The following case illustrates caregiving issues generated in the care of an older man with heart disease that are directly applicable to patients with dementia.

Mark R., a 38-year-old tool-and-die worker, was the primary family caregiver for his parents. His father, Mr. R., was a 72-year-old, retired general contractor with advanced coronary pulmonary disease who was oxygen dependent and could not walk more than 20 feet without going into respiratory distress. His mother, Mrs. R., was a 68-year-old woman with rheumatoid arthritis and obesity, who could ambulate only with difficulty and the help of a walker. Mark had three older siblings: John Jr. (48 years old), Elizabeth (46), and Peter (40). All of the other offspring were married and living with their own families. Mark, who was single, had moved into his parents' home one year previously in order to provide more assistance to them. Mr. R.'s visiting nurse requested family consultation because she thought that "family stress" was exacerbating Mr. R.'s pulmonary distress and contributing to a probable depression in Mrs. R.

The first interview included only Mark, his parents, and the nurse. The other siblings reported at the last minute that they were unable to make the meeting. All six sessions were held in the R. family home, a modest ranch house with pictures of children and grandchildren covering the living room walls. As the first meeting began, Mr. R., who was wearing an oxygen mask and soiled pajamas, stated that he did not understand the reason for the meeting because "we can handle things ourselves." Mrs. R. disagreed, saying that she was worried about how their care was affecting Mark, who had missed two days of work the previous week in order to take them to doctors' appointments. When Mr. R. started to argue with his wife, the therapist gently interrupted with a statement that it was normal for family members to have different perspectives, but that she would like to be able to hear everyone's point of view.

Mark stated that the most difficult aspect of the situation for him was not knowing how best to meet his parents' needs. He very much wanted to help, but got "mixed messages" about what was okay to do for them. His mother frequently asked him for assistance in caring for Mr. R, especially when he had bouts of respiratory distress. However, Mr. R. would get angry if Mark tried to administer medication or reposition him, insisting that he did not want to be a "burden" on his children. At this point in the discussion, Mr. R. interrupted and in angry tones stated: "The other three (children) only care about themselves anyway!" Mark grew visibly red in the face at this remark and shouted back at his father: "That's not true! You push them away!" at which point Mrs. R. began to cry softly.

The therapist quickly recognized the need to interrupt the negative interaction between Mark and his father before the situation became more explosive. Not knowing whether this level of conflict reflected a long-standing pattern of negative communication or simply a response to the acute stress of Mr. R.'s condition, the therapist redirected the conversation onto questions that would help her assess the history and quality of the family's relationships. She interrupted the two men and acknowledged that they both had very strong opinions that needed to be heard.

Recognizing the importance of Mr. R.'s patriarchal role in the family and the likelihood that they were all having difficulty adjusting to his decline, the therapist knew it would be important to validate his role of authority and give him some sense of control over the flow of the meetings. First, she acknowledged that as the "family leader" his input and opinions were essential to the family's well-being. She framed the family meetings as a potential vehicle for "helping you better help yourselves, now that so much has changed," and asked Mr. R. if she might continue to ask some questions in order to better understand the rest of the family.

Mr. R. grudgingly agreed that the meeting could continue. The therapist then asked about the other family members depicted in the photos on the wall. Mrs. R. "introduced" the absent family members by pointing to their pictures and telling fond stories about each of their children and grandchildren. She also noted how Mr. R. had helped many of them with carpentry tasks and making toys for his grandchildren before his illness. Mr. R. softened visibly during this discussion, repeatedly mentioning in sad tones how long it had been since he had seen his other children and their families.

From this discussion, the therapist concluded that there were generally strong bonds of attachment among most of the family members and that this was probably not a "wounded" family in need of extensive therapeutic interventions. However, they had a fixed patriarchal pattern of intergenerational authority that had not changed in a manner consistent with the seriousness of Mr. R.'s decline. They were unaccustomed to discussing difficult topics (see "closed" families above) and solving problems collaboratively, so they had not had any discussion as a family about the seriousness of Mr. R.'s illness. Mark and his siblings had not established adult-to-adult relationships with their father, and this prevented effective caregiving. The therapist recommended a time-limited course of family therapy, focused on opening the lines of communication and helping them reorganize patterns of authority and problem solving. She framed the recommendation in terms that would empower both Mark and Mr. R. to assume new, more appropriate roles of authority in the family.

Turning first to Mr. R., she stated that his children needed "a different kind of help" from him now that his illness was becoming more severe. Noting that this might be the hardest lesson he would ever teach them, she asked Mr. R. if he was ready to help them face the seriousness of his illness and "step up to the plate" to become helpers themselves. She then turned to Mark and asked if he wanted to follow in his father's footsteps as a family leader and decision maker. As Mark was nodding in the affirmative, she further reiterated how important it would be for Mark to continue to seek his father's guidance in this role.

After this discussion, the family agreed to five more family meetings focused on "helping the family transition to a new stage of family life." Mark agreed to fill his other siblings in on the content of the first meeting and to impress on them the importance of attending the next meetings. At least three of the four siblings attended each meeting, often bringing their spouses. During these sessions, the family discussed the nature of Mr. R.'s illness, his likely prognosis, and his advance directives. They arranged a schedule according to which each of the four siblings would help their parents with household chores, medical appointments, and medical procedures. The therapist's role was to model positive forms of communication, while setting limits on negative or critical exchanges as these arose. She also facilitated family grieving and collaborative decision making, often encouraging Mr. R. to "help" his children by letting them become more active in planning for his care and the care of his wife.

THE EFFECTIVENESS OF INTERVENTIONS WITH CAREGIVERS

The effectiveness of interventions must be evaluated from several perspectives. First, it is critical to look at a variety of *outcomes,* because some are more resistant to change than others (George and Gwyther, 1986). Recent meta-analytic research has indicated that interventions are most effective at increasing caregivers' ability and knowledge. Smaller effects are found for caregivers' subjective well-being, perceived uplifts, and burden, and for care recipient symptoms (Sörensen, Pinquart, and Duberstein, 2002). Depression is especially difficult to influence, particularly for dementia caregivers (Pinquart and Sörensen, 2002). Gitlin et al. (2003) report that treatment effects pooled across study sites in the Resources for Enhancing Alzheimer's Caregiver Health (REACH) study were nonsignificant for depression.

Important questions have been raised in recent qualitative reviews of caregiver interventions with regard to whether their effect is not only statistically but also clinically significant (Schulz et al., 2002). Most caregiver interventions do not report clinical diagnoses, but practical effectiveness can be estimated by how much symptom reduction the experimental group experiences, compared to the control group. However, for some measures, such as caregiver satisfaction or distress, the practical significance of even substantial improvement is unclear. Schulz et al. (2002) conclude that clinically significant effects of interventions have been most visible for reduction of caregiver depression and, to a lesser degree, of anxiety and hostility/anger. With regard to quality of life, improvements were found for specific aspects of quality of life, such as burden, perceived stress, and mood, but less so for general subjective well-being. A second approach to understanding the impact of interventions is to evaluate the size of the effect by comparing the levels of distress in caregivers without the intervention and noncaregivers without intervention. Table 10.1 shows this comparison: the difference in psychological distress between caregivers and noncaregivers, for example, is one-half a standard deviation unit. Interventions can reduce this difference by about one-quarter. More impressively, the lower self-efficacy that caregivers typically experience is ameliorated to 87 percent by caregiver interventions.

Interventions vary in their style of administration and content; therefore, certain types of intervention may have stronger effects on some outcomes than others. For example, psychoeducational interventions have a stronger effect on knowledge about the care recipient's condition but a weaker effect on burden. In a meta-analysis of 78 caregiver intervention studies, Sörensen et al. (2002) reported that psychoeducational and psychotherapeutic interventions showed consistent effects on all outcomes, whereas support groups, respite care, and care recipient competence training had more mixed effects. Teaching caregivers to understand the meaning of care recipient symptoms and to provide effective behavioral techniques for approaching these symptoms is definitely helpful. However, for some outcomes, individualized therapy that assists caregivers in reframing stressful events and developing personalized stress management approaches may be important in addressing depression and anxiety.

TABLE 10.1
Comparison of the Amount of Caregiver Distress Relative to the Size of Effects of Caregiver Interventions

	Differences Between Caregivers and Noncaregivers[a]	Effects of Caregiver Interventions[b]	
		Immediate	Long-term
Psychological distress	.55[c]	−.15	−.12
Depression	.58	−.14	−.22
Subjective well-being	−.40	.37	.08
Self-efficacy	−.54	.47	.56

[a]Data adapted from Pinquart and Sörensen, 2003a
[b]Data from Sörensen et al., 2002
[c]All effects are expressed in standard deviation units

In the Sörensen et al. (2002) meta-analysis, multicomponent interventions had the largest effects on ability/knowledge, well-being, and burden. A one-size-fits-all approach to assisting caregivers may not be useful because caregivers have vastly different needs (Knight et al., 1993). In that multicomponent interventions consist of several techniques and target multiple outcome domains, they are best able to address a variety of caregiver needs. Thompson and Gallagher-Thompson (1996) suggest that many intervention approaches complement each other and that, for example, support groups and psychoeducational classes can be particularly effective when offered sequentially. However, no systematic evaluation of specific combination or sequences of intervention has been conducted to date to determine best practices.

The effect of family interventions has not been systematically evaluated across studies. Large variability exists in results from individual studies evaluating family interventions. For example, Caston (1995) reports results from a family-based nursing intervention with African American caregivers, based on the Satir model of family therapy (Satir, Banmen, Gerber, and Gomori, 1991). Compared to a control group, caregiver burnout was reduced and self-esteem was significantly improved. However, Eisdorfer and colleagues report that family intervention alone actually *increased* depressive symptoms for some caregivers (Eisdorfer et al., 2003). Furthermore, these authors found ethnic differences in response to family interventions, such that Cuban American caregivers were more likely to experience a reduction in depression as a result of a family intervention than were white non-Hispanics.

There may be two reasons for these divergent findings. First, caregivers, especially those of persons with dementia, must tackle practical problems that are not always addressed in family therapy approaches. The white, non-Hispanic caregivers in the Eisdorfer study were most likely to benefit from family intervention when it was combined with a communication technology intervention (Czaja and Rubert, 2002), possibly because this technology facilitated more frequent family contact and interaction. Better family communication and interaction patterns may be important to reduce family-generated stressors. For example, combining family counseling with memory training or support group intervention brings about greater reductions in caregiver stress than applying individual or group interventions alone (Brodaty and Gresham, 1989; Whitlatch, Zarit, and von Eye, 1991). However, the studies to date suggest that, in addition to improving family interaction, it is crucial to provide help for coping with the specific care-related problems caregivers face. Many caregivers have relatively well-functioning family systems, but are simply overwhelmed.

The second reason why family interventions may show such divergent results is that different types of caregivers may have very different issues. As with any intervention, family therapy cannot fit every profile. For example, individuals with serious psychopathology may be better served if they receive individual mental health treatment or even medication (Thompson and Gallagher-Thompson, 1996). Family interventions, especially those directed at altering basic family dynamics, may be best suited in cases in which these communication patterns are closed, relationships are fixed, and affectional bonds are strong enough to support a process of change. For example, the caregiver in our second case example was coping with some caregiving-related stress, but most of his distress stemmed from the interactions with the care recipient. He was not so much overwhelmed by the care tasks as he was troubled by problematic patterns of family communication and decision making. Thus, respite or interventions aimed at improving caregiving-related abilities would have been much less effective than an approach aimed at changing the problematic family dynamics.

FACTORS THAT MODIFY THE EFFECTIVENESS
OF INTERVENTIONS

It is important to identify specific populations and situations in which intervention effectiveness is enhanced or reduced, including, for example, (1) characteristics of the caregiver (e.g., spouses or adult children), (2) characteristics of the care recipient (need for physical or dementia care), (3) characteristics of the intervention (individual or group, number of sessions), (4) the extent to which participants adhere to the intervention (regularity of attendance and dropout), (5) reliability and validity of the outcome measures. Additional moderators, which have not been addressed systematically, are (6) the quality of the caregiver–care recipient dyadic relationship and (7) broader family functioning in the care situation.

Characteristics of the Caregiver

Both Sörensen et al. (2002) and Gitlin et al. (2003) report that spouse caregivers benefit less from interventions than do adult children. Adult children probably derive greater advantages from caregiver interventions because they are often less prepared for the strains of caregiving than are spouses. Spouses are more likely to have already cared for their parents and have developed coping strategies or gathered information about community services and supports from their previous experience.

The crucial information that interventions provide is more novel to adult children and therefore more effective at reducing their burden. This may also explain why REACH interventions were more effective with caregivers with lower education (Gitlin et al., 2003). Moreover, adult children often have several additional social roles (e.g., nuclear family responsibilities and work), which may lead to either greater role strain or greater role enhancement (Reid and Hardy, 1999; Stephens, Franks, and Townsend, 1994), both of which may be less affected by present interventions. Further research is necessary to understand which factors are most responsible for spouses' smaller benefit from interventions, so that future interventions can take these factors into account.

Characteristics of the Care Recipient

Because many of the diseases and disabilities leading to the need for care are progressive in nature, the caregivers of older care recipients are likely to encounter more stressors and limitations in their activities (Coen, Swanwick, O'Boyle, and Coakley, 1997). They are thus more likely to benefit from an intervention that either frees up their time or provides them with emotional support. On the other hand, interventions with caregivers of persons with dementia are often less successful than those with other caregivers (Pinquart and Sörensen, 2002). Dementia caregivers cope with unpredictable stressors, such as problem behaviors and personality changes. As these may be more difficult to handle and less modifiable than the stressors common to pure physical care (Birkel and Jones, 1989), it may be more difficult to effect change through intervention with this population.

Characteristics of the Intervention

Regarding the intensity of interventions, there is some evidence that group interventions are less effective at improving caregiver burden and well-being than either individual or mixed interventions, that is, combinations of group and individual programs (Knight et al., 1993; Sörensen et al., 2002; Whitlatch, Zarit, and von Eye, 1991). Generally speaking, interventions that adapt the topics and methods of the intervention to individuals' specific caregiving concerns are most effective. For example, although on average support group interventions may not be as effective as individual-level therapy or psychoeducation, for isolated caregivers group-based approaches may be superior because they serve to increase caregivers' social network and enhance their opportunities to exchange ideas and experiences (Toseland,

Rossiter, and Labrecque, 1989). Combining individual with group interventions may incorporate the best of both worlds.

Caregivers benefit more from longer interventions, especially with regard to depression, possibly because of the supportive aspects of prolonged contact with a group or a professional. Care recipients experience fewer symptoms as a result of longer interventions because it takes more time for caregivers to learn, place their trust in, and subsequently implement new response patterns that can affect change in care recipients' behavior. Longer interventions also allow time for multiple approaches, which are more effective in changing care recipients' symptoms (Ostwald et al., 1999).

Adherence to the Intervention

One interesting finding from meta-analysis is that programs with higher dropout rates differ in their effectiveness on various outcomes. On the one hand, psychoeducational interventions involve fewer sessions and have a lower dropout rate. They are also very effective at increasing knowledge and abilities. On the other hand, interventions with high dropout rates tend to show smaller increases in knowledge but larger improvements on care recipient outcomes, caregiver burden, and depression. This may be due primarily to the highly motivated "stayers." Intervention "dose" may be directly related to reduction in depressive symptoms: In order to achieve a three-point reduction of depression scores, caregivers in the REACH study required an additional 3 hours and 22 minutes of behavioral intervention (Belle et al., 2003).

Reliability and Validity of Outcome Measures

For many practitioners, methodological issues are far less relevant than questions of content and format of the interventions. Nevertheless, if outcome measures are not valid or reliable, they can make an ineffective intervention look more effective. This wastes valuable resources and does not help the caregivers' well-being. In contrast, poorly chosen measures may make an effective intervention look ineffective. This can perpetuate the belief that interventions are ineffective and lead to funding cuts for interventionists and service providers. Therefore, careful choice of instruments to evaluate effectiveness is very important. Measures of satisfaction with an intervention have long been discredited as showing positive bias and not indicating whether material was learned or improvements in well-being were achieved. On the other hand, demonstrating an objective increase in knowledge about care recipients' conditions or a decrease in burden and depressive symptoms is likely to be highly useful in the evaluation of interventions.

IMPLICATIONS FOR CLINICAL PRACTICE

Consistent with the recommendations of the American Association for Geriatric Psychiatry and the American Medical Association, we believe it reflects optimal practice to implement interventions with family caregivers (American Association for Geriatric Psychiatry, 2004; American Medical Association, 2004). However, although caregiver outcomes can be improved to some degree, it is rarely possible to effect change in all areas of caregiver need at once. Based on this premise, we make the following recommendations:

1. *Decide what is the desired outcome.* Clinicians and practitioners must decide in advance whether specific targeted outcomes or whether general improvement of well-being is the goal of their intervention. Each of these goals may require a different set of intervention techniques, implementation strategies, and attention to different potential moderators. For example, if the goal is to reduce care recipient symptoms, psychoeducational group interventions may be more effective than individual approaches. On the other hand, if caregiver burden is the target outcome, psychoeducation, social support, respite care, or an individualized combination of these treatments with family consultation are recommended.

2. *Match the length of the intervention to the goal of the program.* It is important to pilot the effectiveness of an intervention that lasts only a short time. Interventions of seven to nine sessions should be adequate to increase ability / knowledge but may be too limited to improve depression. Psychotherapy, while costly, requires more sessions but may still be a preferred method to approach depression and anxiety in caregivers. It should be verified that caregivers actually apply newly acquired knowledge, for example, through booster sessions, involvement of additional family members, or telephone check-in.

3. *Follow-up measurements should extend at least 12 months.* Although a majority of the intervention effects persist after an average of seven months postintervention (Sörensen et al., 2002), it is not clear whether they have lasting effects. Because caregiving often lasts years, it is vital to ensure that the gains experienced by caregivers are not short-lived. Several interventionists build in booster sessions, by phone or by home visit, and ad hoc counseling sessions to assist caregivers in putting the skills and knowledge they gained into practice and maintaining coping strategies over time.

4. *Develop an outreach plan.* Interventions often do not reach the people who need them the most, in part because of the approaches taken, accessibility of interven-

tion sites, and cultural issues regarding the receipt of outside help. For example, minority groups may be less likely to avail themselves of interventions if they do not involve active outreach. A variety of barriers exist to minority involvement in interventions. Programs are often not community based and therefore are more difficult to access; interventionists often are from the majority culture and lack the skills to address particular cultural issues; university-based programs are often viewed with distrust. Dementia caregivers in particular are often underserved because they may be unable to attend sessions based outside their homes. They may lose motivation because they tend to benefit less than other caregivers (Sörensen et al., 2002). Therefore, practitioners need to consider closely the population they intend to work with and develop strategies to reduce barriers to participation and retention.

   5. Pay attention to issues surrounding family transitions. Families are most likely to evidence problematic patterns during periods of transition. Therefore, great attention should be directed to the family-wide stressors that are created by changes in caregiving patterns. This challenge presents a special opportunity for family therapists to intervene more broadly than with just the caregiver. However, to date caregiver interventions rarely target an entire family system, despite the fact that past "baggage" may prevent effective caregiving. A small number of studies have evaluated family interventions or combinations of individual and family interventions, but more research is needed to clarify who would most benefit from family approaches. Theory in this area suggests that family interventionists should first establish what level of difficulty the family is facing. The practitioner needs to explore whether the family (1) is simply in need of more education about how to cope with dementia-related behaviors and limitations, (2) is overwhelmed by the emotional intensity evoked by the disease or the complexity of the decisions that need to be made, (3) has deficits in relational competence or has closed family patterns that need to be addressed, or (4) is "wounded" and would benefit from a more long-term therapeutic treatment plan. Although family intervention by itself is often not sufficient to reduce caregiver burden and depression, adding family therapy to other intervention strategies may be particularly useful in situations in which long-standing problematic family communication patterns prevent effective problem solving.

   6. Accentuate the positive. Many interventions focus on reducing negative effects of caregiving but do not address increasing positive emotion and focusing on aspects of caregiving that increase subjective well-being. Theoretically, a distinction exists between positive and negative dimensions of emotional health (e.g., Bradburn, 1969; Diener and Emmons, 1984; Zautra and Reich, 1983). If emotional health is more than the absence of psychological distress, individuals may experience negative affect simultaneously with positive affect. Positive and negative affect emerge as two relatively independent dimensions of emotions when measured over longer periods (e.g., Bradburn, 1969; Watson and Tellegen, 1985). Thus, with regard to caregiving, many individuals may report burden and symptoms of depression while also experiencing adequate levels of psychological well-being such as positive affect and life-satisfaction (Chappell and Reid, 2002; Pinquart and Sörensen, in press). We recommend incorporating elements into an intervention that systematically assist in developing positive appraisal, finding meaning, and recognizing enjoyable aspects of caregiving.

7. Combine treatment approaches. Although the evidence base for the effectiveness of multiple-method intervention approaches is still somewhat inconsistent (Pinquart and Sörensen, in press), we do recommend combining several intervention types. To enhance caregiver knowledge initially, practitioners should always provide relevant information through psychoeducational approaches plus skills training in coping with disease-specific issues. Multiple-component approaches that combine individual or family counseling/psychoeducation, support groups, cognitive-behavioral interventions, and continuous follow-up increase the caregiver's ability to cope with care recipient behavior problems and are effective for alleviating burden and enhancing well-being (Sörensen, Pinquart, and Duberstein, 2002). In some studies, the effectiveness of these approaches has been demonstrated for reducing depression as well (e.g., Mittelman, Roth, Coon, and Haley, 2004; Schulz et al., 2003). Still, these findings need to be replicated more broadly. Because not all caregivers will respond to the same approaches, using combinations is more likely to reach a larger group of people. Including family consultation or mediation may be helpful, especially when multiple caregivers disagree on effective caregiving approaches or are unable to modify existing decision-making hierarchies. However, the evidence base is not as solid for these interventions. Since caregivers in poorly functioning families will likely be less responsive to standard interventions, combining single approaches that are known to reduce caregiver burden and depression with family consultation, which can improve overall family functioning, is promising.

CONCLUSION

Unfortunately, data on the effectiveness of interventions with dementia caregivers, especially for reducing depression, are still quite limited. More studies that systematically compare multimodal to single-approach interventions are needed. Belle et al. (2003; see also Czaja et al., 2003) suggested that analyzing the influence of specific intervention components may provide information that is inaccessible when entire interventions are compared to each other. For example, Belle et al.

(2003) found that targeting caregiver knowledge, skills, and affect is not significantly related to improvement in depression, whereas validating whether caregivers actually apply newly learned cognitive and behavioral strategies does significantly reduce depressive symptoms. Dementia caregivers and spousal caregivers have thus far benefited less from interventions than have caregivers of persons with other chronic diseases. It remains to be seen whether novel caregiver interventions, especially ones involving multiple approaches and family therapy, can be modified to be more effective. We recommend that clinicians participate in multisite research trials to answer this question.

REFERENCES

American Association for Geriatric Psychiatry. 2004, May 30. Family and caregivers counseling in dementia: Medical necessity. Health care professionals: Position statements. www.aagponline.org/prof/position_dementia.asp.

American Medical Association. 2004, May 30. Issues in family caregiving. www.ama-assn.org/ama/pub/category/5032.html.

Beck, C. J., and Sales, B. D. 2001. *Family mediation: Facts, myths, and future prospects.* Washington, D.C.: American Psychological Association.

Belle, S. H., Czaja, S. J., Schulz, R., Zhang, S., Burgio, L. D., Jones, R., Mendelsohn, A. B., and Ory, M. G. 2003. Using a new taxonomy to combine the uncombinable: Integrating results across diverse interventions. *Psychology and Aging* 18:396–405.

Birkel, R. C., and Jones, C. J. 1989. A comparison of the caregiving networks of dependent elderly individuals who are lucid and those who are demented. *Gerontologist* 29:114–19.

Blenkner, M. 1965. Social work and family in later life, with some thoughts on filial mortality. In E. Shanas and G. Streib (Eds.), *Social structure and the family: Generational relations* (pp. 46–59). Englewood Cliffs, N.J.: Prentice-Hall.

Boss, P., and Couden, B. 2002. Ambiguous loss from chronic physical illness: Clinical interventions with individuals, couples and families. *Journal of Clinical Psychology* 58:1351–60.

Bradburn, N. M. 1969. *The structure of psychological well-being.* Chicago, Ill.: Adline.

Brodaty, H., and Gresham, M. 1989. Effect of a training programme to reduce stress in carers of patients with dementia. *British Medical Journal* 299:1375–79.

Burdz, M. P., Easton, W. O., and Bond, J. B. 1988. Effect of respite care on dementia and nondementia patients and their caregivers. *Psychology and Aging* 3:38–42.

Carpenter, B. D. 2001. Attachment bonds between adult daughters and their older mothers: Associations with contemporary caregiving. *Journals of Gerontology: Psychological Sciences* 56B:P257–66.

Caston, C. 1995. Self-directed Skills nursing model: Decrease burnout in African-American caregivers. *Dissertation Abstracts International: Section B: The Sciences and Engineering* 55(8B): 3235.

Chappell, N. L., and Reid, C. 2002. Burden and well-being among caregivers: Examining the distinction. *Gerontologist* 42:772–78.

Cicirelli, V. G. 1991. Attachment theory in old age: Protection of the attached figure. In K. A. Pillemer and K. McCartney (Eds.), *Parent-child relations throughout life* (pp. 25–42). Hillsdale, N.J.: Erlbaum.

Cicirelli, V. G. 1993. Attachment and obligation as daughters' motives for caregiving behavior and subsequent effect on subjective burden. *Psychology and Aging* 8:144–55.

Coen, R. F., Swanwick, G. R., O'Boyle, C. A., and Coakley, D. 1997. Behaviour disturbance and other predictors of carer burden in Alzheimer's disease. *International Journal of Geriatric Psychiatry* 12:331–36.

Czaja, S. J., and Rubert, M. P. 2002. Telecommunications technology as an aid to family caregivers of persons with dementia. *Psychosomatic Medicine* 64:469–76.

Czaja, S. J., Schulz, R., Lee, C. C., and Belle, S. H. 2003. A methodology for describing and decomposing complex psychosocial and behavioral interventions. *Psychology and Aging* 18:385–95.

Diener, E., and Emmons, R. A. 1984. The independence of positive and negative affect. *Journal of Personality and Social Psychology* 47:1105–17.

Drummond, M. F., Mohide, E. A., Tew, M., Streiner, D. L., Pringle, D. M., and Gilbert, J. R. 1991. Economic evaluation of a support program for caregivers of demented elderly. *International Journal of Technology Assessment in Health Care* 7:209–19.

Eisdorfer, S. J., Czaja, D. A., Loewenstein, M. P., Rubert, S. A., Mitrani, V. B., and Szapocznik, J. 2003. The effect of a family therapy and technology-based intervention on caregiver depression. *Gerontologist* 43:521–31.

Farran, C. J., Miller, B. H., Kaufman, J. E., Donner, E., and Fogg, L. 1999. Finding meaning through caregiving: Development of an instrument for family caregivers of persons with Alzheimer's disease. *Journal of Clinical Psychology* 55:1107–25.

Gallagher-Thompson, D., Lovett, S., Rose, J., McKibbin, C., Coon, D., Futterman, A., et al. 2000. Impact of psychoeducational interventions on distressed family caregivers. *Journal of Clinical Geropsychology* 6:91–110.

George, L. K., and Gwyther, L. P. 1986. Caregiver well-being: A multidimensional examination of family caregivers of demented adults. *Gerontologist* 26:253–59.

Gitlin, L. N., Belle, S. H., Burgio, L. D., Czaja, S. J., Mahoney, D., Gallagher-Thompson, D., Burns, R., Hauck, W. W., Zhang, S., Schulz, R., and Ory, M. G. 2003. Effect of multicomponent interventions on caregiver burden and depression: The REACH multisite initiative at 6-month follow-up. *Psychology and Aging* 18:361–74.

Goldberg, R. J., and Wool, M. S. 1985. Psychotherapy for the spouses of lung cancer patients: Assessment of an intervention. *Psychotherapy and Psychosomatics* 141–50.

Gonyea, J. G., and Silverstein, N. M. 1991. The role of Alzheimer's disease support groups in families' utilization of community services. *Journal of Gerontological Social Work* 16:43–55.

Hargrave, T. D., and Anderson, W. T. 1992. *Finishing well: Ageing and reparation in the intergenerational family.* New York: Brunner/Mazel.

Hargrave, T. D., and Hanna, S. M. 1997. *The aging family: New visions in theory, practice and reality.* New York: Brunner/Mazel.

Hepburn, K., Caron, W., and Mach, J. R. 1991 Caregivers of persons with chronic illnesses or impairments: Strategies and interventions. In W. A. Myers (Ed.), *New techniques in the psychotherapy of older patients* (pp. 39–59). Washington, D.C.: American Psychiatric Press.

Hinchliffe, A. C., Hyman, I. L., Blizard, B., and Livingston, G. 1995. Behavioural complications of dementia: Can they be treated. *International Journal of Geriatric Psychiatry* 10:839–47.

Hinrichsen, G. A., and Pollack, S. 1997. Expressed emotion and the course of late-life depression. *Journal of Abnormal Psychology* 106:336–40.

Kaplan, L., and Boss, P. 1999. Depressive symptoms among spousal caregivers of institutionalized mates with Alzheimer's: Boundary ambiguity and mastery as predictors. *Family Process* 38:85–103.

King, D. A. 2001. The case of the "expendable elder": Family therapy with an older depressed man. In S. H. McDaniel, D. D. Lusterman, and B. Seaburn (Eds.), *A casebook for integrating family therapy* (pp. 157–68). Washington, D.C.: American Psychological Association.

King, D. A., Bonacci, D. D., and Wynne, L. C. 1991. Families of cognitively impaired elders: Helping children confront the filial crisis. *Clinical Gerontologist* 10:3–15.

Kinney, J. M., Stephens, M. A. P., Franks, M. M., and Norris, V. K. 1995. Stresses and satisfaction of family caregivers to older stroke patients. *Journal of Applied Gerontology* 14:3–21.

Knight, B. G., Lutzky, S. M., and Macofsky-Urban, F. 1993. A meta-analytic review of interventions for caregiver distress: Recommendations for future research. *Gerontologist* 33: 240–48.

Knight, B. G., and McCallum, T. J. 1998. Psychotherapy with older adult families: The contextual, cohort-based maturity/specific challenge model. In I. H. Nordhus, G. R. VandenBos, S. Berg, and P. Fromholt (Eds.), *Clinical Geropsychology* (pp. 313–28). Washington, D.C.: American Psychological Association.

Kramer, B. J. 1997. Gain in the caregiving experience: Where are we? What next? *Gerontologist* 37:218–32.

Lawton, M. P., Rajagopal, D., Brody, E., and Kleban, M. H. 1992. The dynamics of caregiving for a demented elder among black and white families. *Journal of Gerontology* 47: S156–64.

LoGiudice, D., Waltrowicz, W., Brown, K., Burrows, C., Ames, D., and Flicker, L. 1999. Do memory clinics improve the quality of life of carers? A randomized pilot trial. *International Journal of Geriatric Psychiatry* 14:626–32.

Lovett, S., and Gallagher, D. 1988. Psychoeducational interventions for family caregivers: Preliminary efficacy data. *Behavior Therapy* 19:321–30.

Mitrani, V. B., and Czaja, S. J. 2000. Family-based therapy for dementia caregivers: Clinical observations. *Aging and Mental Health* 4:200–209.

Mittelman, M. S., Ferris, S. H., Shulman, E., Steinberg, G., Ambinder, A., Mackell, J., and Cohen, J. 1995. A comprehensive support program: Effect on depression in spouse-caregivers of AD patients. *Gerontologist* 35:792–802.

Mittleman, M. S., Roth, D. C., Coon, D. W., and Haley, W. E. 2004. Sustained benefit of supportive intervention for depressive symptoms in caregivers of patients with Alzheimer's disease. *American Journal of Psychiatry* 161:850–56.

Montgomery, R. J., and Borgatta, E. F. 1989. The effects of alternative support strategies on family caregiving. *Gerontologist* 29:457–64.

National Alliance for Caregiving (NAC) and American Association of Retired Persons (AARP). 1997. Family caregiving in the U.S.: Findings from a national survey. Washington, D.C.: NAC.

Ostwald, S. K., Hepburn, K. W., Caron, W., Burns, T., and Mantell, R. 1999. Reducing caregiver burden: A randomized psychoeducational intervention for caregivers of persons with dementia. *Gerontologist* 39:299–309.

Pinquart, M., and Sörensen, S. 2002. Interventionseffekte auf Pflegende Dementer und andere informelle Helfer: Eine Meta-Analyse [Effects of interventions with caregivers for demented elderly and other frail older adults: A meta-analysis]. *Zeitschrift für Gerontopsychologie und-psychiatrie* 15:85–100.

Pinquart, M., and Sörensen, S. 2003a. Differences between caregivers and noncaregivers in psychological health and physical health: A meta-analysis. *Psychology and Aging* 18:250–67.

Pinquart, M., and Sörensen, S. 2003b. Associations of stressors and uplifts of caregiving with caregiver burden and depressive mood: A meta-analysis. *Journals of Gerontology: Psychological Sciences and Social Sciences* 58B:P112–28.

Pinquart, M., and Sörensen, S. 2004. Associations of caregiver stressors and uplifts with subjective well-being and depressive mood: A meta-analytic comparison. *Aging and Mental Health* 8:438–39.

Qualls, S. 1999. Realizing power in intergenerational families hierarchies: Family reorganization when older adults decline. In M. Duffy (Ed.), *Handbook of counseling and psychotherapy with older adults* (pp. 228–41). New York: John Wiley & Sons.

Qualls, S. 2000. Therapy with aging families: Rationale, opportunities and challenges. *Aging and Mental Health* 4:191–99.

Reid, J., and Hardy, M. 1999. Multiple roles and well-being among midlife women: Testing role strain and role enhancement theories. *Journals of Gerontology: Social Sciences* 54B: S329–38.

Roth, D. L., Haley, W. E., Owen, J. E., Clay, O. J., and Goode, K. T. 2001. Latent growth models of the longitudinal effects of dementia caregiving: A comparison of African American and white family caregivers. *Psychology and Aging* 16:427–36.

Satir, V., Banmen, J., Gerber, J., and Gomori, M. 1991. *The Satir model: Family therapy and beyond*. Palo Alto, Calif.: Science and Behavior Books.

Schulz, R., Burgio, L., Burns, R., Eisdorfer, C., Gallagher-Thompson, D., Gitlin, L. N., and Mahoney, D. F. 2003. Resources for Enhancing Alzheimer's Caregiver Health (REACH): Overview, site-specific outcomes, and future directions. *Gerontologist* 43:514–20.

Schulz, R., O'Brien, A., Czaja, S., Ory, M., Norris, R., Martire, L. M., Belle, S. H., Burgio, L., Gitlin, L., Coon, D., Burns, R., Gallagher-Thompson, D., and Stevens, A. 2002. Dementia caregiver intervention research: In search of clinical significance. *Gerontologist* 42:589–602.

Semple, S. J. 1992. Conflict in Alzheimer caregiving families: Its dimensions and consequences. *Gerontologist* 32:648–55.

Shields, C. G. 1992. Family interaction and caregivers of Alzheimer's disease patients: Correlates of depression. *Family Process* 31:19–33.

Shields, C. G., King, D. A., and Wynne, L. C. 1995. Interventions with later-life families. In Mikesell, D. D., Lusterman, D. D., and McDaniel, S. H. (Eds.), *Integrating family therapy: Handbook of family psychology and systems theory* (pp. 141–58). Washington, D.C.: American Psychological Association.

Sörensen, S., Pinquart, M., and Duberstein, P. 2002. How effective are interventions with caregivers? An updated meta-analysis. *Gerontologist* 42:356–72.

Speice, J., Shields, C. G., S. G., and Blieszner, R. 1998. The effects of family communication patterns during middle-phase Alzheimer's disease. *Families, Systems and Health* 16:233–48.

Stephens, M. A. P., Franks, M. A., and Townsend, A. L. 1994. Stress and rewards in women's multiple roles: The case of women in the middle. *Psychology and Aging* 9:45–52.

Szapocznik, J., and Kurtines, W. M. 1989. *Breakthroughs in family therapy with drug-abusing problem youth.* New York: Springer.

Teri, L., Logsdon, R. G., Uomoto, J., and McCurry, S. M. 1997. Behavioral treatment of depression in dementia patients: A controlled clinical trial. *Journal of Gerontology: Psychological Sciences* 52B:P159–66.

Thompson, L. W., and Gallagher-Thompson, D. 1996. Practical issues related to maintenance of mental health and positive well-being in family caregivers. In L. L. Carstensen, B. A. Edelstein, and L. Dornbrand (Eds.), *The practical handbook of clinical gerontology* (pp. 129–50). Thousand Oaks, Calif.: Sage.

Toseland, R. W., Rossiter, C. M., and Labrecque, M. S. 1989. The effectiveness of peer-led and professionally led groups to support family caregivers. *Gerontologist* 29:465–71.

Townsend, A. L., and Franks, M. M. 1995. Binding ties: Closeness and conflict in adult children's caregiving relationships. *Psychology and Aging* 10:343–51.

Vitaliano, P. P., Russo, J., Young, H. M., Becker, J., and Maiuro, R. D. 1991. The screen for caregiver burden. *Gerontologist* 31:76–83.

Watson, D., and Tellegen, A. 1985. Toward a consensual structure of mood. *Psychological Bulletin* 98:219–35.

Whitbeck, L. B., Hoyt, D. R., and Huck, S. M. 1994. Early family relationships, intergenerational solidarity, and support provided to parents by their adult children. *Journal of Gerontology* 49:S85–94.

Whitlatch, C. J., Zarit, S. H., and von Eye, A. 1991. Efficacy of interventions with caregivers: A reanalysis. *Gerontologist* 31:9–14.

Williamson, D. 1991. *Intimacy paradox: Personal authority in the family system.* New York: Guilford.

Wright, L. K. 1993. *Alzheimer's disease and marriage: An intimate account.* London: Sage.

Wynne, L. 1984. The epigenesis of relational systems: A model for understanding family development. *Family Process* 23:297–318.

Zarit, S. H., Stephens, M. A. P., Townsend, A., and Greene, R. 1998. Stress reduction for family caregivers: Effects of adult day care use. *Journal of Gerontology: Social Sciences* 53B:S267–77.

Zarit, S. H., Zarit, J. M., and Reever, K. E. 1982. Memory training for severe memory loss: Effects on senile dementia patients and their families. *Gerontologist* 22:373–77.

Zautra, A. J., and Reich, J. W. 1983. Life-events and perceptions of life quality: Developments in a two-factor approach. *Journal of Community Psychology* 11:121–32.

CHAPTER ELEVEN

Social Supports for the Caregiver

DAVID A. CHIRIBOGA, PH.D.

The idea that social supports can be helpful to caregivers is not a surprise to anyone familiar with research on stress. After all, for more than forty years the empirical literature on stress has been pointing out that social resources—including social supports—act as mediators in the classic stress paradigm. The gist of this literature is that for nearly every stressful situation imaginable, including both chronic and acute conditions, having supportive relationships can be helpful and can reduce stress. What may be surprising is that there is increasing evidence that social relationships on occasion may not only not provide support but may be detrimental to well-being.

This chapter focuses on the informal supports available to caregivers and how these supports help—and sometimes hinder—as caregivers struggle to continue providing care while maintaining the quality of their own lives. Previous chapters in this volume presented the various ways in which the more formal support system provides care to caregivers. As these chapters make clear, caregiving does not occur in a vacuum. The caregiver lives and operates in a surround of social others, some of whom are prominent on the research radar screen and some of whom are not. Some of them may be perceived by the caregiver as providing social support and some may not. This chapter begins with general comments about social supports and relevant theoretical frameworks. It then reviews critical aspects of available social supports but emphasizes the less-studied aspects, including the characteristics and significance of social supports for minority caregivers and what might be called the "invisible" supports. It concludes with some comments about the possible need for a shift in how we study the supports of caregivers.

CONCEPTUALIZING SOCIAL SUPPORTS

There is agreement in the literature that the more social support is available or perceived, the less problematic the life of the caregiver. The actual findings vary in terms of outcomes and strength of associations, but the direction of association is generally consistent. For example, Chappell and Reid (2002) found that social supports were related to psychological well-being but not to reported caregiver burden. Edwards and Scheetz (2002) found an association between more social supports and less burden among caregivers of persons with Parkinson disease. At least one large randomly sampled survey has found that helping others is a strong predictor of self-reported mental health (Schwartz, Meisenhelder, Ma, and Reed, 2003). In other words, the act of helping others—whether the recipient be a caregiver or care recipient—has its own rewards.

To consider the "whys" and "wherefores" of support, we can begin by noting that social relationships entail all sorts of interactions, some related to leisure, some to emotional and sexual expression, and some to assistance and guidance. The phrase "social support" is generally used when the focus of attention is on the role of family, friends, and acquaintances in providing each other with assistance. This role, of course, sounds very much like caregiving. A key distinction between the assistance provided in what is designated as social support and in caregiving lies in the degree of reciprocity involved. When the assistance simply refers to that which is commonly part of everyday transactions between people, it is more likely to be perceived simply as support. In other words, as long as there is give and take and assistance flows freely in both directions, the situation is viewed as part of the normal, to-be-expected exchanges that occur between people.

On the other hand, when one individual is unable to reciprocate for sustained periods of time, the support being provided is more likely to be characterized as caregiving. From this perspective, the distinction between support to caregivers and support provided by caregivers becomes blurred. Consider, for example, the situation in which assistance that friends and relatives provide to more burdened caregivers is both sustained and unreciprocated for months, if not years, because of the proverbial "36-hour day" that surrounds caregiving (Mace and Rabins, 1999). This loss of reciprocity can have serious consequences and in part may be responsible for the reduction in social supports and social contacts often reported by caregivers (e.g., Coen, O'Bolye, Swanwick, and Coakley, 1999; Wallston, 2000) as well as greater conflict with providers of support. Indeed, one website for caregivers advises the latter to be prepared for "loss of friends and strained family relations" (Keys to Successful Caregiving, 2003). This loss of friends may also reflect the simple time demands created by the role of caregiving or even a fear of dementia (a stigmatization) on the part of older friends.

Social supports can be subdivided into informal and formal categories. "Informal supports" is a phrase used to distinguish unpaid assistance by families and friends from the "formal" paid assistance provided by professionals and semiprofessionals such as social workers, nurses, visiting homemakers, and the clergy. Naturally, formal social support will more likely focus on impairment-based information related to how to seek assistance, complete forms, assist with ADLs such as toileting and bathing, etc. (O'Connell, Baker, and Prosser, 2003). Several studies have shown that caregivers often have no idea how to cope with health-related issues and need help in this arena (e.g., Hudson, Aranda, and McMurray, 2002).

As is the case with support versus caregiving, at times the differences between formal and informal become blurred. For instance, one of the earliest gerontological studies of supports found that even contacts with seemingly peripheral persons like a favorite grocery store clerk or bank teller may provide a buffer against the impact of stressors (Lowenthal and Haven, 1968). Because such individuals are not paid to provide support, presumably they would be classified as informal agents of support. Perhaps the most important point to emphasize here is that the distinction based on payment status is arbitrary: it ignores the fact that paid and unpaid supports may provide similar help to the caregiver, especially with regard to furnishing information, respite, and in some cases emotional support as well (e.g., Loke, Liu, and Szeto, 2003; Schulz et al., 2003). We will return to this similarity of roles in a later section.

What do social supports actually consist of? Generally the term is used to refer to behaviors that provide emotional, instrumental, self-esteem enhancing, or informational support (Martire, Schulz, Mittelmark, and Newsom, 1999; Unger et al., 1999). Validation and assistance in caregiving issues is another form of support (e.g., Deimling, Smerglia, and Schaefer, 2001). In addition to the many studies that consider simply the relative presence of such supports, satisfaction or the actual or perceived adequacy of support has also been examined (Jang et al., 2003), where the focus of attention may be the support provided by just one person or by an entire social network (e.g., Antonucci, 1994). It may be helpful to bear in mind that quality and quantity of informal support depend heavily on characteristics of the network, such as size, frequency of contacts, and quality of relationships (Thoits, 1999; Lin, 1999).

Measurement

One factor encouraging the general growth of social support research has been the availability of an extensive array of assessment instruments applicable to the study of caregiver support, many of which have been around for years and thus have a wealth of validating information. Among the most widely used is the venerable six-item Social Support Questionnaire (Sarason et al., 1987), which assesses support availability and satisfaction, as do the support scales developed by Krause and Borawski-Clark (1995). Moving to another dimension, the Social Network Index (Cohen et al., 1997) documents how many people are seen on a regular basis and the social roles occupied by these people (e.g., spouse, child). The Social Network Scale of Lubben (1988) covers similar territory.

Support as a Mediator of Stress

Although literally hundreds of studies have reported a positive influence of supports on the well-being of individuals, most research has focused on the well-established idea that supports have the potential to act as a mediator or "buffer" against the impact of stressful conditions. Buffering may result from the direct provision of needed resources, be they emotional or financial support, services, or information (House, Umberson, and Landis, 1988). Less obvious is that the presence of social supports may work to counteract the deleterious impact of stress on the immune system or on self-esteem (e.g., Cohen et al., 1997; Kiecolt-Glaser, 1999). Of course, one should not forget that secondary caregivers also provide support—but in this case the support is often very specific to the caregiving task, and as such is not really covered by the term "social support." Moreover, secondary caregivers have been themselves reported as a primary source of conflict for the caregiver, often because of disagreements concerning either how to provide care or the amount required (e.g., Sanchez-Ayendez, 1998).

The Importance of the Type of Dependency-creating Situation

The level of disease severity and the trajectory of decline clearly has an impact on the burden placed on the caregiver, and therefore on the latter's general as well as specific needs for social support (Bass, McClendon, Deimling, and Mukherjee, 1994). Progressive neurological diseases in particular create exacerbated dependency needs. Alzheimer disease, multiple sclerosis, and Parkinson disease all have varying but progressively debilitating courses, but medical and social needs of patients vary. Caregiving for persons with dementia, especially those with Alzheimer disease (AD), has been a particular focus of attention because dementia impairs the patient's ability to reciprocate and to express appreciation (e.g., Janevic and Connell, 2001). With the limitations on reciprocity that come with AD, it is probably no surprise that caregivers of persons with dementia report greater burden than those providing care to the nondemented (e.g., Ory et al., 1999).

The Caregiver as a Person in Need

It is appropriate to consider the caregiver as someone who, like the care recipient, is potentially in sustained need of social support. There are at least three reasons. First, caregivers to older adults are often themselves older and frail enough that they themselves have needs for help, though these needs may be overshadowed by those of the more obviously dependent family member. A second reason is that the sheer burden of caring for a dependent family member may in itself jeopardize the health and well-being of the caregiver (see chapter 4). In this respect, an important question must be posed: How likely is it that a caregiver will actually ask for assistance? Nadler (1997) made a useful distinction between those who are relatively independent but appropriately seek help and those who make inappropriate and excessive use of help from others. The latter may result in less effective caregiving as well as burnout of supports. Still others may need help but for various reasons may hesitate to ask. It is well documented that women are more likely to reach out for help and advice (and driving directions!) than are men, and they typically have and maintain larger networks of friends than do men.

The third reason is that caregivers are facing not simply time-consuming demands but a multitude of stressors that arise in consequence of the caregiving situation— as well as the stressors normally encountered by noncaregivers. In this regard, social supports have been found helpful to people experiencing nearly all conditions of stress: feeling involved in relationships or networks perceived to be supportive generally has a positive influence on well-being. On the other hand, lower levels of perceived support are linked to a variety of poor outcomes, including death (Berkman, Leo-Summers, and Horvitz, 1992). There is evidence that the importance of social relationships may even be accentuated for the elderly. For example, compared to younger adults, 17-year all-cause mortality rates in one large hospital system were more strongly associated with smaller social networks for persons aged 60 and older (Seeman et al., 1987).

Such results suggest that focusing on the social supports specific to caregiving may present just one part of the overall picture of what the caregiver is experiencing. Moreover, social supports are obviously just part of the answer to the question "How do I go on?" Coen, O'Boyle, Swanwick, and Coakley (1999), for example, report that while social support was statistically associated with lower burden of caring for persons with Alzheimer disease, the variables perceived by caregivers to be most associated with their overall quality of life included the general presence of children and siblings, opportunities to socialize and pursue leisure activities, etc. What they saw as important to their lives were relationships and opportunities to relate to others in situations having little or nothing to do with the need to provide care to a family member.

SOCIAL SUPPORT FOR CAREGIVERS

Now I would like to discuss in more detail the various kinds of informal and formal support providers, as well as a class of people that might be referred to as "invisible" supports. As we proceed it may be helpful to keep in mind the sociological idea that individuals can develop "social capital" as a result of interactions with others, but this capital is most often in limited supply and can be expended quickly in the absence of reciprocity, a sense of shared goals, or self-interest (e.g., Uphoff, 2000).

Informal Support: Who Actually Provides It?

Studies have generally suggested that families provide the bulk of social support for the elderly and caregivers to the elderly. As indicated by Deimling, Smerglia, and Schaefer (2001), a family's overall index of adaptability, cohesion, and conflict may facilitate or attenuate family efforts at support. Of interest is that some minority groups have an apparent advantage with regard to the availability of support: the extended and even nuclear family is generally more extensive among those of Hispanic American and African American heritage (Hogan and Spencer, 1993; Jackson and Antonucci, 1992). In addition, people associated with religious organizations may figure prominently in the social network of African Americans (McRae, Thompson, and Cooper, 1999).

On the other hand, when sustained support is needed, the heterogeneity of families, even within particular groups such as Hispanics or African Americans, suggests that the mere existence of a family does not guarantee adequate care (Bengtson and Silversteen, 1993). Historical increases in life expectancies and divorce, along with a trend toward having fewer children, further emphasize the need to avoid generalizations concerning the support potential of families, and also have implications for who is available to provide social supports within the family.

The "Why" of Informal Support Efficacy in the Context of Caring

Why then do supports help the caregiver, to the extent that in fact they do help? One finding of relevance is a study by Toseland, McCallion, Gerber, and Banks (2002) that looked at caregivers to community-resident individuals afflicted with a dementia. In this study, social supports were found to be an enabling force that was associated with greater access to health and human services. They were therefore influential in meeting the actual needs of the dependent elder, as well as lightening the load on the caregiver.

Social networks analyses add a broader perspective to the study of supports, because such analyses often divide networks into components that include but are not necessarily limited to support. For example, Magliano and colleagues (2003) studied the social networks of more than 700 caregivers of persons with schizophrenia. Network components studied included social contacts, practical support, psychological support, and help in emergencies involving caregiving. One rather striking finding was that substantial proportions of the sample did not report ample support resources. More than 50 percent reported that friends and relatives were only sometimes available to talk to or meet with regarding various problems. From 37 to 43 percent reported only sometimes getting psychological support; from 22 to 31 percent felt practical support was available only sometimes; 27 to 28 percent reported help was available during problems and emergencies. In general, the older caregivers in this study had fewer social resources available to them than did the younger, and this was also true for the less educated caregivers and those whose care recipient exhibited greater symptomatology.

Limitations to Informal Support

Ironically, many of the same studies documenting the value of supports to caregivers often report a decline in the size of the latter's social network, either because of the stigmatizing qualities of the dependency-creating problems (for example,

Alzheimer disease) or because the time demands imposed by the caregiver role reduce the opportunity for time spent with family and friends (Acton, 2002). There
are other limiting factors, however.

Harrington (2000) points out that with the greater equality of women, and their
increasing penetration into the work force, the burden of caregiving has also become greater. Though the burden in some sense may be eased with this increased
participation in the work force, given the greater income and policies such as family leave, the advantages are not evenly distributed. Those with lower incomes, who
are also more likely to be minorities, may not only receive minimal pay but may
(1) be single parents and hence not reap the benefits of a dual income family, (2) not
be eligible for the fringe benefits associated with higher-status jobs: sick leave and
family leave (Aranda and Knight, 1997).

Changing policies and reimbursements to more formal systems of caregiving
also contribute to burden, because the availability of formal supports may reduce
the perceived needs of the caregiver, as judged by the caregiver's support system, as
well as change the types of support that are actually needed from informal sources
(Williams et al., 2003). When, for example, respite care or necessary information is
readily available, the technical needs of the caregiver may be reduced—which in
turn may permit a greater focus on emotional support.

The context of caregiving should also be considered. For example, someone
who lives in comparative isolation and/or in poverty may have greater difficulty obtaining either informal or formal supports (Williams et al., 2003). Distance from
family members, as well as the number of family members available to help, becomes a matter of particular importance. Here minority status may prove an advantage, because several researchers have pointed out that not only do African
Americans tend to have larger extended families but the families tend to live closer
together than non-Hispanic whites (e.g., Dilworth-Anderson, Williams, and Cooper,
1999; Dilworth-Anderson, Williams, and Gibson 2002; Sanchez-Ayendez, 1998). As
will be discussed later, this does not necessarily lead to more or effective support
provision.

In the future the sources of social support for caregivers may undergo a profound change. As a result of forces such as the dramatic increases in divorce that began with the end of World War II, the rise of so-called blended or reconstituted and
single-parent families, and an increasing number of never-marrieds, we are moving
to more nontraditional systems of support in which generational and relational lines
are mixed and crossed. The need for more formal provision of support may therefore become greater.

Formal Support as Part of the Overall Support System

As already mentioned, informal providers are not the only source of support. The formal support system not only provides direct and supplemental help to care recipients but on occasion may perform some of the same functions made available to caregivers through informal supports. These functions may be very specific to the type of intervention or provider. For example, Lincoln et al. (2003) employed a randomized controlled trial to examine the effect of a government-provided support program for stroke patients and their caregivers in England. Results indicated that while there were no differences in the mood and independence of patients and caregivers receiving or not receiving the intervention, those receiving the intervention were better informed about who to contact for help, which strategies to use to reduce the risk of further strokes, and where to turn for emotional support.

Very little information is available on how much support, other than informational, derives from formal caregivers. Secrest (2002) reports on a small qualitative study of perceived support provided by nurses to stroke patients and their primary caregivers. The respondents generally characterized the nurses along a continuum ranging from helpful to more conflicted, and did not report any emotional or therapeutic support. Thomas et al. (2002) found that caregivers generally sought information about the dependency-creating illness and available services and options from physicians; the physician, however, was not found to be the caregiver's primary source for information. The health professional should expect the unexpected: one study found that a major help to older caregivers was the provision of hearing aids (Tolson, Swan, and Knussen, 2002). In another study, van den Heuvel et al. (2002) found that, in contrast to home visits by paid staff, group support improved the self-confidence and coping skills of caregivers, and younger female caregivers increased in levels of social support. However, as Wiles (2003) points out, changing policies and decreasing funds available for reimbursement are increasing the difficulties of informal caregivers in gaining access to the formal caregiving system.

Respite and related services, including institutionalization, also need to be considered in terms of impact on the need and receipt of social supports. Zank and Schacke (2002) report that the use of a day care program by dependent elders was perceived as personally helpful by caregivers. In one repeated measures study that followed Taiwan caregivers from point of placement of elder into a nursing home to four months later, the caregivers significantly reduced their reports of low family support, and their scheduling demands and health problems decreased (Yeh, Johnson, and Wang, 2002).

Finally, it is also important to consider the support needs of formal caregivers. The needs of these individuals are rarely considered: after all, one might think, this is their job and they are getting paid for their efforts. Unfortunately, hands-on formal caregivers who actually spend the most time with clients—and may provide the only personal attention received by clients—are both poorly paid and less educated than the more "professional" level providers such as nurses or social workers. It is therefore not surprising that jobs such as the home care worker or nursing aide have high turnover rates. The informational and instrumental needs of these formal caregivers can be—and sometimes are—addressed through formal training. However, few if any guidelines exist for what such training should entail, and few programs actually exist. Those that do exist tend to be focused on specific issues such as creating a positive relationship with the client (e.g., Kuipers and Moore, 1995), pain management (e.g., Wright, Varholak, and Costello, 2003), communication skills (e.g., Bourgeois, Dijkstra, Burgio, and Allen, 2003), or behavioral intervention skills (e.g., Glenwick, Slutzsky, and Garfinkel, 2001). With some rare exceptions (Smith, 1983), few programs exist to satisfy the psychosocial needs of formal caregivers. Clearly this is an area with a strong need for research and development.

"Invisible" Social Support

In the study of caregiving and the supports available to caregivers, many potential sources of support may not appear on the official "radar screen." As already mentioned, one potential source is the host of clerks and salespeople and bank tellers and mail deliverers and meter readers with whom one may have regular though infrequent contact (e.g., Lowenthal and Haven, 1968). As discussed next, there are other sources of support that generally go unrecognized, but which may play a vital role.

1. *The Care Recipient.* The recipient is rarely studied as a provider of social support, possibly because of the tendency to believe that the recipient is unable to reciprocate. The ability to provide support to the caregiver obviously depends on the cognitive as well as physical capacity of the recipient. In a qualitative study of Dutch spousal caregivers to persons with multiple sclerosis, Boeije, Duijnstee, and Grypdonck (2003) found that feelings of shared problems, marital loyalty, and commitment to the relationship all contributed to a continuation of the caregiving role. Spruytte, van Audenhove, Lammertyn, and Storms (2002) found that children and spouses of mentally ill family members, or those with dementia, generally reported low levels of conflict and high levels of emotional warmth in their relations with the care recipient. Deviant behavior and the caregiver's adverse reaction to this behavior

eroded the quality of the relationship. The authors concluded that future research should pay more attention to the caregiver-recipient relationship.

Martire et al. (2002) also looked at the quality of the caregiver-recipient relationship. They found that women with osteoarthritis were likely to be more negative in their reaction to their husbands' instrumental support, if they placed a high value on functional independence. On the other hand, in a study of 24 dyads consisting of elders with osteoarthritis and their caregivers, it was found that a couples-oriented intervention was more effective than a patient-only intervention in terms of symptom management (Martire et al., 2003). These studies suggest the value of considering the potential of the caregiver–care recipient dyad as a functional mutual support system. In other words, the recipient of care may still be capable of providing at least token support and help to the caregiver—what Lewinter (2003) calls "symbolic" reciprocity.

Left relatively unexplored is any systematic study of how support (as opposed to dependency needs) from the recipient of caregiving may change over time. As might be expected, and as discussed in the section dealing with conceptual frameworks, caregiver burden increases as the degree of dementia increases (e.g., Deimling, Smerglia, and Schaefer, 2001). This may of course be due to multiple factors, including the cumulative toll on the caregiver, "wear and tear" on the caregiver's support system (an idea that suggests that more attention should be paid to how to nourish and maintain this system), and possibly the gradual loss of support from the care recipient. Langer, Abrams, and Syrjala (2003) found that for certain cancer patients requiring stem cell transplantation, the correspondence between patient-spouse levels of marital satisfaction decreased as measured six months before surgery and one year after surgery.

2. Spirituality. There is evidence that for some caregivers greater spirituality, described as a sense of connectedness with a higher power, helped them cope with the burden of care (e.g., Acton and Miller, 2003). This is not specific to caregiving, because the literature suggests that spirituality in various forms helps older people cope with life's problems in general (e.g., Jang et al., 2003). In a study of African American women providing care to an asthmatic child, Sterling and Peterson (2003) found that religious beliefs played an important role in the caregiving relationship. In a small descriptive study of African Americans and European Americans, Theis et al. (2003) also found that participation in religious activities was helpful to many respondents, and they concluded that health care professionals should work with clergy. Given their greater involvement in general with religion, religious beliefs and spirituality may play a greater role in the lives of African American caregivers (Jang et al., 2003).

3. *Pets.* There is evidence that in specifically focusing on the idea of human sources of support for the caregiver we may be casting too narrow a net. While arguably pets do not provide "social" support, and their range of supportive behavior may be limited to making the caregiver feel valued or loved, there clearly is evidence that pets can and do make life more livable for their human companions (e.g., Allen, 1996).

4. *Other Invisible Sources.* The wide realm of internet chat rooms, cyberpals, and listservs may also play a supportive role, although these are just beginning to receive empirical attention with regard to older adults (e.g., White et al., 2002). They may be akin in function to the organized self-help groups that exist at local, regional, and national levels and that themselves often maintain an internet presence.

SUPPORT AND THE MINORITY CAREGIVER

The prevailing assumption in the literature is that minority caregivers are blessed with an abundance of social supports (e.g., Calderon and Tennstedt, 1998; Jackson, Antonucci, and Gibson, 1995) and that such caregivers not only have a decreased burden but also are less likely to institutionalize family members because of this support. Burton and Stack (1993) characterized caregiving in the African American family in terms of what they call "multigenerational collectives," wherein kin-related tasks are systematically assigned according to family ideology and norms and roles. In several publications, Burton and colleagues make the point that the structure and function of such multigenerational collectives depends in great part on timing within the family of such transitions as parent and grandparenthood, as well as the role of context (e.g, Burton and Sörensen, 1993).

At least in part due to the availability of family supports, African American caregivers have often reported less burden than other groups (Haley et al., 1996)—in spite of the fact that they spend more time caregiving than do white Americans (McNeil, 1999). In studies in which African and non-Hispanic white caregivers reported roughly equivalent levels of burden, there is a suggestion that a lack of social-support resources played a role (Young and Kahana, 1995). On the other hand, it is important for health professionals to recognize that there is a danger in equating ample resources with positive outcomes. The literature suggests that the more solid and close the family network is, the more likely the family is to reject outside help until the burden of caring becomes extremely high (e.g., Williams and Dilworth-Anderson, 2002).

More solid and close family networks may therefore present with unrecognized risks, especially for minority families, because the latter often are often viewed as strong in family supports. Such risk is reflected in the results of researchers like

Calderon and Tennstedt (1998), who report that African American and Puerto Rican caregivers relied more on family and less on formal services. This may also explain why Williams, Dilworth-Anderson, and Goodwin (2003) found a relationship between role strain and depressive symptomatology among African American caregivers, despite strong family ties. Their conclusion was that any perception that African American caregivers are less vulnerable to burden does not fit the data.

A related point is that while there is agreement in the literature that African American caregivers have ample social supports and benefit from them, the evidence stemming from research with other ethnic/racial groups is mixed. The differing contexts faced by other groups may pose a greater challenge to minority caregivers, regardless of greater family solidarity. For example, while they may have larger extended families than do non-Hispanic white Americans, older Mexican Americans are likely to be markedly less educated and of lower income than non-Hispanic whites; immigration history may also affect a family's ability to provide support (e.g., Chiriboga et al., 2002). In addition, the differential prevalence of disabling conditions can affect caregiving. For example, Hispanics have higher rates of dementia and diabetes than do whites, and both Hispanics and African American elders may become dependent at earlier ages (Aranda and Knight, 1997; Gurland et al., 1999; Fitten, Ortiz, and Ponton, 2001; Wallsten, 2000).

A particularly critical issue is whether the caregiver has adequate proficiency with English. Familiarity with the host language (in this case, English) is a central component of acculturation. In the absence of linguistic proficiency, a deciding factor concerning the efficacy of the social support network may be whether there is anyone who can facilitate interactions with the more formal systems of care (e.g., Doty, 2003). Chiriboga et al. (2002) reported that among older Mexican Americans, the more often Spanish was used in family gatherings, the greater the depression of the subjects. This finding supports the hypothesis that when an extended family as a whole lacks English proficiency it is less able to support individual family members in need because of problems in accessing the health care system.

Such differing socioeconomic and disease contexts place differing demands not only on the caregiver but also on the informal and formal support systems. The importance of traditional family values, including solidarity, may in fact unduly heighten the expectations of caregivers. Perhaps for reasons such as these, there is evidence that relations between Mexican American caregivers and their social supports may be more strained than is the case for African American and even Anglo caregivers (Adams et al., 2002; Aranda and Knight, 1997).

The great variability by ethnicity and race also can be found in cross-cultural research. For example, Kim and Lee (2003) found that Korean caregivers of cognitively or functionally impaired parents reported levels of depression and health problems that were higher than those reported in studies of Western caregivers. Karasawa, Hatta, Gushiken, and Hasegawa (2003) found that a perceived lack of support from family members was associated with higher levels of caregiver depression in Japanese caregivers.

WHEN SOCIAL RELATIONSHIPS ARE NOT SUPPORTIVE

While we generally assume that exchanges with the social network are positive and supportive, the caregiver's network may in fact create or exacerbate problems (Haley et al., 2003). Based on open-ended questions asked of 176 dementia care-givers, Lilly, Richards, and Buckwalter (2003) report that only slightly more than 50 percent of references to friends were positive. There is a growing literature on the problems resulting from relationships, with the problems coming in several forms. One is relationships that have become strained due to the very fact of caregiving. Due to severe emotional and time constraints, caregivers' ability to maintain and nourish potentially helpful, supportive relationships can be eroded. Anderson, Par-menter, and Mok (2002), for example, found that caregivers of family members with more severe traumatic brain injury reported higher levels of family dysfunction than did caregivers to the less severely injured. Clark, Shields, Aycock, and Wolf (2003) de-veloped a 15-item Family Caregiver Conflict Scale (FCCS) that covers communica-tion, problem solving, overall functioning, and perceived criticism within the family. One finding based on this scale was that spousal caregivers reported less family con-flict than the nonspousal caregivers.

Another risk profile is typified by a long history of troubled relations with sib-lings or relatives who are currently acting as supports to a caregiver. Moreover, there is some evidence that at least when the support to the primary caregiver is coming from a relative who is also a caregiver, there is an egocentric bias operating, such that the secondary caregiver may perceive the primary caregiver as exagger-ating the need and difficulty of the caregiving situation (Lerner et al., 1991).

Other support problems and issues have been identified. Neufeld and Harrison (2003) described a subset of eight women caregivers from a longitudinal study who reported that family or friends did not provide supportive relationships. Two types of problems were described. The first was unmet expectations for help (see also Song, Biegel, and Milligan, 1997). Unmet expectations may result from the need to maintain high levels of support to caregivers over such lengths of time that the supporters become tired and burned out. Studying adult children and parents who were involved in reciprocal but not caregiving relationships, Silverstein, Chen, and

Heller (1996) found that the need to maintain high levels of support was associated with an increase in depressive symptoms. Presumably the same phenomenon would be found in adult children providing support to a caregiving parent, and to other caregiver-support relationships as well.

The second type of problem identified by Neufeld and Harrison consisted of negative exchanges, in which the social other criticized or belittled the caregiver's efforts. When secondary caregivers perceive the problems of the dependent family member as less severe than described by the primary caregiver, this can lead to conflict. A small qualitative study of 17 caregivers to persons with AD in India indicated that family conflict was not uncommon, including reports of criticism by other family members (Shaji, Smitha, Lal, and Prince, 2003). In part, the level of family conflict may reflect the fact that many of the study participants were younger women, including daughters-in-law, who may have been forced by their gender and role to provide care.

Is There a "Dark Side" to Social Support?

Up to this point we have been discussing how supports to caregivers may not work because of conditions and conflicts specific to the caregiving situation. On a more general level, social scientists are beginning to pay attention to the potential of close social relationships to have negative effects, regardless of the context. Indeed, there is evidence that, over time, negative social exchanges have greater consequences than positive exchanges (e.g., Newsom, Nishishiba, Morgan, and Rook, 2003). Witness the high rate of divorce in America, elder abuse, and the general phenomenon of family violence. While some of the negativity in relationships may be deliberate, there is research suggesting that even well-intended efforts at support may have negative consequences (e.g., Coyne, Wortman, and Lehman, 1988; Lewis and Rook, 1999). The clinician and/or researcher who is interested in the problem side of social supports for caregivers should be aware of additional issues, as outlined below:

1. *Burnout*. Social supports may not prove adequate to the demands created by certain situations, especially when demands are chronic and unrelenting. The vast literature on caregiver burden is conceptually related to the older concept of burnout. Of particular interest: as alluded to in the section dealing with minority caregiving, larger and more cohesive families may be more resistant to seeking support from outside sources and may experience greater burden as a result. Moreover, because of the greater numbers of people involved, larger networks may generate greater interpersonal conflict (Riley and Eckenrode, 1986). The health professional

should attend to signs of burnout not only in the primary caregiver but also among her or his social supports. Advising the caregiver about respite care and homemaker programs, encouraging her to expand her support system, and enabling the caregiver to take a vacation all represent strategies to help relieve burnout for all parties.

2. *Undermining.* The actions and attitudes of family and friends, because of their importance to the individual, can undermine an individual's sense of self-esteem. Support and undermining have been found to be relatively independent, with both affecting mental health (Vinokur and van Ryn, 1993). To the extent that the caregiver has begun to feel inadequate or ineffective, the health professional may need to work with the client's feelings of self-worth.

3. *Desolation.* The death of close and valued members of one's social network has a strong, and usually negative, effect on people at any age (e.g., Carnelley, Wortman, and Kessler, 1999). Ironically, those with large and/or more closely knit families may suffer more losses, and the consequences of losses, because in effect they have more to lose. Those with histories of social isolation may in later life be spared the stresses associated with social loss, although they also may lack a well-established personal support system. In the case of a caregiver, loss of supports through bereavement may be particularly distressing if they occur during the later and more demanding stages of the caregiving career. In this sense, having strong bonds to supportive people may leave the caregiver in a position of vulnerability. Hence, the health professional may wish to determine whether clients have a recent history of social loss that may impact their own ability to provide care and support.

4. *Timing.* Those who provide support to caregivers have their own lives and demands that deserve consideration: a call for help when the support provider is overwhelmed may lead to a less than enthusiastic response. Even subtle issues can affect the quality of support. Rook, Pietromonaco, and Lewis (1994) report that the emotional mood of individuals helped determine whether their interactions with another person were positive or negative. A critical factor in the influence of mood seemed to be whether or not people's levels of dysphoria were matched or not, suggesting that in the case of caregivers who are feeling somewhat depressed because of the burdens of caring, the most supportive others might be those who themselves are not on an emotional high.

5. *Social Control.* In fields other than aging, there is growing interest in one corollary of being embedded in a social support system: the potentially greater presence of social control. In a viable family system, for example, parents exert a strong influence (i.e., demonstrate social control) on their children's behavior, and the peer network of a child is well known to influence that child's behavior. Similarly, caregivers may begin to influence the dependent elder, as may agents of formal sup-

port, and the same influence may begin to be exerted by those who are called on to support the caregiver. One area of growing interest is whether social control can result in reductions in health risk behaviors (e.g., Lewis and Rook, 1999).

Although social control may have a beneficial intent, the potential for harm as well as benefit is clearly present. In the field of gerontology, this potential has often been studied under the rubric of "paternalism" or expert bias. Well-intended family members and formal providers may assume more responsibility than necessary for an older person's day-to-day life, whether caregiver or care recipient, resulting in a loss of independence disproportionate to the older person's actual functional limitations (Bootsma-van der Wiel et al., 2001). The health care provider should avoid the appearance of dictating strategies and solutions to those involved in the caregiving situation and should identify overly controlling behavior in caregivers. In both instances, the end result may be greater dependency of the care recipient and greater burden on the entire caregiving support system.

Overall, because of the potential for support burnout and increased interfamily strain, it is not surprising that interventions aimed at family functioning have proved effective for relieving caregiver burden (Lincoln et al., 2003). The main issue here is to recognize and be alert for problems that are arising not only because of the caregiving situation but also because of long-standing interpersonal strains and conflicts.

Support Stability and the Evolving Demands of Caregiving

It has already been noted that the demands placed on the caregiver and his or her support system often change over time. Aneschensel et al. (1995; see also Chiriboga, 1994) found that caregiving is an evolving role that often has an insidious onset and grows more demanding over time. The idea that there is a trajectory of caregiving— what Aneshensel and colleagues call a "career"—that is associated with the trajectory of the illness makes common sense, and indeed there is ample evidence for this. In one study of caregivers to stroke patients, caregiver strain was found to increase over the period from three to six months poststroke (Blake, Lincoln, and Clarke, 2003). This temporally evolving association of greater burden or strain with greater severity of disease has also been noted with dementia (Gaugler, Davy, Pearlin, and Zarit, 2000). Such findings suggest that the need for social supports, and for particular kinds of support (i.e., instrumental, emotional), may vary over the course of the disease.

Several studies have specifically looked at process issues. For example, using a grounded-theory qualitative approach, Perry (2002) found that wives of persons with Alzheimer disease described an unfolding of recognizable changes in their husbands, had to readjust their activities to accommodate this, and had to modify their own personal identities to ones more appropriate to the new and evolving situation. Sörensen and Zarit (1996) used a conceptual framework to guide research into the degree to which caregiving was anticipated and planned for in multigenerational families, with results suggesting that while cross-generational discussion around possible caregiving needs was not uncommon, actual planning was unusual. Sörensen and Pinquart (2000) also found that the extent of social resources potentially available through the family influenced plans for future caregiving.

Finally, one intriguing study suggests that there is a need to consider not only the staging of the disease as it determines the caregiving career but also the timing of the caregiving demands in terms of the caregiver's stage of life and role status. In a study of 278 women who simultaneously occupied several demanding roles, Stephens, Townsend, Martire, and Druley (2001) found that various age/role combinations had different implications for parent care. For example, women who experienced conflict between the roles of parent care and child care were more likely to be younger and less educated and to have younger children—factors that may have adversely affected their ability to maintain a socially supportive network. Such results indicate the potential value in considering the "career" (the natural history of the support system) of the social support systems of the caregivers: the support needs evolve in correspondence with the evolving demands placed on the caregiver. The results also demonstrate that the translational process of moving from theory to research is justified and is proving fruitful to investigators seeking to understand how social supports influence caregivers and their behavior (Pillemer, Suitor, and Wethington, 2003).

TWO THEORIES RELEVANT TO SUPPORT

In addition to the career framework, several other conceptual models may help to package and explain the significance of social supports for caregivers. Some of these models may help in understanding specific elements of the support-caregiver relationship. Role identity models emphasize the diverse roles that individuals occupy, as well as the fact that these roles may on occasion come into conflict (e.g., Siebert, Mutran, and Reitzes, 1999). Resource models emphasize the utility of the individual's social resources when dealing with relationships such as that of the caregiver and significant other (e.g., Lin, 1999). Stress models emphasize supports as mediators or buffers (e.g., Thoits, 1999; Cohen et al., 1997). At a deeper level, there are two theories that may help to put the support literature in perspective: the theory of exchange or equity and the theory of distributive justice.

Exchange Theory

According to contemporary theories of social exchange or equity, people are primarily concerned with minimizing their costs or maximizing their profits, as defined by commonly desired resources (Tyler et al., 1997). Central to defining costs and benefits is the level of reciprocity of any sequence of exchanges, where the costs and benefits of any exchange incurred by individual A are balanced by the costs and benefits incurred by individual B. As noted by von dem Knesebeck and Siegrist (2003, p. 209), violation of the social norm of reciprocity "elicits strong negative emotions of anger and frustration among those concerned, resulting in a sense of being treated unfairly and in an unjust way. If experienced recurrently, nonreciprocity in social exchange may have a profound impact on human well-being and health." Interestingly, in a study of randomly selected older subjects in Germany and the United States, von dem Knesebeck and Siegrist (2003) report that degree of nonreciprocity and perceived adequacy of emotional support made independent contributions to depressive symptomatology. Hence, reciprocity presents as a separate and distinct component of social exchanges.

Such findings have obvious implications for caregiving. When confronted with someone who is chronically in need of support, for example, a caregiver or indeed a care recipient, the potential supporter is put in an "avoidance-avoidance" conflict in which the costs of nonintervention are weighed against those of intervention. When operating within a longer time frame, people may be willing to incur immediate costs in anticipation of an ultimately profitable exchange: a gift, an inheritance, a mother's love, even the continuing friendship of someone who is valued.

On the other hand, implicit to most exchange theories is the notion that while people usually express allegiance to publicly accepted norms of fairness and entitlement, they use these rules to optimize their own share of commonly desired resources. Indeed, if the outcome is judged to be sufficiently profitable, or costly, they may ignore the dictates of traditional values or justice (e.g., Horwitz, Reinhard, and Howell-White, 1996). Translated into the context of this chapter, they may be reluctant to provide care or provide support to a caregiver unless "there is something in it for them."

Distributive Justice

In contrast to exchange theory, models based on the notion of distributive justice (Lerner, Ross, and Miller, 2002) present rules of entitlement as playing a central rather than a secondary and dependent role in the organization of a person's goals and governing his or her transactions with others. According to this model, people become invested in their own view of how things do and should happen in their world. One assumption is that people are guided not by self-profit maximization but by the question of "Who is entitled to what from whom?" In one study of adult child caregivers to parents with Alzheimer disease, it was found that the burden of care was perceived as greater when the parent was rated as having in the past been a kinder and more considerate parent. The conclusion was that the child caregivers felt more obligated to care for the more positively viewed parent, which resulted in more care but greater burden (Chiriboga, Yee, and Weiler, 1992).

IMPLICATIONS FOR CLINICAL PRACTICE

In wrapping up this chapter, we come again to the question "How do I go on?" We have seen that social supports have consistently been associated with a reduced burden of care, but we also noted that this association should not be taken for granted. Health care assessments should reflect this understanding that having more people around who are potential sources of support is not necessarily enough. While both African and Hispanic Americans tend to have larger and closer extended families, this does not necessarily translate into adequate help, at least for Hispanic caregivers. Evaluation of the quality as well as the quantity of support is therefore necessary for the planning of psychological interventions.

The answer to the question of "How do I go on?" obviously has direct implications not only for the primary caregiver but also for her or his support system, because in most cases the well-being of the caregiver is equated with reduced burden on those who are supporting the caregiver. Another way of saying this is that caregiving does not occur in isolation but takes place in an often complex social context—a context in which the health professional should be attentive not only to the needs of the caregiver but also to those who provide support to the caregiver. One obvious clinical strategy is to take a social history as early as possible, a history that documents not only the social resources available to the caregiver but also potential strains and recent departures or bereavements that may have disrupted the caregiver's network. Consistent reminders to caregivers of the need to use, manage, nurture, and maintain this social support may yield therapeutic dividends.

A related issue that has received little if any attention has to do with the social environment. One may well speak of a "caregiving-in-place" scenario, in which the caregiver is living and caring in a long-familiar home and neighborhood. In such instances, the provider of care is more likely to have a well-developed and functional support system. At the other extreme are family caregivers who have not lived in their homes or localities for any length of time and therefore have not developed a good social support system. Residential stability may be a key ingredient in determining the level of burden, as well as the overall success, of caregiving. A thorough psychosocial evaluation addressing such housing/environmental domains is necessary for optimal functioning of the entire caregiver system.

Finally, another question is how the assumption of the caregiving role affects the caregiver's relationship to supports, in both the short and the long term. Just as most of the attention in caregiving research has focused on the giver rather than the receiver of care, little or no attention has been paid to the potentially disruptive effect of having someone in your support network become a caregiver. How often, for example, does the social support system itself "burn out," and what steps might be taken to minimize the risk of such burnout? I recall an instance when a colleague found herself the primary caregiver to her seriously ill mother and carefully divided her network into what amounted to two "teams," alternated in her support seeking so as to reduce the strain on either team. Such strategies may be useful for those caregivers faced with the prospects of a sustained and time-intensive period of helping a family member.

CONCLUSION

It is clear that the study of social supports provided to caregivers is now reaching a stage in which greater depth of study is required and a more complex framework for analysis is needed that will yield reliable data that can be translated into effective evidence-based intervention strategies.

REFERENCES

Acton, G. I. 2002. Self-transcendent views and behaviors: Exploring growth in caregivers of adults with dementia. *Journal of Gerontological Nursing* 28(12):22–30.

Acton, G. J., and Miller, E. W. 2003. Spirituality in caregivers of family members with dementia. *Journal of Holistic Nursing* 21(2):117–30.

Adams, B., Aranda, M., Kemp, B., and Takagi, K. 2002. Ethnic and gender differences in distress among Anglo American, African American, Japanese American and Mexican American spousal caregivers of persons with dementia. *Journal of Clinical Geropsychology* 8(4):279–301.

Allen, K. 1996. Social support from people and pets: Effects on automatic stress responses. *Society for Companion Animal Studies* 3:34–36.

Anderson, M. I., Parmenter, T. R., and Mok, M. 2002. The relationship between neurobehavioural problems of severe traumatic brain injury (TBI), family functioning and the psychological well-being of the spouse/caregiver: Path model analysis. *Brain Injury* 16(9):743–57.

Aneshensel, C. S., Pearlin, L. I., Mullan, J. T., Zarit, S. H., and Whitlatch, C. J. 1995. *Profiles in caregiving: The unexpected career.* San Diego: Academic Press.

Antonucci, T. C. 1994. A life-span view of women's social relations. In B. F. Turner and L. E. Troll (Eds.), *Women growing older* (pp. 239–69). Thousand Oaks, Calif.: Sage.

Aranda, M., and Knight, B. 1997. The influence of ethnicity and culture on the caregiver stress and coping process: A sociocultural review and analysis. *Gerontologist* 37:342–54.

Bass, D. M., McClendon, M. J., Deimling, G. T., and Mukherjee, S. 1994. The influence of a diagnosed mental impairment on family caregiving strain. *Journal of Gerontology: Social Sciences* 49(3):S146–55.

Bengtson, V. L., and Silverstein, M. 1993. Families, aging and social change: Seven agendas for 21st century researchers. In G. L. Maddox and M. P. Lawton (Eds.), *Annual review of gerontology and geriatrics,* Vol. 13 (pp. 15–38). New York: Springer.

Berkman, L. F., Leo-Summers, L., and Horwitz, R. I. 1992. Emotional support and survival after myocardial infarction. *Annals of Internal Medicine* 117:1003–9.

Blake, H., Lincoln, N. B., and Clarke, D. D. 2003. Caregiver strain in spouses of stroke patients. *Clinical Rehabilitation* 17(3):312–17.

Boeije, H. R., Duijnstee, M. S., and Grypdonck, M. H. 2003. Continuation of caregiving among partners who give total care to spouses with multiple sclerosis. *Health and Social Care in the Community* 11(3):242–52.

Bootsma-van der Wiel, A., Gussekloo, J., de Craen, A. J. M., van Exel, E., Knook, D. L., Lagaay, A. M., et al. 2001. Disability in the oldest old: "Can do" or "do do"? *Journal of the American Geriatrics Society* 49:909–14.

Bourgeois, M. S., Dijkstra, K., Burgio, L. D., and Allen, R. S. 2003. Communication skills training for nursing aides of residents with dementia: The impact of measuring performance. *Clinical Gerontologist* 27(1–2):119–28.

Burton, L. M., and Sörensen, S. 1993. Temporal context and the caregiving role: Perspectives from ethnographic studies of multigeneration African-American families. In S. H. Zarit, L. I. Pearlin, and K. W. Schaie (Eds.), *Caregiving systems: Informal and formal helpers: Social structure and aging* (pp. 47–66). Hillsdale, N.J.: Lawrence Erlbaum Associates.

Burton, L. M., and Stack, C. B. 1993. Conscripting kin: Reflections on family, generation and culture. In P. A. Cowan and D. Field (Eds.), *Family, self and society: Toward a new agenda for family research.* Hillsdale, N.J.: Lawrence Erlbaum.

Calderon, V., and Tennstedt, S. T. 1998. Ethnic differences in the expression of caregiver burden: Results of a qualitative study. *Journal of Gerontological Social Work* 30(1/2):159–78.

Carnelley, K. B., Wortman, C. B., and Kessler, R. C. 1999. The impact of widowhood on depression: Findings from a prospective survey. *Psychological Medicine* 29(5):1111–23.

Chappell, N. L., and Reid, R. C. 2002. Burden and well-being among caregivers: Examining the distinction. *Gerontologist* 42:772–80.

Chiriboga, D. A. 1994. Of career paths and expectations: Comments on Pearlin and Aneshensel's "Caregiving: The Unexpected Career." *Social Justice Research* 7(4):391–400.

Chiriboga, D. A., Black, S. A., Aranda, M., and Markides, K. 2002. Stress and depressive symptoms among Mexican American elderly. *Journal of Gerontology: Psychological Sciences* 57B(6):P559–68.

Chiriboga, D. A., Yee, B. W. K., and Weiler, P. G. 1992. Stress in the context of caring. In L. Montada, S-H Filipp, and M. Lerner (Eds.), *Life crises and experiences of loss in adulthood* (pp. 95–118). New York: Plenum.

Clark, P. C., Shields, C. G., Aycock, D., and Wolf, S. L. 2003. Preliminary reliability and validity of a family caregiver conflict scale for stroke. *Progess in Cardiovascular Nursing* 18(2): 77–82, 92.

Coen, R. F., O'Boyle, C. A., Swanwick, G. R. J., and Coakley, D. 1999. Measuring the impact on relatives of caring for people with Alzheimer's disease. *Psychology and Health* 14(2): 253–61.

Cohen, S., Doyle, W. J., Skoner, D. P., Rabin, B. S., and Gwaltney, J. M. 1997. Social ties and susceptibility to the common cold. *Journal of the American Medical Association* 277:1940–44.

Coyne, J. C., Wortman, C. B., and Lehman, D. R. 1988. The other side of support: Emotional over-involvement and miscarried helping. In B. H. Gottlieb (Ed.), *Social support: Formats, processes, and effects* (pp. 305–30). Beverly Hills: Sage.

Deimling, G. T., Smerglia, V. L., and Schaefer, M. L. 2001. The impact of family environment and decision-making satisfaction on caregiver depression: A path analytic model. *Journal of Aging and Health* 13(1):47–71.

Dilworth-Anderson, P., Williams, S. W., and Cooper, T. 1999. Family caregiving to elderly African Americans: Caregiver types and structures. *Journals of Gerontology: Psychological Sciences and Social Sciences* 54(4):S237–41.

Dilworth-Anderson, P., Williams, I. C., and Gibson, B. E. 2002. Issues of race, ethnicity and culture in caregiving research: A 20-year review (1980–2000). *Gerontologist* 42:237–72.

Doty, M. M. 2003. *Hispanic patients' double burden: Lack of health insurance and limited English*. Publication No. 592 (February 2003). New York: The Commonwealth Fund. Also available at www.cmwf.org.

Edwards, N. E., and Scheetz, P. S. 2002. Predictors of burden for caregivers of patients with Parkinson's disease. *Journal of Neuroscience Nursing* 34(4):184–90.

Fitten, L. J., Ortiz, F., and Ponton, M. 2001. Frequency of Alzheimer's disease and other dementias in a community-outreach sample of Hispanics. *Journal of the American Geriatrics Society* 49:1301–8.

Gaugler, J. E., Davy, A., Pearlin, L. I., and Zarit, S. H. 2000. Modeling caregiver adaptation over time: The longitudinal impact of behavioral problems. *Psychology and Aging* 15(3):437–50.

Glenwick, D. S., Slutzsky, M. R., and Garfinkel, E. 2001. Teaching a course in abnormal psychology and behavior intervention skills for nursing home aides. *Teaching of Psychology* 28(2):133–36.

Gurland, B. J., Wilder, D. E., Lantigua, R., Stern, Y., Chen, J., Killeffer, E. H. P., and Mayeux, R. 1999. Rates of dementia in three ethnoracial groups. *International Journal of Geriatric Psychiatry* 14(6):481–93.

Haley, W. E., LaMonde, L. A., Han, B., Burton, A. M., and Schonwetter, R. 2003. Predictors of depression and life satisfaction among spousal caregivers in hospice: Application of a stress process model. *Journal of Palliative Medicine* 6(2):215–24.

Haley, W. E., Roth, D. L., Coleton, M. I., Ford, G. R., West, C. A. C., Collins, R. P., and Isobe, T. L. 1996. Appraisal, coping and social support as mediators of well-being in black and white family caregivers of patients with Alzheimer's disease. *Journal of Consulting and Clinical Psychology* 64:1221–29.

Harrington, M. 2000. The American Mindset on Social Supports for Families and Children. On website for "Grantmakers for Children, Youth & Families," www.gcyf.org/pubs/circles/harrington.pdf (accessed 10/9/03).

Hogan, D. P., and Spencer, L. J. 1993. Kin structure and assistance in aging societies. In G. L. Maddox and M. P. Lawton (Eds.), *Annual review of gerontology and geriatrics* (pp. 169–86). New York: Springer.

Horwitz, A. V., Reinhard, S. C., and Howell-White, S. 1996. Caregiving as reciprocal exchange in families with seriously mentally-ill members. *Journal of Health and Social Behavior* 37:149–62.

House, J. S., Umberson, D., and Landis, K. R. 1988. Structure and processes of social support. *Annual Review of Sociology* 14:293–318.

Hudson, P. L., Aranda, S., and McMurray, N. E. 2002. Intervention development for enhanced lay palliative caregiver support: The use of focus groups. *European Journal of Cancer Care* 11:262–70.

Jackson, J. S., and Antonucci, T. C. 1992. Social support processes in the health and effective functioning of the elderly. In M. L. Wykle and E. Kahana (Eds.), *Stress and health among the elderly.* New York: Springer, pp. 72–95.

Jackson, J. S., Antonucci, T. C., and Gibson, R. S. 1995. Ethnic and cultural factors in research on aging and mental health: A life-course perspective. In D. K. Padgett (Ed.), *Handbook of ethnicity, aging and mental health* (pp. 22–46), Westport, Conn.: Greenwood Press.

Janevic, M. R., and Connell, C. M. 2001. Racial, ethnic, and cultural differences in the dementia caregiving experience: Recent findings. *Gerontologist* 31:334–47.

Jang, Y., Borenstein-Graves, A., Haley, W. E., Small, B. J., and Mortimer, J. A. 2003. Determination of a sense of mastery in African American and white older adults. *Journal of Gerontology: Social Sciences* 58B(4):S221–24.

Karasawa, K., Hata, T., Gushiken, N, and Hasegawa, J. 2003. Depression among Japanese informal caregivers for elderly people. *Psychology, Health and Medicine* 8(3):371–76.

Keys to Successful Caregiving. www.cchs.net/health/health-info/docs/2200/2242.asp?index=9226 (accessed 10/17/03).

Kiecolt-Glaser, J. K. 1999. Stress, personal relationships, and immune function: Health implications. *Brain, Behavior, and Immunity* 13(1):61–72.

Kim, J. S., and Lee, E. H. 2003. Cultural and noncultural predictors of health outcomes in Korean daughter and daughter-in-law caregivers. *Public Health Nursing* 20(2):111–19.

Krause, N., and Borawski-Clark, E. 1995. Clarifying the functions of social support in later life. *Research on Aging* 16(3):251–79.

Kuipers, E., and Moore, E. 1995. Expressed emotion and staff-client relationships: Implications for community care of the severely mentally ill. *International Journal of Mental Health* 24(3):13–26.

Langer, S., Abrams, J., and Syrjala, K. 2003. Caregiver and patient marital satisfaction and affect following hematopoietic stem cell transplantation: A prospective, longitudinal investigation. *Psychooncology* 12(3):239–53.

Lerner, M. J., Ross, M., and Miller, D. T. (Eds.). 2002. *The justice motive in everyday life*. Cambridge: Cambridge University Press.

Lerner, M., Somers, D., Reid, D., Chiriboga, D., and Tierney, M. 1991. Adult children as caregivers: Egocentric biases in judgments of sibling contributions. *Gerontologist* 31:746–55.

Lewinter, M. 2003. Reciprocities in caregiving relationships in Danish elder care. *Journal of Aging Studies* 17(3):357–77.

Lewis, M. A., and Rook, K. S. 1999. Social control in personal relationships: Impact on health behaviors and psychological distress. *Health Psychology* 18(1):63–71.

Lilly, M. L., Richards, B. S., and Buckwalter, K. C. 2003. Friends and social support in dementia caregiving: Assessment and intervention. *Journal of Gerontological Nursing* 29(1):29–36.

Lin, N. 1999. Social networks and status attainment. *Annual Review of Sociology* 25:467–87.

Lincoln, N. B., Francis, V. M., Lilley, S. A., Sharma, J. C., and Summerfield, M. 2003. Evaluation of a stroke family support organiser: A randomized controlled trial. *Stroke* 34(1):116–21.

Loke, A. Y., Liu, C. F., and Szeto, Y. 2003. The difficulties faced by informal caregivers of patients with terminal cancer in Hong Kong and the available social support. *Cancer Nursing* 26(4):276–83.

Lowenthal, M. F., and Haven, C. 1968. Interaction and adaptation: Intimacy as a critical variable. *American Sociological Review* 33:20–30.

Lubben, J. 1988. Assessing social networks among elderly populations. *Family and Community Health* 11:42–52.

Mace, N. L., and Rabins, P. V. 1999. *The 36-hour day: A family guide to caring for persons with Alzheimer disease, related dementing illnesses, and memory loss in later life* (3rd ed.). Baltimore: Johns Hopkins University Press.

Magliano, L., Fiorillo, A., Malangone, C., Marasco, C., Guarneri, M., and Maj, M. 2003. The effect of social network on burden and pessimism in relatives of patients with schizophrenia. *American Journal of Orthopsychiatry* 73(3):302–9.

McNeil, J. M. 1999. Preliminary estimates on caregiving from wave 7 of the 1996 survey of income and program participation. No. 231. Washington, D.C.: U.S. Department of Commence, Bureau of the Census. Also available at website: www.census.gov/dusd/MAB/wp231.pdf (accessed 9/9/03).

McRae, M. B., Thompson, D. A., and Cooper, S. 1999. Black churches as therapeutic groups. *Journal of Multicultural Counseling and Development* 27(4):207–20.

Martire, L. M., Schulz, R., Keefe, F. J., Starz, T. W., Osial, T. A. Dew, M. A., and Reynolds, C. F. 2003. Feasibility of a dyadic intervention for management of osteoarthritis: A pilot study with older patients and their spousal caregivers. *Aging and Mental Health* 7(1):53–60.

Martire, L. M., Schulz, R., Mittelmark, M. B., and Newsom, J. T. 1999. Stability and change in older adults' social contact and social support: The Cardiovascular Health Study. *Journals of Gerontology: Social Sciences* 54B(5):S302–11.

Martire, L. M., Stephens, M. A. P., Druley, J. A., and Wojno, W. C. 2002. Negative reactions to received spousal support: Predictors and consequences of miscarried support. *Health Psychology* 21(2):167–76.

Nadler, A. 1997. Personality and help seeking. In G. R. Pierce, B. Lakey, I. G. Sarason, and B. R. Sarason (Eds.), *Sourcebook of social support and personality* (pp. 379–407). New York: Plenum.

Neufeld, A., and Harrison, M. J. 2003. Unfulfilled expectations and negative interactions: Non-support in the relationships of women caregivers. *Journal of Advanced Nursing* 41(4):323–31.

Newsom, J. T., Nishishiba, M., Morgan, D. L., and Rook, K. S. 2003. The relative importance of three domains of positive and negative social exchanges: A longitudinal model with comparable measure. *Psychology and Aging* 18(4):746–54.

O'Connell, B., Baker, L., and Prosser, A. 2003. The educational needs of caregivers of stroke survivors in acute and community settings. *Journal of Neuroscience and Nursing* 35(1):21–28.

Ory, M. G., Hoffman, R. R. III, Yee, J. L., Tennstedt, S., and Schulz, R. 1999. Prevalence and impact of caregiving: A detailed comparison between dementia and nondementia caregivers. *Gerontologist* 39:177–85.

Perry, J. 2002. Wives giving care to husbands with Alzheimer's disease: A process of interpretive caring. *Res Nurs Health* 25(4):307–16.

Pillemer, K., Suitor, J. J., and Wethington, E. 2003. Integrating theory, basic research, and intervention: Two case studies from caregiving research. *Gerontologist* 43 (Special Issue 1): 19–28.

Riley, D., and Eckenrode, J. 1986. Social ties: Subgroup differences in cost and benefits. *Journal of Personality and Social Psychology* 51:770–78.

Rook, K. S., Pietromonaco, P. R., and Lewis, M. 1994. When are dysphoric individuals distressing to others and vice versa? Effects of friendship, similarity, and interaction task. *Journal of Personality and Social Psychology* 67(3):548–59.

Sanchez-Ayendez, M. 1998. Middle-aged Puerto-Rican women as primary caregivers to the elderly: A qualitative analysis of everyday dynamics. *Journal of Gerontological Social Work* 30(1/3):75–97.

Sarason, I. G., Sarason, B. R., Shearin, E. N., and Pierce, G. R. 1987. A brief measure of social support: Practical and theoretical implications. *Journal of Social and Personal Relationships* 4:497–510.

Schulz, R., Burgio, L., Burns, R., Eisdorfer, C., Gallagher-Thompson, D., Gitlin, L. N., and Mahoney, D. F. 2003. Respite for Enhancing Alzheimer's Caregiver Health (REACH): Overview, site-specific outcomes, and future directions. *Gerontologist* 43:514–20.

Schwartz, C., Meisenhelder, J. B., Ma, Y., and Reed, G. 2003. Altruistic social interest behaviors are associated with better mental health. *Psychosomatic Medicine* 65(5):778–85.

Secrest, J. S. 2002. How stroke survivors and primary support persons experience nurses in rehabilitation. *Rehabilitation Nursing* 27(5):176–81.

Seeman, T. E., Kaplan, G. A., Knudsen, L., Cohen, R., and Guralnik, J. 1987. Social network ties and mortality among the elderly in the Alameda County Study. *American Journal of Epidemiology* 126(4):714–23.

Shaji, K. S., Smitha, K., Lal, K. P., and Prince, M. J. 2003. Caregivers of people with Alzheimer's disease: A qualitative study from the Indian 10/66 Dementia Research Network. *International Journal of Geriatric Psychiatry* 18(1):1–6.

Siebert, D. C., Mutran, E. J., and Reitzes, D. C. 1999. Friendship and social support: The importance of role identity to aging adults. *Social Work* 44(6):522–33.

Silverstein, M., Chen, X., and Heller, K 1996. Too much of a good thing? Intergenerational social support and the psychological well-being of older parents. *Journal of Marriage and the Family* 58(4):970–82.

Smith, M. 1983 (November). Problem-solving and support groups for nurses and aides in a nursing home. Paper presented at the annual meeting of the Gerontological Society of America.

Song, L-Y., Biegel, D. E., and Milligan, S. E. 1997. Predictors of depressive symptomatology among lower social class caregivers to persons with chronic mental illness. *Community Mental Health Journal* 33(4):269–86.

Sörensen, S., and Pinquart, M. 2000. Vulnerability and access to resources as predictors of preparation for future care needs in the elderly. *Journal of Aging and Health* 12(3):275–300.

Sörensen, S., and Zarit, S. H. 1996. Preparation for caregiving: A study of multigeneration families. *International Journal of Aging and Human Development* 42:43–63.

Spruytte, N., van Audenhove, C., Lammertyn, F., and Storms, G. 2002. The quality of the caregiving relationship in informal care for older adults with dementia and chronic psychiatric patients. *Psychology and Psychotherapy* 75(3):295–311.

Stephens, M. A., Townsend, A. L., Martire, L. M., and Druley, J. A. 2001. Balancing parent care with other roles: Interrole conflict of adult daughter caregivers. *Journal of Gerontology: Psychological Sciences* 56(1):24–34.

Sterling, Y. M., and Peterson, J. W. 2003. Characteristics of African American women caregivers of children with asthma. *American Journal of Maternity and Child Nursing* 28(1):32–38.

Theis, S. L., Biordi, D. L., Coeling, H., Nalepka, C., and Miller, B. 2003. Spirituality in caregiving and care receiving. *Holistic Nursing Practice* 17(1):48–55.

Thoits, P. A. 1999. Self, identity, stress, and mental health. In C. S. Aneshensel, J. C. Phelan, et al. (Eds.), *Handbook of sociology of mental health* (pp. 345–68). New York: Kluwer Academic.

Thomas, P., Chantoin-Merlet, S., Hazif-Thomas, C., Belmin, J., Montagne, B., Clement, J. P., Lebruchec, M., and Billon, R. 2002. Complaints of informal caregivers providing home care for dementia patients: The Pixel Study. *International Journal of Geriatric Psychiatry* 17(1):1034–47.

Tolson, D., Swan, I., and Knussen, C. 2002. Hearing disability: A source of distress for older people and carers. *British Journal of Nursing* 11(15):1021–25.

Toseland, R. W., McCallion, P., Gerber, T., and Banks, S. 2002. Predictors of health and human service use by persons with dementia and their family caregivers. *Social Science and Medicine* 55(7):1255–66.

Tyler, T. R., Boeckman, R. J., Smith, H. J., and Huo, Y. Z. 1997. *Social justice in a diverse society.* Boulder, Colo.: Westview Press.

Unger, J. B., McAvay, G., Bruce, M. L, Berkman, L., and Seeman, T. 1999. Variations in the impact of social network characteristics on physical functioning in elderly persons: MacArthur Studies of Successful Aging. *Journal of Gerontology: Social Sciences* 54B(5):S245–51.

Uphoff, N. 2000. Understanding social capital: Learning from the analysis and experience of participation. In P. Dasgupta and I. Serageldin (Eds.), *Social capital: A multifaceted perspective* (pp. 215–52). Sociological Perspective on Development Series. Washington, D.C.: World Bank.

van den Heuvel, E. T. P., de Witte, L. P., Stewart, R. E., Schure, L. M., Sanderman, R., and Meyboom-de Jong, B. 2002. Long-term effects of a group support program and an individual support program for informal caregivers of stroke patients: Which caregivers benefit the most? *Patient Education Counsel* 47(4):291–99.

Vinokur, A. D., and van Ryn, M. 1993. Social support and undermining in close relationships: Their independent effects on the mental health of unemployed persons. *Journal of Personality and Social Psychology* 65(2):350–59.

von dem Knesebeck, O., and Siegrist, J. 2003. Reported nonreciprocity of social exchange and depressive symptoms: Extending the model of effort-reward imbalance beyond work. *Journal of Psychosomatic Research* 55:209–14.

Wallsten, S. S. 2000. Effects of caregiving, gender, and race on the health, mutuality, and social supports of older couples. *Journal of Aging and Health* 12:90–111.

White, H., McConnell, E., Clipp, E., Branch, L. G., Sloane, R., Pieper, C., and Box, T. L. 2002. *Aging and Mental Health* 6(3):213–21.

Wiles, J. 2003. Informal caregivers' experiences of formal support in a changing context. *Health and Social Care in the Community* 11(3):189–207.

Williams, A. M., Forbes, D. A., Mitchell, J., Essar, M., and Corbett, R. 2003. The influence of income on the experience of informal caregiving: Policy implications. *Health Care for Women International* 24(4):280–91.

Williams, S. W., and Dilworth-Anderson, P. 2002. Systems of social support to families who care for dependent African American elders. *Gerontologist* 42:224–36.

Williams, S. W., Dilworth-Anderson, P., and Goodwin, P. Y. 2003. Caregiver role strain: The contribution of multiple roles and available resources in African American women. *Aging and Mental Health* 7(2):103–12.

Wright, J., Varholak, D., and Costello, J. 2003. Voices from the margin: The nurse aide's role in pain management of institutionalized elders. *American Journal of Alzheimer's Disease and Other Dementias* 18(3):154–58.

Yeh, S. H., Johnson, M. A., and Wang, S. T. 2002. The changes in caregiver burden following nursing home placement. *International Journal of Nursing Studies* 39(6):591–600.

Young, R., and Kahana, E. 1995. The context of caregiving and well-being outcomes among African and Caucasian Americans. *Gerontologist* 35:225–32.

Zank, S., and Schacke, C. 2002. Evaluation of geriatric day care units: Effects on patients and caregivers. *Journal of Gerontology: Psychological Sciences* 57(4):P348–57.

PART 5

Societal Issues of Caregiving

Part V addresses overarching social concerns. Diversity issues, the legal and health care environment, and the current delivery system for dementia health care are investigated. In chapter 12, Margaret P. Norris explores various health policies and their impact on caregiving in America today. She reviews federal policies such as the Family Medical Leave Act, Medicare reimbursement and hospice policies, Medicaid policies for spending down, and the Medicare Catastrophic Coverage Act. She emphasizes the fact that most federal policies do not in fact protect caregivers very well, with the exception of the Medicaid spend-down policies that shield some assets of spouses of patients with dementia entering nursing homes, thus preventing total impoverishment of healthy spouses. Regarding the private system of health care, managed care largely fails those older adults who receive most of their care from family members. Dr. Norris notes that short lengths of stay and failure to reimburse long-term care place the burden on family members who receive no payment for their assistance, and thereby de facto consign the economic, health, and social burden predominantly to women. The badly underfunded Community Mental Health Care Act has likewise kept the burden of dementia care on informal caregivers.

In chapter 13, F. M. Baker discusses the role of ethnic elders in caregiving and how caregiving differs across cultures. She reviews the history of caregiving in African American, Asian American, and Latino American cultures and uses clinical cases to illustrate the special challenges involved in providing such caregivers and care recipients with culturally sensitive care. Dr. Baker makes a special effort to address the challenges faced by caregivers of immigrants in her presentation of a vignette describing two generations of a Japanese American immigrant family in the scenario of a family elder developing dementia. Another case discussion centers on the impact of historical events in the life of a Native American ethnic elder. Dr. Baker promotes use of the LEARN model to facilitate the communication between health professionals and ethnic elders and their families.

In chapter 14, Michele J. Karel and Jennifer Moye discuss ethical implications often faced by caregivers and strategies to guide ethical decision making. They discuss basic ethical principles such as autonomy and beneficence and how these have a role to play in the care of the person with dementia. They address the thorny topics of impairment in decision-making capacity and surrogate decision making. They identify tools for advance directive planning, including values histories, advance proxy plans, durable powers of attorney, wills, and caregivers plans. For protecting the incompetent adult, they discuss the use of conservatorships, guardianships, and alternatives to guardianship. Finally, they describe the role of the health care team, ethics committees, adult protective services, ombuds programs, guardians ad-litem, and the courts in protecting the interests of persons with dementia. The myriad issues in this chapter (and indeed the entire volume) highlight the multiple contexts of ethical debate and the need for overarching principles to guide health professionals' nuanced response to ever-changing clinical situations in the care of older adults with dementia.

CHAPTER TWELVE

Health Care Policies and Caregivers

MARGARET P. NORRIS, PH.D.

As described by the Alzheimer's Association and the National Alliance for Caregiving, "families are the backbone of the long term care system" (Alzheimer's Association and National Alliance for Caregiving, 1997). It is estimated that approximately 25 percent of households provide care for a family member over age 50 (Nguyen, 2000), and roughly 75 percent of older adults residing in the community and needing care from others receive that care from family or other unpaid sources (Liu, Manton, and Liu, 1985). This chapter will review policies that affect the largest system providing care to older adults—the family. First, public policies that affect family caregivers will be covered. This public policy review will be limited to federal policies. Although many states have laws in place that address the needs of caregivers, review of such a large number of policies is beyond the scope of this chapter. Excellent legislative updates for all 50 states are available at the web page for the Family Caregiving Alliance, www.caregiver.org. In addition to the federal policies, this chapter will address private policies, such as those established by the private insurance industry via managed care and national private organizations. As seen below, some of these public and private policies provide support and assistance to caregivers, such as the Family Medical Leave Act. Unfortunately, other policies restrict or prohibit assistance to caregivers. For example, the managed care system of the private insurance industry has had a detrimental impact on families providing the majority of care to elders. Currently the onus of responsibility for supporting family caregivers primarily lies with private organizations.

Numerous federal policies affect family caregivers. As reviewed below, these include (1) the Family Medical Leave Act, (2) Medicare policies restricting psychotherapy services for families, (3) Medicare hospice end-of-life care, (4) Medicaid policies for "spending down" and the Medicare Catastrophic Coverage Act, and (5) federal research programs. These initiatives, which both provide and withhold assistance to family caregivers, especially affect families caring for persons with dementia.

THE DEMAND AND COSTS OF CAREGIVING

No other group has been so directly affected by caregiving policies as caregivers of persons with dementia. The estimated number of caregivers of persons with dementia in the United States ranges from 2.4 to 3.1 million (Schulz, O'Brien, Bookwala, and Fleissner, 1995). Because of the cognitive, behavioral, physical, and emotional impairments characteristic of dementia, the care for persons with dementia is thought to be more demanding and stressful than the care for persons with other chronic illnesses and disabilities. This difference is well documented. Compared to other caregivers, dementia caregivers have significantly worse physical and mental health, emotional stress, financial strain, and employment conflicts due to their caregiver responsibilities (Ory et al., 1999). Dementia caregivers also spend more time in their caregiving duties, which are more emotionally demanding. They have fewer relatives and friends available to assist them, and they report more family conflict over the care of the patient. Not surprisingly, dementia caregivers also are more likely than others to avail themselves of support services such as respite care, outside meal delivery, and personal care or nursing service. Despite having more support services, dementia caregivers nevertheless receive very little assistance. Only a small minority (14–20%) report receiving services such as respite care, transportation, or assistance with housework. Surprisingly, the least commonly used service was support groups; only 9.7 percent had taken part in a caregiver support group (Ory et al., 1999). This figure is especially troubling given the benefits of caregiver support and counseling services. For example, caregivers receiving group and individual counseling kept their spouses at home for 329 days longer, on average, than those in the control group (Mittelman et al., 1996). While the cost savings of delayed institutionalization are substantial, little research directly questions whether the emotional cost of postponing nursing home placement is a worthy goal. Delayed nursing home placement may have substantial negative outcomes, such as decline in the emotional and physical health of both the patient and the caregiver. Our reliance on family caregivers may prevent us from asking whether postponing nursing home placement is worth the trade-off of reducing economic costs if it also means increasing family burden and risking more rapid health decline of patients and caregivers.

The cost of caring for persons with Alzheimer disease in the United States is estimated to be $90–$100 billion annually (Freed, Elder, Lauderdale, and Carter, 1999; Riggs, 2001). This figure is roughly half the estimated value of the care provided by families, $196 billion per year (Arno, Levine, and Memmott, 1999). Nonprofessional caregivers are providing approximately 75 percent of the care, and their unpaid services constitute enormous "invisible" costs. Clearly, replacing family caregiving with formal systems and institutions would cause costs to soar (Arno et al., 1999; Riggs, 2001).

Medicare per capita expenditure for persons with Alzheimer disease is 70 percent more than for care recipients without Alzheimer disease (Eppig and Poisal, 1997). These high costs are especially astonishing given that they do not include the long-term care and prescription drugs that are among the highest care costs for these patients. Yet it is not surprising that persons with Alzheimer disease incur costly medical expenses. Memory deficits interfere with accurate medication use and healthy nutrition. Poor judgment and awareness diminish recognition of signs of infection or other changes in physical condition. Injuries are also more common as a result of declining judgment. These mental and physical impairments result in more frequent and lengthier hospitalizations for persons with Alzheimer disease, many of which could be prevented if Medicare paid for personal care and maintenance therapies that would greatly reduce the risk of these crises (Riggs, 2001).

Family caregivers of persons with dementia are not, of course, the only group bearing the burdens of caring for loved ones. Considerable negative burdens have been documented in examining the impact on families of persons with other serious illnesses—for example, respiratory failure, congestive heart failure, chronic obstructive pulmonary disease, cancer, Parkinson disease, and other neurological illnesses (Covinsky et al., 1994). In the latter study, 20 percent had a family member who had to quit work to care for the patient, 31 percent lost most or all of the family savings, and 29 percent lost the family's major source of income. These financial losses occurred despite the fact that 96 percent of the patients had medical insurance, reflecting the fact that much of the home care expenses are not covered by private or public insurance. Other burdens included moving to a less expensive home, delaying medical care for another family member, and altering education plans for a family member. Because older individuals with Alzheimer disease are more likely to have comorbid medical problems such as delirium and/or neurological problems such as Parkinson disease, the cumulative cognitive and medical impairments will have a further detrimental impact on the burden of their caregivers.

PUBLIC POLICIES AFFECTING CAREGIVERS
The Family and Medical Leave Act (FMLA)

The FMLA is designed to prevent employees from losing their jobs as a result of taking leave of absence to care for an ill family member. Signed in 1993, it is one of the few federal policy initiatives that directly address the needs of family caregivers. The impetus to create such legislation was a dramatic shift in employment patterns: large numbers of women had entered the work force creating the dual responsibilities of work duties and caring for dependents (Ripple, 1999). A brief history of the bill reveals a reluctant reception for supporting family caregivers. The initial iteration of the FMLA failed approval by Congress under the Reagan administration. Although the ensuing Congress approved a family leave bill, President George Herbert Bush then vetoed it. The current FMLA then became the first piece of domestic legislation signed by President Clinton (Hudson and Gonyea, 2000). The primary benefit offered by the FMLA is guaranteed job reinstatement following a leave defined under the provisions of the law.

The FMLA provides for 12 weeks of unpaid leave for spouses or children caring for the patient. Reasons for the leave permitted under the law include birth and care of a newborn child, placement of an adopted or foster child into the family, illness of the employee, and care for his or her spouse, child, or parent with a serious health condition. The law defines "serious health condition" in extensive detail. The FMLA limitations are numerous: (1) It allows only for unpaid leave, rendering it irrelevant to many middle and lower-middle-class families. (2) It is limited to 12 weeks; thus its relevance to the care of persons with dementia is quite limited. (3) It is limited to spouses and children of the patient and does not apply to other family members or friends who may be willing to provide the care. (4) There are numerous eligibility restrictions; for example, it does not apply to employers with 50 or fewer employees. As a result, it is estimated that only 55 percent of Americans are covered under its provisions (Gordon, 1997). Given these limitations, how much assistance does the FMLA provide? For example, a woman earning a limited income from a small company may be willing to care for her sister with dementia, but the FMLA fails her on account of all the restrictions listed above: she is not likely to be able to afford to take unpaid leave; a maximum 12-week leave does not address the long-term course of dementia; she is not covered under the law because her relation to the patient is sister; she works for a small company. Thus the FMLA provides no assistance in this situation, which is a rather common one. Individual state laws, collective bargaining agreements, or corporate policies may offer additional provisions and flexible work arrangements such as flextime, "banking" sick leave, telecommuting, reduced work hours, and job sharing (Nguyen, 2000). Overall, the FMLA is a first step toward federal government recognition of the assistance needed if family caregivers are going to assume the main burden of caring for frail older adults. Nevertheless, the benefits (and costs) of the FMLA are considered modest. It has been perceived as a symbolic effort that is a case of "policy minimalization," that is, the needs originally intended to be addressed by the law are largely missing from the final product (Hudson and Gonyea, 2000).

Medicare Policies

Medicare, the federal health insurance program for older Americans, has reimbursement policies that are unfavorable to caregivers and persons with dementia. One of the reactions to the escalating medical costs of Medicare has been a large-scale program to reduce fraud, waste, and abuse in billing (Operation Restore Trust). While such programs are irrefutably necessary, there are tragic examples of the pendulum swinging too far in the direction of excluding appropriate services. An unfortunate example of this was the automatic denial (until September 2001) of psychological and restorative therapies for persons with a diagnosis of dementia, based on an unsubstantiated assumption that such patients would be unable to benefit from such services. Certainly, the denial of these services for persons with dementia made many caregiving situations more strained and difficult. The Center for Medicare and Medicaid Services (CMS) no longer allows such arbitrary exclusions, but this recent ruling took years of effort by the American Bar Association, the Alzheimer's Association, and professional organizations representing psychiatry and psychology. Carriers may still deny payment following audits of records that fail to document evidence that the patient has the potential to benefit from services. This may be a fair compromise, since only persons with mild to moderate deficits in the earlier stages of dementia are able to benefit from those services. Unscrupulous providers who are providing psychotherapy to severely impaired persons with dementia should be forced to alter their practices by refusal of payment for such inappropriate services.

One of the most troublesome federal policies to family caregivers is the exclusion of Medicare benefits for services in which the patient is not physically present. For psychology and psychiatry services, this means that counseling the family with the patient present (procedure code 90847) is reimbursable, whereas counseling the family without the patient present (procedure code 90846) is not reimbursed. (A handful of individual Medicare carriers override this exclusion and reimburse for 90846 services.) Consultations with family caregivers are critical for appropriate and safe management of the patient. Presumably almost all geropsychologists have treated or assessed persons with dementia for whom there was a need to meet alone with the patient's family to have candid discussions about the patient's prognosis and management. It must be rare for a geropsychologist to conduct all family consultations with the patient present. To hold these discussions in a frank manner, to allow the caregivers to honestly address their questions and struggles, and to preserve the dignity of the patient, at least some of these consultations must be conducted without the patient present. Furthermore, this exclusion prohibits payment for cost-effective psychoeducational group therapy provided to caregivers. As a result, peer caregivers, trainees in graduate programs, or volunteer mental health professionals provide most of these group-support services for no fee.

Hospice Policies

In the late stage of illness, Alzheimer patients may be considered terminal and qualify for hospice services. Unfortunately, end-of-life care is another arena in which federal policies can impede assistance given to caregivers. Hospice care is available to Medicare beneficiaries if their physicians have determined that they are likely to die within six months. These patients must then choose between receiving medical services through the traditional Medicare system or palliative care provided by hospice and paid for by Medicare (Peres, 2003). Dying patients opting for hospice are limited to the services provided by hospice, including bereavement counseling offered only through hospice. Hospice patients are no longer eligible to receive mental health services provided by a private mental health provider of their choice. Other health care services are also denied to hospice patients. Skilled nursing home care is available only if the patient is receiving care unrelated to their terminal illness, a stipulation that may be atypical and hard to document because it is rare that multiple illnesses are completely discrete conditions (Peres, 2003). The same disqualification occurs for hospice patients who would otherwise be eligible for home health benefits. These restrictive Medicare rules for terminal patients result in families being able to rely only on hospice services, forfeiting the many other services provided by traditional Medicare, and often being left without health care professionals of their choice to help them at this emotionally painful time.

Medicaid Policies for "Spending Down" and the Medicare Catastrophic Coverage Act

Not all care for elderly persons takes place at home. Many families face the time when 24-hour care is better provided in a nursing home. Clearly, the cost of skilled nursing care is far higher than most families can afford to pay. Approximately 47 percent of nursing home costs are paid by Medicaid (Levit et al., 1997). Medicaid is the health care insurance program funded by the federal and state governments to provide insurance to indigent individuals. Without Medicaid assistance, low-income patients would not have access to nursing home care. Many elders qualify for Medicaid by "spending down," depleting assets down to eligibility levels established in their state. Before the Medicare Catastrophic Coverage Act (MCCA) of 1988, depletion of assets resulted in large-scale impoverishment of the spouses of nursing home residents. The laudable purpose of this policy is to prevent spouses of nursing home residents from becoming impoverished by "spending down" all their assets in order for the ailing spouse to qualify for Medicaid. Within one year after the MCCA was passed, provisions that protected larger amounts of the patient's assets were repealed; however, provisions to prevent spousal impoverishment were preserved (Walker, Gruman, and Robison, 1999). Currently, spouses of institutionalized care recipients are allowed to keep one-half of the couple's assets up to certain limits, which vary across states (Cohen, Kumar, and Wallack, 1993; Walker et al., 1999).

There are common misunderstandings about the Medicaid payment for nursing home care. First, only 33 to 40 percent of individuals entering nursing homes are immediately eligible for Medicaid (Cohen et al., 1993). Most enter nursing homes as private payers and spend down quickly; 40 percent deplete assets within one year (Walker et al., 1999) and three-fourths spend down within two years of admission (Cohen et al., 1993). Even after all the patient's assets have been spent, residents continue to pay a significant portion of their nursing home care because private pensions and social security income are used to pay the nursing home first, followed by Medicaid paying the difference. Hence, far more private resources of lower- and middle-class residents go into nursing home care than is commonly recognized. Without further legal protection for spouses' income and assets, some caregivers will continue to face dire economic devastation.

Federal Research Programs

The federal government supports caregivers through large-scale funded research. The Resources for Enhancing Alzheimer's Caregiver Health (REACH) is an excellent example of such support. Established in 1995, this multisite research program, sponsored by the National Institute on Aging and the National Institute on Nursing Research, conducts social and behavioral research on interventions directed toward caregivers for Alzheimer and related dementia disorders (Schulz et al., 2003). Federal grant projects examine a myriad of caregiver programs, including the effectiveness of interventions to reduce caregiver depression, behavioral techniques to improve caregiver and patient well-being, methods to reduce caregiver distress, systems to increase service use in caregivers, strategies to improve caregivers' physical health, and many others. Readers can obtain lists of past and current studies funded by the National Institute of Health on the web page for CRISP (Computer Retrieval of Information on Scientific Projects): www.crisp.cit.nih.gov/. These research projects play a vital role in improving the quality of care for our elders, especially for that majority who are cared for at home by nonprofessionals. Unfortunately, it is also important to recognize that research funding for caregiver intervention pales in comparison to that spent by the pharmaceutical industry to develop drugs that have very modest benefits in mitigating dementia symptoms.

PRIVATE SYSTEMS AFFECTING CAREGIVERS

The managed-care delivery system for health care embraced by the private insurance industry often fails older adults who are receiving much of their care from family members (Boland, 1996; Gordon, 1997). Primary methods used by managed care to contain costs are decreased use of hospitalizations and reduced length of stay. In fact, these goals have been realized with hospital admissions and lengths of stay both down 20 percent, resulting in a 40 percent decline in hospital days (Gordon, 1997). These reductions are not, of course, the result of miraculous recoveries; on the contrary, managed care is now depending on the unpaid assistance from family caregivers to step in where nursing staff in hospitals provided care in the past. The inevitable although rarely recognized outcome of managed care's containment efforts is that patients are discharged in more acute and unstable physical conditions to their homes, where family and friends assume responsibility for their recovery care (Barter, 1996; Gordon, 1997). Gordon (1997) further points out that the repercussions have inordinately affected women. The nurses whose employment conditions have been tightened and downsized by managed care are predominantly female, and those caring for these more acutely ill patients at home are roughly 75 percent female.

Rooted in an assumption that most health care targets acute medical problems (Boland, 1996), managed care is an inherent mismatch with treatment of chronic health problems that are most common in late life (e.g., heart disease, diabetes, and dementia). These conditions are much more difficult to appropriately manage with a cost effectiveness priority. Chronic conditions need a multidisciplinary approach to coordinate home-based and community-based care that depends heavily on family caregivers (Boland, 1996).

This current atmosphere of managed care and overreliance on family caregivers is an about-face from the past days of institutional care for persons with mental illness. During the era in which psychoanalysis and classical behaviorism dominated the theories and treatment of mental illness, families were often viewed as central causes of emotional disturbance. Thus systematic isolation from families was often seen as a therapeutic component to long-term hospitalizations. Families of the mentally ill were sorely stigmatized. The zeitgeist changed dramatically in the 1950s when institutional care came under fire for providing less than humane, albeit expensive care. By the 1960s, passage of the Community Mental Health Act reflected the transformed values for ending long-term hospitalizations and returning patients to their communities. Quite unfortunately, however, the Community Mental Health Act was badly underfunded, rendering its goals unobtainable. Prevention and community care were never fully realized. "So, after years of forced isolation and a decade of blame, families were asked to do what expensive institutions and health care professionals failed to do—provide care for persons with serious mental illness" (Camann, 1996, p. 482). The initial resistance to the FMLA and its ultimately modest benefits to family caregivers suggest the zeitgeist in forty years has not yet entirely changed.

Numerous private organizations provide a great deal of the caregiver support that government systems fail to provide. Among the leading caregiver support organizations are the National Alliance for Caregiving, the Alzheimer's Association, the National Family Caregivers Association, the Well Spouse Foundation, and the National Association of Area Agencies on Aging. These organizations provide many functions, including public awareness, advocacy, access to resources, training and educational materials, national conferences, research funding, referral services, and various means of connecting caregivers via support groups, list serves, and letter writing. Most of these organizations are nonprofit, although some (e.g., the Well Spouse Foundation) require membership dues. The National Alliance for Caregiving is a coalition organization that includes more than thirty national organizations. Such coalition efforts are critical for effective advocacy and lobbying efforts. Nevertheless, in the absence of federal governance, private organizations can reflect piecemeal approaches without authority and weight.

IMPLICATIONS FOR CLINICAL PRACTICE

This review points toward numerous pragmatic actions for clinicians to undertake in their work with caregivers. These recommendations include educating caregivers and working with professional organizations to advocate on behalf of caregivers.

Since many of the public policies reviewed above are typically unknown to caregivers, clinicians can provide much assistance by informing caregivers about the FMLA, the limitations of opting into Medicare hospice, or how to gain information about spending down and protecting the assets and income of the spouse. In addition, clinicians should inform caregivers about the risks of exceeding realistic caregiving limits, including the health declines, emotional stress, financial strain, and employment problems that often accompany demanding caregiver responsibilities. Much of this education can be accomplished by providing pamphlets and brochures from associations such as the Alzheimer's Association and the National Family Caregivers Association. Caregivers also need to be encouraged to take advantage of assistance from others, both informally through family and friends who are able to assist, as well as through formal systems that provide respite care, meal delivery, and home health care. Many caregivers either do not know about the availability of such programs or are reluctant to use them without the recommendation and sanction of their health care providers. Caregivers need to be strongly encouraged to attend to their own physical and mental health; referrals to other health care providers are often central to this effort. Further, many caregivers do not know that psychotherapy is a benefit of either their own medical insurance or through their spouse's insurance. Such information is often key to putting the plan into action. Finally, some caregivers need realistic perspectives on nursing home care. Many individuals have out-of-date and erroneous perceptions of nursing homes. Caregivers need to be counseled about the advances that have been made in the quality of care in nursing homes, the critical role that the caregiver continues to provide after nursing home placement, and the detriments to the patient's and caregiver's health when home care extends for longer than it should.

In addition to educating caregivers, health care professionals can more broadly support them by extending their direct services to advocacy efforts. It is vital to advocate for caregivers by staying abreast of laws, regulations, and public policies that affect these issues. Both national and state legislative updates are available at the previously cited web address, www.caregiver.org, in the Public Policy and Research page. For example, the Lifespan Respite Care Act awaits approval by the House of Representatives; health care professionals should be on the alert for developments of this and future laws that need grassroots efforts to support their passage. Also, most professional organizations have public policy committees to keep their members informed about upcoming legislation and policies that either hinder or assist the people served by the profession, such as caregivers. The American Association of Geriatric Psychiatry, the American Psychological Association's clinical geropsychology section, and Psychologists in Long Term Care are examples of professional organizations with proactive public policy committees that advocate on behalf of patients and their caregivers. These and other organizations have been successful in past advocacy efforts. Convincing the Center for Medicare and Medicaid Services to prohibit automatic denial of payment for some therapy services provided to all persons with a diagnosis of dementia is a good example of such successes. Caregiver associations, such as those mentioned above, are also vehicles for providing systemic support for caregivers. Health care professionals who provide services to caregivers can make a more potent impact on the health and well-being of caregivers by supporting these large-scale advocacy efforts.

CONCLUSION

If the current caregiver support policies are inadequate, the forecast for the future is ominous (Riggs, 2001). Several demographic shifts will further strain the reliance on families for most caregiving. There will be a large increase in the number of older adults in need of assistance as the baby boom generation ages. Simultaneously, the decrease in the birth rate means there will be fewer children to provide this care. The trend for family members to reside in different geographical locations will also reduce the number of caregivers who are locally available. The redefinition of families resulting from divorce and remarriages will challenge assumptions of who is responsible for the aging parent. Finally, the overreliance on women to provide parental care while also working full-time and raising children (and grandchildren) may run its course and meet resistance and burnout. All these factors suggest that the availability of family for elder care is likely to erode in the future.

This review of policies that affect caregivers clearly indicates that our societal and political systems have created some policies that lend a helping hand to caregivers, whereas other policies turn a blind eye on them. Health care policies are, of course, an evolving state of affairs. Reform may lie ahead. The Lifespan Respite Care Act (Senate Bill 538) was passed in the Senate in 2003 and awaits approval by the House of Representatives. If passed, this legislation will provide $90 million for competitive grants to states and eligible agencies to fund respite care programs such as emergency respite care, training and recruitment for respite workers and caregivers, and program evaluation (Elmore, 2003). Unlike the FMLA, this law would apply to any unpaid adult caregiver, not just parents or children. In addition to the Lifespan Respite Care Act, further legislative and regulatory changes in Medicare and Medicaid are inevitable. Certainly, there is better public recognition of the needs of caregivers than there was only twenty years ago.

Our elder care system is highly dependent on family caregivers. This is not merely an economic factor. Most older adults who are in need of assistance prefer to stay in their homes and receive their care from family members (Forti, Johnson, and Graber, 2000). Yet we must recognize that this comes at significant financial, physical, and emotional costs to the caregivers (Schulz et al., 1995). As the geriatric population expands in the future with the aging of the baby boomer generation, policy makers are likely to face demands from the public and health care sector to adopt low-cost support systems to aid families in their care for the aged population. We will have to address such questions as: (1) At what point are we expecting too much of the families? (2) Under what circumstances do families do better than formal systems in caring for older, disabled patients, and vice versa? (3) Relatedly, now that research has identified factors that help prevent or delay institutionalization, should we also ask when patients are better cared for in nursing homes than at home? Are there circumstances in which keeping the person at home is not in the best interest of the patient? Certainly there are such circumstances but there is a dearth of research in this area because we have accepted the assumption that home care is better than institutionalized care. (4) How do the costs and outcomes of recent drug therapies for Alzheimer disease compare to family support services? While ample funding is available to research drugs that may offer modest hope for efficacy, there are relatively minimal funds to provide caregivers with the psychoeducational support that we know is of great benefit. It is reasonable to speculate that family support services are significantly less expensive and more effective than current drug therapy (Freed et al., 1999). Such debates about how to allocate financial resources for providing health care for older Americans will intensify in the years ahead. Clearly, health care policies have not yet adjusted to the dependence we have cultivated on family and unpaid caregivers.

REFERENCES

Alzheimer's Association, and National Alliance for Caregiving. 1997. Who cares? Families caring for person's with Alzheimer's disease. Retrieved October 2003 from www.alz.org/ resource center/by topic/basic facts.htm#statistics.

Arno, P. S., Levine, C., and Memmott, M. M. 1999. The economic value of caregiving. *Health Affairs* 18:182–88.

Barter, M. 1996. Unlicensed assistive personnel and lay caregivers in the home. *Home Care Provider* 1:131–33.

Boland, P. 1996. The role of reengineering in health care delivery. *Managed Care Quarterly* 4:1–11.

Camann, M. A. 1996. Family-focused mental health care policy. *Issues in Mental Health Nursing* 17(5):479–86.

Cohen, M. A., Kumar, N., and Wallack, S. S. 1993. Simulating the fiscal and distributional impacts of Medicaid eligibility reforms. *Health Care Financing Review* 14:133–50.

Covinsky, K. E., Goldman, L., Cook, E. F., Oye, R., Desbiens, N., Reding, D., Fulkerson, W., Connors, A. F., Lynn, J., and Phillips, R. S. 1994. The impact of serious illness on patients' families. *Journal of the American Medical Association* 272:1839–44.

Elmore, D. L. 2003, September. Reaching the underserved. *Monitor on Psychology* 34:32–33.

Eppig, F. J., and Poisal, J. A. 1997. Mental health of Medicare beneficiaries: 1995. *Health Care Financing Review* 18:207–10.

Forti, E. M., Johnson, J. A., and Graber, D. R. 2000. Aging in America: Challenges and strategies for health care delivery. *Journal of Health and Human Services Administration* 23:203–13.

Freed, D. M., Elder, W. W., Lauderdale, S., and Carter, S. 1999. An integrated program for dementia evaluation and care management. *Gerontologist* 39:356–61.

Gordon, S. 1997. The impact of managed care on female caregivers in the hospital and home. *Journal of the American Medical Women's Association* 52:75–77.

Hudson, R. B., and Gonyea, J. G. 2000. Time not yet money: The politics and promise of the Family Medical Leave Act. *Journal of Aging and Social Policy* 11:189–200.

Levit, K. R., Lazenby, H. C., Braden, B. R., Cowan, C. A., Sensenig, A. L., McDonnell, P. A., Stiller, J. M., Won, D. K., Martin, A. B., Sivarajan, L., Donham, C. S., Long, A. M., and Stewart, M. W. 1997. National health expenditures, 1996. *Health Care Financing Review* 19:161–200.

Liu, K., Manton, K M., and Liu, B. M. 1985. Home care expenses for the disabled elderly. *Health Care Financing Review* 7:51–58.

Mittelman, M. S., Ferris, S. H., Shulman, E., Steinberg, G., and Levin, B. 1996. A family intervention to delay nursing home placement of patients with Alzheimer's disease. *Journal of the American Medical Association* 276:1725–31.

Nguyen, B. 2000. When care is needed at home: Your rights under the Family and Medical Leave Act. *American Journal of Nursing* 100:107.

Ory, M. G., Hofffman, R. R., Yee, J. L., Tennstedt, S., and Schulz, R. 1999. Prevalence and impact of caregiving: A detailed comparison between dementia and nondementia caregivers. *Gerontologist* 39:177–85.

Peres, J. R. 2003. End-of-life care: How do we pay for it? *Public Policy & Aging Report* 13:1–6.

Riggs, J. A. 2001. The health and long-term care policy challenges of Alzheimer's disease. *Aging and Mental Health* 5:138–45.

Ripple, M. L. 1999. Supervisors beware: The Family and Medical Leave Act may be hazardous to your health. *Journal of Contemporary Health Law and Policy* 16:273–303.

Schulz, R., Belle, S. H., Czaja, S. J., Gitlin, L. N., Wisniewski, S. R., and Ory, M. G. 2003. Introduction to the special section on resources for enhancing Alzheimer's caregiver health (REACH). *Psychology and Aging* 18:357–60.

Schulz, R., O'Brien, A. T., Bookwala, J., and Fleissner, K. 1995. Psychiatric and physical morbidity effects of dementia caregiving: Prevalence, correlates, and causes. *Gerontologist* 35:771–91.

Walker, L., Gruman, C., and Robison, J. 1999. Medicaid eligibility workers discuss Medicaid estate planning for nursing home care. *Gerontologist* 39:201–08.

CHAPTER THIRTEEN

Ethnic Elders and Caregiving

F. M. BAKER, M.D., M.P.H., DISTINGUISHED F.A.P.A.

The United States is facing the beginning of a new paradigm. By 2030, the majority of people age 65 and older will be people of color (Angel and Hogan, 1991). The combined population of persons age 65 and older who are African American, American Indian / Alaska Native, Asian American / Pacific Islander, and Hispanic American will be larger than the population of Caucasian American persons age 65 and older (see figure 13.1; Siegel, 1999).

DEFINITIONS

Aranda (2001) provided important clarifications of race, ethnicity, culture, and minority group. These terms have been used interchangeably and therefore inappropriately (Wilkerson, 1986). Aranda (2001) noted that ethnicity refers to "a shared sense of 'peoplehood'" or "identification by a group due to their shared unique social and cultural heritage that is passed on from one generation to another." The definition of culture as "a group's way of life: the values, beliefs, traditions, symbols, language, and social organization that are meaningful to the group" was favored for use in dementia caregiving research in the United States (Aranda, 2001). Minority group status was defined as "shared cultural values, lifestyles, and/or physical characteristics" of stigmatized groups and groups "barred" from full participation in American society (Aranda, 2001, p. S122). Thus the term *ethnic elders* will be used in this chapter to define persons age 65 and older who are people of color, whose ethnicity and culture are different from those of persons age 65 and

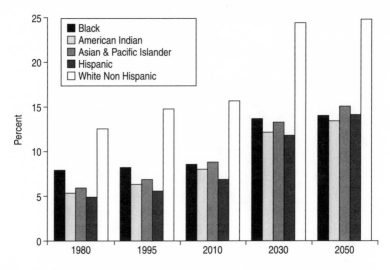

Figure 13.1 Proportion of the Total Population 65 Years and Over, for Major Race/Hispanic-origin Groups, 1980 to 2050.
SOURCE: Siegel, 1999, p. 3. Copyright © The Gerontological Society of America. Reproduced by permission of the publisher.

older who are Caucasian and of European ethnicity and culture (Baker and Lightfoot, 1993).

MACROHISTORY, MICROHISTORY, AND BIRTH COHORT

Neugarten (1979) wrote of time, age, and the life cycle, emphasizing that each individual accomplishes his or her progression through the stages of the life cycle at the person's unique pace. Colarusso and Nemiroff (1987), Engle (1980), and Baker (1982, 1987, 2000) emphasized the importance of understanding the macrohistory (the societal events that affect the individual) and the microhistory (the unique events specific to the individual that affect the individual's life). A brief review of the macrohistory of ethnic elders will provide an important context for a review of the existing literature on the caregivers of these elders.

The ethnic elders of the twenty-first century are a diverse population. Persons age 65 in 2005 were born in 1940 during the beginning of World War II. They would have been age 16 in 1956, a time of legalized segregation and the release of Japanese Americans from their internment in camps in the western United States. During the period of the civil rights movement—the time of the assassinations of President John F. Kennedy, the Rev. Dr. Martin Luther King Jr., and the former head of the Department of Justice Robert Kennedy—and the conflict in American society over the Vietnam War, these elders would have been in their twenties. Many were involved in the civil rights movement and participated in demonstrations for equal rights for African Americans and Native Americans, and better wages, housing, and health benefits for Hispanic American farm workers. With the repeal of the Asian exclusion acts in 1965, many older Asians joined their families in America.

In their thirties, these ethnic elders would have seen the beginning rollback of affirmative action initiatives and the rise of political conservatism in America during the 1970s. Many had married and were addressing the dual concerns of advancing their careers and obtaining the best education for their children. In the 1980s, these ethnic elders would have been in their forties. Worried about their job security, these ethnic elders as parents were concerned as their children competed to enter college, to find work, and to establish their own life structures. Some were concerned that their children not get caught up in the alternative lifestyle of the streets: drug abuse and its downward spiral.

In the 1990s, when this birth cohort of ethnic elders were in their fifties, American society was experiencing significant industrial growth: the computer industry was burgeoning with commercial opportunities and the growth of stocks seemed unlimited. These individuals were beginning to seriously contemplate retirement, to notice their expanding waistlines, and to become reflective about the opportunities available to them during their life course and, perhaps, the accomplishments of their children.

In 2000, as this birth cohort of ethnic elders went into their sixties, they were beginning to be concerned about their health problems, particularly hypertension, diabetes mellitus, arthritis, glaucoma, obesity, heart disease, and stroke (Baker et al., 1993; Braithwaite and Taylor, 1992; Cuellar, 1990). Some would be stricken with cancer or facing the effects of chronic physical illnesses such as end-stage renal disease from diabetes and cardiovascular disease, or cirrhosis from alcohol dependence. A sense of the time remaining for some ethnic elders would strengthen the normal developmental life review and interest in mentoring the next generation (Baker, 1987). Many ethnic elders were worried that they might need to become the parent for their grandchild owing to the early death of their children due to accidents, substance abuse, and/or human immunodeficiency virus (HIV) infection (Braithwaite and Taylor, 1992).

Consideration of the birth cohort of ethnic elders is very important because of the impact that societal attitudes and societal prohibitions have had on their opportunities for education, employment, housing, and financial resources (Baker, 2000). Ethnic elders age 65 in 2005 differ from ethnic elders who were age 65 in 1965. Limited education, few employment opportunities for nonwhite Americans even with a college education, and legalized segregation and exclusion were realities faced by ethnic elders born in 1900. Many of the ethnic elders of the twenty-first century will have benefited from the increased opportunities in education, employment, and housing resulting from the societal upheaval generated by the civil rights movement of the 1960s and the increasing range of opportunities available to their children. However, some of the other ethnic elders of the twenty-first century of African Caribbean, Asian, and Latino origin are recent immigrants to the United States who are still in the process of acculturation, or are U.S. residents attempting to care for their parents, whom they have brought to the United States. (For further details of the macrohistory of African American, American Indian / Alaska Native, Asian American / Pacific Islander, and Latino American ethnic elders see Baker, 2000.)

THE DIVERSITY OF ETHNIC ELDERS

The diversity among the groups that comprise ethnic elders makes generalization across groups and sometimes within groups a difficult task (Aranda, 2001; Baker and Lightfoot, 1993; Cuellar, 1990). African Americans, African Caribbean, and Africans may be lumped together, but they have distinct ethnic and cultural identities (Allen, 1988; Baker, 1988).

Gover (2000) noted that there were 556 federally recognized Native American tribes speaking more than two hundred different languages with varying degrees of acculturation to the dominant culture (Trimble, 2000). Manson (1995) described differences between rural-resident and urban-resident American Indians, particularly economic differences, as an illustration of further complexity in attempting to make statements about this population. Studies of Alaska Natives are difficult because of their remote residences (Jervis and Manson, 2002).

There have been two waves of immigration of Asians to the United States. Chinese, Japanese, and Filipino immigrants came to provide cheap manual labor from the late 1880s to 1924. The Chinese Exclusion Act of 1882 and the Oriental Exclusion Act of 1924 stopped immigration and naturalization. These early immigrants, predominantly male, became a bachelor cohort because of legal and informal sanctions against intermarriage. In 1965 the Asian exclusion acts were repealed, resulting in a second wave of immigration that included many Asian women. The most recent Asian immigrants have come from Southeast Asia. Angel and Hogan (1991) reported the Asian elderly population by nation of origin as being made up of Filipino (26.7%), Chinese (26.6%), Japanese (24.7%), Asian Indians (14.6%), Korean (4.2)%), Vietnamese (2.2%), and other Asian (1%).

The first Hispanic immigrants to the Unites States came from Mexico and Puerto Rico. Salvadorans, Nicaraguans, and Columbians followed Cubans who fled the Castro revolution. Although the term *Hispanic Americans* was dominant in the 1980s, *Latinos* is the preferred term in the twenty-first century to describe the diverse population of Spanish-speaking persons residing in the United States. The Latino elderly population (Angel and Hogan, 1991) is composed of Mexican Americans (47.6%), Cuban Americans (18.1%), Puerto Rican Americans (10.9%), Central and South Americans (8.4%), and other Hispanics (15%).

Among African American, Asian American, and Latino American cultures, the family is an extended family of aunts, uncles, and cousins. Among African Americans and Latinos, nonbiologically related persons may be "adopted" into the family because of the bonds that the person has established with family members. These extended family networks facilitate caregiving tasks and serve as an expanded network of human resources for the caregiver. Several authors have noted the importance of this informal network of extended family members for caregivers of ethnic elders (Baker, 1994; Boyd-Franklin, 2003; Cuellar, 1990; Gallagher-Thompson and Steffen, 1994; Lewis and Ausberry, 1996; Martinez, 1988).

African Americans

By the 2000 U.S. Census, African Americans accounted for 12 percent of the U.S. population (Baker, 2000). The old-old, persons aged 85 and older, is the fastest growing segment of the elderly African American population. Based on population projections comparing population growth from 1980 to 2000, there has been a 103.7 percent increase in African American men aged 85 and older and a 179.6 percent increase in African American women aged 85 and older (Manuel, 1988). The longer an African American elder lives, the greater age he or she can expect to reach. This has been termed the "crossover" effect: African Americans, particularly men, tend to die before age 60, but if they live until age 70, African Americans live longer than Caucasians. It has been hypothesized, but not studied, that those African Americans surviving into their seventh decade are "hardy survivors" who will live to their ninth decade. When Manuel (1988) separated life expectancy data by age, by year, by race, and by gender, the crossover point was found to be age 65 in 1960, but not until age 85 in 1980. Further studies are needed to clarify whether this crossover effect will be observed in the old-old of the twenty-first century.

African American elders are a diverse population, with those residing in New York, Los Angeles, and Atlanta (urban cities) having experiences and resources very different from those of African American elders living in rural areas of Mississippi and Arkansas.

Although nine generations removed from the time of legalized slavery in the United States (during which persons from many different African nations were brought in chains to America), African cultural values of collectivity, sharing, affiliation, obedience to authority, belief in spirituality, respect for the elderly, and respect for the past (Pinderhughes, 1982) remain core values for many African Americans today. An obligation to one's elders is instilled from childhood in most African American families. Although adult children are moving away from their parents for better job opportunities, it is not unusual for one sibling to "move home" in order to be close to an aging elder (parent, aunt) who is becoming frail and in need of increasing assistance.

A number of studies have looked at African American caregivers; these were summarized first by Gonzales et al. (1995) and then by Lewis and Ausberry (1996). Cuellar (2002) compared a convenience sample composed of 36 African American and 38 Caucasian caregivers in a rural sample in southern Mississippi. All provided care to bed-bound elderly adults who were diagnosed with cerebrovascular accident and were receiving additional care from home health agencies. African American caregivers had a mean age of 57 and were predominantly daughters. Caucasian caregivers had a mean age of 62 and were predominantly spouses. African American caregivers reported lower self-efficacy or confidence in their capabilities, lower stress, and lower depression. African American caregivers in this rural Mississippi setting had a higher life satisfaction and more diverse support network compared to Caucasian caregivers. Rural Caucasian caregivers were more likely to depend on formal networks for respite care. Although Caucasian American caregivers reported higher self-efficacy, the author questioned whether these caregivers might be unable to access respite care services when needed. The author also questioned whether the higher depression scores among Caucasian American caregivers were related to these older caregiver spouses considering themselves as drawing nearer to the end of their lives as they noted the increasing frailty of their spouses (Cuellar, 2002).

Lampley-Dallas et al. (2001) conducted a study of urban (Oklahoma City) African American caregivers. Data were obtained from two focus groups whose members were solicited from adult day care settings, nursing home staff, local churches, family, and friends. All caregivers (N = 13) were caring for persons with cognitive impairment diagnosed as Alzheimer disease, multi-infarct dementia, or an organic brain syndrome. Eighty-seven percent of these caregivers were women, with a mean age of 54 years. Eighty percent had some college or were college graduates, with 54 percent living with the elder care recipient. These urban, well-educated, African American caregivers acknowledged that caregiving produced disruption in their living arrangement and negative effects on their physical, mental, and emotional health. These authors reported that the caregivers "accepted their caregiving role and viewed it as a duty or obligation owed to their family members." Although they found joy in their situation, a few caregivers admitted that they suffered from denial, guilt, anger, and frustration. This qualitative focus group study identified four main categories of caregiving topics: informal social support network, formal social support network, other health care or service providers, and prevention. In this urban sample, family, friends, and church members were a supportive and active informal social support network that these caregivers found effective for themselves (Lampley-Dallas et al., 2001). Other authors have also reported the importance of church members and the extended family of African Americans as important informal social support (Dilworth-Anderson and Gibson, 1994; Taylor and Chatters, 1986a; Taylor and Chatters, 1986b; William et al., 2003). Formal social supports noted by Lampley-Dallas et al. (2001) included adult day services and nursing homes.

A major concern of these urban, ethnic caregivers was that the demented elder be treated respectfully and with dignity. These caregivers expected nursing home, home health care, and adult day services to provide "sensitive" care, to be of "good quality," and to have "well-trained staff." One caregiver described her disappointment and discomfort with nursing home placement. She heard the staff say, "Here comes Mrs. P, you better check on Mr. P." Mrs. P. was concerned because other nursing home residents did not have family members or friends to visit, and this comment implied that care was dependent on the family's monitoring the staff. When this older, male elder with dementia became the only male in the nursing home, his family brought him home (Lampley-Dallas et al., 2001).

These urban caregivers identified the absence of knowledge about the formal network of services as a barrier to care. Demeaning attitudes were disincentives to use these services, and assumptions about the caregiver's ability to pay for services were viewed as examples of subtle racism. Rude behavior by staff, policy hassles, and the absence of follow-through were identified as barriers to care. At the same time, these African American, urban caregivers acknowledged their procrastination and need to maintain control and privacy about family matters contributing to their not using formal social service resources (Lamprey-Dallas et al., 2001).

Several researchers have spoken about the role of spirituality in African American caregivers' ability to cope with the tasks of caregiving (Cuellar, 2002; Lamprey-

Dallas et al., 2001; Theis et al., 2003). The role of spirituality for African Americans (Boyd-Franklin, 2003) and particularly African American caregivers (Kaye and Robinson, 1994; Lewis and Ausberry, 1996; Picot et al., 1997, Taylor and Chatters, 1991) continues to be a consistent finding in the literature, with Theis et al. (2003) noting its importance to the care recipient also. "God wouldn't give me more than I can bear," "God is good all the time!" "Leaning on the Lord," and "Give it to the Lord" are phrases shared by African American elders summarizing the role of faith in helping them to deal with the task of caregiving in the context of their lives.

Asian Americans

Caregiving by ethnic communities reflects the diversity of these populations. Persons who are immigrants bring to the United States the values of their homelands, although definition of roles, generational responsibilities, and expectations of good quality of life may change from one generation to the next. Care issues for the Japanese elder illustrate this point (Tempo and Saito, 1996). In contrast to other Asian American groups, only the Japanese have given specific names to the different generations residing in the United States. The first generation (Issei) brought the values of Japan with them. The majority of settlers came from the southern prefectures of Japan—Yamaguchi and Hiroshima (Tempo and Saito, 1996). The father or eldest son made decisions within the family. The importance of not bringing shame on the family, hard work, loyalty, and acceptance of what fate dealt one were core values of this generation. Emotional self-restraint (gaman) and deferential behavior (enryo) were other core values of the Issei generation.

The Nisei (second) generation, children of the Issei, experienced the rupture of their families with Executive Order 9066. Japanese families were removed from their homes and businesses and placed in internment camps. Many families were moved from California to midwestern camps. These Nisei children proved their loyalty to the United States by serving in the 4424 Regimental Combat Team and the 100th Infantry Battalion. These two units became the most highly decorated units in U.S. history, receiving 18,143 individual decorations for valor (Tempo and Saito, 1996).

The third generation in the United States, the Sansei, continued to implement the standards of their grandparents and continued the tradition of the senior male making decisions for the family.

When the father (from the Issei generation) became demented and was aggressive to his wife, the eldest son refused to consider placement of his father in a nursing home. Although his mother and siblings (two brothers

and one sister) who lived with the father supported nursing home placement, the eldest son focused on exercising his role not to abandon his
responsibility for his father. Formal caregivers involved with this family organized a family meeting to explore options. The involvement of the father
in an adult day care program provided some respite for the family.

Awareness of the cultural standards and the definition of responsibilities of the
culture of origin can help the health professional's interventions with ethnic elders
and their caregivers. Such appreciation can enable the health professional to be sensitive to the cultural context and mores, whether they are fully operational or have
been modified in succeeding generations (Tempo and Saito, 1996).

The engagement of the Asian elder and his family in treatment requires an appreciation of a different expectation of a visit with a health professional. The intense
eye contact, liberal physical gestures, and direct questions about intimate matters is
considered offensive and intrusive by Japanese Americans. Communication can be
facilitated by the use of nonverbal and indirect styles of communications. Acknowledgment of the importance of the family group or community in the Japanese elder's
life can demonstrate a level of cultural awareness on the part of the interviewer.
Helping the Japanese American elder and his family to understand the process and
to feel comfortable in asking questions, as well as allowing them time to reach a decision as a family and an extended community, are important approaches to working with these families (Tempo and Saito, 1996; Yamamoto, 1986).

There are few population-based studies of Asian American elders (Elliott et al.,
1996; Janevic and Connell, 2001; Mollica and Lavelle, 1988). Although Chinese
Americans, Japanese Americans, and Filipino Americans have been present in the
United States from the 1800s, recent Asian populations have emigrated along with
their elders. Cambodians, Laotians, Vietnamese, and Hmong will bring unique
concerns based on their life experiences, which may have included time in a refugee
camp. Incarceration and torture of former non-Communist military personnel and
civilians and sexual abuse of Indochinese women by Thai pirates increase the risk
for post-traumatic stress disorder among members of this immigrant population
(Mollica and Lavelle, 1988). It is to be hoped that studies of caregiving for these ethnic elders will be conducted in the future.

Latinos

Studies about Latino caregivers have increased in recent years. Valle (1994) wrote
one of the early papers that emphasized the importance of a culture-fair approach

to the assessment of neuropsychiatric symptoms in dementia and in the diagnosis of dementia. Several authors reported that Latino caregivers had higher rates of depression than Caucasian caregivers (Cox and Monk, 1990; Harwood et al., 1998; Mintzer et al., 1992). Because the Latino population is very diverse, it is often necessary to study the separate groups included within this population. However, this necessity can lead to methodological constraints such as small sample size. In addition, the validity of generalization from some studies is limited, as they were not based on population-based samples of Mexican American, Cuban American, Puerto Rican, and Central and South American persons, the major Latino groups in the United States (Cuellar, 1990).

Hinton et al. (2003) studied a sample of noninstitutionalized Latino elderly who were enrolled in the Sacramento Area Latino Study on Aging (SALSA) and their informal caregivers. The sample was drawn from five counties and was divided into those with dementia and those with cognitive impairment without dementia. Latino caregivers of demented elderly with neuropsychiatric symptoms were more likely to report symptoms of depression on the Center for Epidemiologic Studies Depression Scale (CES-D) (Radloff, 1977). Specific factors identified as modifying the level of depression in the caregiver included whether the caregiver was a spouse and the age and dementia status of the care recipient. Suggested explanations for this included the fact that older Mexican American spouses were more likely to hold onto their cultural values that strengthened them in the caregiver role. These wives may have drawn strength from being able to carry out their roles as caregiver and received strength from their religious beliefs. The authors also questioned whether Latino spouses who had been caregivers for a longer period compared to nonspouses had developed an adaptation to the role of caregiver and were a more resilient group (Hinton et al., 2003).

Navaie-Waliser et al. (2001) studied an urban sample. Using a random-digit dialing technique, they contacted a representative sample of 2,241 households in New York City. To be included in the study, individuals had to have been directly involved in caregiving within the 12 months preceding the study and to be age 18 or older. Randomly selected members of eligible households completed a structured, pretested survey questionnaire over the telephone. This sample was composed of 164 Caucasian, 129 African American, and 87 Latino families. African American caregivers were providing more activities of daily living (ADLs) care (dressing, feeding, transferring, and toileting) than Latino caregivers. Latino caregivers provided more care than Caucasian caregivers. Both African American and Latino American caregivers reported unmet needs with care provision. Latinos were more likely to receive help from formal caregivers. Both African American and Latinos reported increased religiosity since becoming a caregiver (Navaie-Waliser et al., 2001).

The National Institutes of Health funded a national, five-year, multisite study to investigate the effectiveness of innovative interventions to support family caregivers (i.e., the Resources for Enhancing Alzheimer's Caregiver Health, or REACH) (Coon, Schulz, and Ory, 1999). The sample was obtained from the Palo Alto site of this REACH study (Gallagher-Thompson et al., 2003). These investigators looked at the impact of a ten-week psychoeducational program, Coping with Caregiving (CWC), compared to an Enhanced Support Group for 122 Caucasian and 91 Latino female caregivers drawn from the REACH study. Several authors had demonstrated that psychoeducational groups were effective in reducing depression and burden among caregivers (Gallagher-Thompson, et al., 2000; Zarit et al., 1987), as well as frustration and anger (Gallagher-Thompson and DeVries, 1994). In this sample, Latino female caregivers were younger (mean age = 51) and more likely to be daughters and daughters-in-law compared to Caucasian caregivers, who were older (mean age = 62) and more likely to be wives. Care recipients for both groups of caregivers were approximately age 76, with Latino caregivers caring for more women and Caucasian caregivers caring for more men. There was no difference between groups in ADLs and level of cognitive impairment of the care recipients. A Cognitive Behavior Therapy approach (Gallagher-Thompson and Steffen, 1994; Teri and McCurry, 2000; Torres-Matrullo, 1982) was used in the Coping with Caregiving psychoeducational program. The authors modified it to be sensitive to the stigma toward psychotherapy among Latinos and to avoid the appearance of self-indulgence. The Coping with Caregiving program emphasized education (homework assignments and chalkboards) and "the importance of participating in pleasurable activities for the purpose of becoming a better caregiver" (Gallagher-Thompson et al., 2003). Both Caucasian and Latino caregivers in the CWC group reported decreased depression, increased use of positive coping strategies, the tendency to use fewer negative coping strategies, and fewer negative interactions in their social network (Gallagher-Thompson et al., 2003). Both the CWC and the Enhanced Support Group members reported being less bothered by care recipient memory and behavior problems at the end of the ten-week group experience. No significant differences between Latino and Caucasian caregivers were found (Gallagher-Thompson et al., 2003). As Latino female caregivers in this study (predominantly Mexican American) had less education (average 11 years) compared to Caucasian female caregivers (average 14 years), the success of the intervention provides important information about a culturally sensitive approach that may be helpful to other populations of Latino caregivers in regions outside of northern California.

These studies are of particular interest because there have been few studies of representative samples of ethnic caregivers, particularly in urban settings. The difference in Latino populations across the nation needs to be acknowledged. Studies of Cuban Americans in Florida, Mexican Americans in the Southwest and West, and persons from Puerto Rico, Santo Domingo, El Salvador, and Nicaragua in New York City should explore populations of caregivers with different levels of acculturation, socioeconomic advancement, and knowledge of resources. Sensitivity to these differences and, particularly, the unique cultural heritage of the country of origin will need to be incorporated into any study design.

Native Americans

Qualitative and quantitative studies of caregiving among Native American families were very few until the 1990s. Strong (1984) compared caregiver burden and coping among 10 Northwest Indians and 10 Caucasian American caregivers matched on the variable of sex, income, and rural residence. These Northwest Indian caregivers perceived themselves as having less control over the caregiver situation and placed more emphasis on the positive dimensions of managing the needs of a dependent elder. The coping strategy used by these Northwest Indian caregivers was termed "passive forbearance" (Strong, 1984). These caregivers emphasized acceptance and adaptation to the caregiving situation rather than control over it.

Hobus (1990) reported on the concerns of family caregivers for a frail Lakota elder who returned home periodically from an off-reservation Anglo nursing home. The nurse helping this family noted several major problems that emerged from the family assessment. Problems identified were knowledge deficits in how to provide care to the elder and how to obtain outside help, and lack of familiarity with the consumer rights of nursing home residents. Additional concerns were guilt related to not providing care to the elder at home; fear about the eventual death of the elder in an alien surrounding; resentment toward previous health care providers; and concern for the health of the primary family caregiver during the elder's home visits.

Hennessy and John (1996) studied family caregivers among five tribes and found multiple sources of burden, including stresses resulting from competing responsibilities between work or other family duties and caregiving, along with perceived negative effects of this competition on caregiving duties and on personal health and well-being. John et al. (2001) contrasted the studies of Hennessy and John (1995, 1996) and Hennessy, John, and Anderson (1999) with the studies of Steinmetz (1988) on caregiver strain. The Native American caregivers, in contrast to Anglo caregivers, emphasized the effect of caregiver strain on the group (i.e., family and tribe) rather than strains that infringed on caregiver's personal or individual needs (such as privacy or time for self) (John et al., 2001). American Indian families actively attempted to enlist support from their formal and informal networks to create an effective daily routine and to seek information from potential resources to assist them with caregiver responsibilities (John et al., 2001).

John et al. (2001) described a study of 69 Pueblo Indian caregivers (10 families) who were identified between 1995 and 1997 initially as part of the American Indian Aging Program in New Mexico with funding from the National Institute on Aging. Caregivers were identified from local American Indian senior service (Title VI) programs. Those who entered into the study provided care to recipients who were age 65 and older and required help with at least one activity of daily living (ADL) or at least two independent activities of daily living (IADLs).

The identified Pueblo Indian caregivers were 86 percent female (54 percent daughters, 11 percent wives) and a median age of 49. Some 47 percent were married, 36 percent were single, 13 percent were widowed, and 4 percent were divorced or separated. The care recipients' diagnoses were not given, but their characteristics suggested moderate to severe cognitive problems, with 92 percent of care recipients wandering, being restless, agitated, or engaging in dangerous activities at least once in the preceding month. Urinary incontinence was an occasional problem for 40 percent of care recipients and a frequent problem for 13 percent. The mean age of care recipients was 81 years, with 67 percent requiring some assistance with each of the IADLs and 25 percent needing assistance with each ADL (John et al., 2001). Using a modified version of the Caregiver Burden Scale (Zarit et al., 1990) whose face validity in this population had been established in a prior study (John, 1995), an in-person interview of Pueblo caregivers was completed.

A trained indigenous service provider administered the instrument in the caregiver's home or other acceptable location by reading each question. This was done because "this more conversational mode is more culturally appropriate and because among elderly caregivers literacy in English might be limited" (John et al., 2001, p. 213). This study found that caregiver burden among Pueblo Indian caregivers was multidimensional. Four factors emerged from the exploratory factor analysis: role conflict, negative feeling, caregiver efficacy, and guilt. These four dimensions or types of burden differed from those reported by Zarit and Zarit (1990), who identified role strain and personal strain. For Pueblo caregivers, role conflict reflected the impact of caregiving on their lives: lack of privacy, the absence of time for self, adverse effect on health, and being pulled between the elders and other responsibilities, with the caregiver's social life suffering. Most caregivers experienced these types of burden (Zarit et al., 1980).

The negative feeling factor was found to correlate with previous pilot studies. Green et al. (1982) identified three items related to their negative feeling factor, and

Novak and Guest (1989) identified a five-item negative factor. Although Novak and Guest (1989) termed their five-item factor emotional burden, John et al. (2001) described it as the negative feelings related to behavioral problems often associated with cognitive impairment. Three of the five items of Novak and Guest (1989) were similar to the items found by John et al. (2001): I feel "embarrassed, uncomfortable having friends over, and angry about interacting with the care recipient" (p. 800).

The caregiver efficacy factor reflected doubts of Pueblo caregivers about their ability to sustain the caregiving task. The guilt factor reflected the Pueblo caregivers' concern that they could do a better job and should be doing more. John et al. (2001) found that the distribution of responses in the study suggested that guilt was the most common form of caregiver burden among Pueblo Indians. These authors noted, "Guilt is a form of caregiver burden that exists even when [the caregiver is] performing a culturally prescribed role." Because Pueblo Indian family caregivers experienced guilt more intensely than did the three other types of caregiver burden, these authors recommended that service providers determine whether the guilt is warranted and that they make interventions as indicated—that is, referral for services, clarification for the caregiver's faulty perceptions, and affirmation of the caregiver's work.

When American Indians were the last group to receive the right to vote in 1924, Mr. Gray Claw was a child. Although the history between the United States government and American Indian tribes had been genocidal and treacherous at times (Baker, 2000; Walker and LaDue, 1986), Mr. Gray Claw's Navajo language and culture helped him to serve the United States with distinction as a Navajo code talker during World War II. Mr. Gray Claw returned to live on the reservation with his family. When his children were sent to boarding school at age 12, he was angry, confused, resentful, and concerned. He wanted his children, particularly his son, to learn the Navajo way.

Because of his wisdom and judgment, Mr. Gray Claw became a tribal chief and tribal members sought his advice. His son moved away to work as a "sky walker," building tall steel structures on the West and East coasts. When his son and his family returned to visit his parents during annual Pow Wows (tribal meetings), it was the source of much celebration for the Gray Claw family.

When Mr. Gray Claw became forgetful and then progressively more confused, a special healing ceremony was held, "a sing," which required several months of preparation. The medicine man, a traditional healer, prepared special sand paintings and songs. The family prepared food for the five days of the healing ceremony, which was a community event. Because of the significant financial burden on Mr. Gray Claw's wife and his daughter's family, the son contributed financially. Members of the reservation community assisted with the preparations and provided some of the housing for tribal members attending "the sing" and some of the food. After the healing ceremony, Mr. Gray Claw did somewhat better—staying within the village rather than wandering toward the mountains. When he began to become increasingly anxious and irritated, appeared to be talking to spirits and deceased relatives, and no longer slept at night, his wife talked with the medicine man who had conducted the healing ceremony the year before. He suggested that they talk with Dr. Luke at the reservation clinic. When they talked with Dr. Luke, it was established that Mr. Gray Claw had not seen a physician for more than ten years, because he had been well. Dr. Luke indicated that he needed to see Mr. Gray Claw in person, and he asked the medicine man if he could help with this.

After the medicine man encouraged Mr. Gray Claw to visit Dr. Luke with his family, Mr. Gray Claw was seen at the clinic. Over several visits, Mr. Gray Claw became comfortable with Dr. Luke and an examination and blood work were completed. A diagnosis of moderate dementia of the Alzheimer type was made. The family discussed Dr. Luke's recommendation for Western medicine with the medicine man, who talked with Dr. Luke on the family's behalf. A trial of Dr. Luke's medication was begun, along with the use of a herbal remedy to help with sleep prescribed by the medicine man. Both practitioners checked for drug-drug interactions. Mr. Gray Claw's behavior gradually improved over the next few weeks. He was sleeping at night, teaching his grandchildren the Navajo way through stories and crafts, and describing his work as a Navajo code talker during World War II. Mr. Gray Claw returned to his seat in the council of tribal elders.

The social worker at the clinic had begun to share information with the family about resources in the community. Unfortunately, the reservation did not have adult day care services and there were no nursing home facilities on the reservation. If the family became unable to care for Mr. Gray Claw, he would need to be placed in an Anglo facility. If this happened, Mr. Gray Claw would be pulled away, again, from his family at a vulnerable time in his life, just as he had been pulled away from his parents as an adolescent when he was sent to an Indian boarding school—a fate that Mr. Gray Claw was unable to prevent his own children from experiencing.

This vignette illustrates the impact of historical events on the life of an ethnic elder. Mr. Gray Claw's concern about his children's going to Indian boarding school reflected his memories of his own experience. The different efforts of the U.S. government's attempts to "help" American Indian tribes have resulted too often in hurting them. It also illustrates that health care professionals need to remember that Western medicine may not be the first choice for ethnic elders and that a community healer may need to validate the practitioner of Western medicine for Native American elders. The dual approach of the two practitioners may facilitate a more positive relationship and limit the risk of drug interactions.

It is good that investigators are beginning to study caregiving among Native American populations. It is to be hoped that future studies will provide information contrasting caregiving among reservation-resident and urban-resident Native American populations. Data from the Indian Bureau are based only on Native Americans resident on reservations; Native Americans resident in urban settings are less well studied and may be expected to have different concerns. Studies of caring among Alaska Natives as well as Pacific Islander caregivers and care recipients will require qualitative and quantitative studies to identify the specific and unique concerns of these populations.

IMPLICATIONS FOR CLINICAL PRACTICE

Clinical strategies to engage these diverse populations in research and in clinical settings require investigators and clinicians to gain familiarity with the specific populations of ethnic elders with whom they will be working. It is important to begin with a review of texts and papers that provide some information about the ethnic elder and his or her family. Talking with a social worker, religious leader, or a native healer (medicine man, curandera, herbalist, or root doctor) working in the ethnic elder's community will provide important information about how the elder defines health and illness. One will learn about the ethnic elder's expectations of roles in later life (e.g., remaining active and involved with housekeeping or farming although crippled with arthritis; being active in the church and the community as a source of knowledge and comfort; serving in the capacity of community leader as the oldest person in an extended kinship network). The investigator and clinician can learn how the ethnic elder and the elder's family seeks treatment; who is defined as providing health care (from the ethnic elder's culture); and when Western medicine will be consulted. Information about the scope of the ethnic elder's informal network and who is defined as "family" will also be obtained from these contacts.

Lewis and Ausberry (1996) suggested a helpful mnemonic to remember as an approach to working with ethnic elders and their families, the LEARN model of Berlin and Fowkes (1983). The mnemonic reads as follows: L = learn, E = explain, A = acknowledge, R = recommend, and N = negotiate. Lewis and Ausberry encourage those working with ethnic elders and their families to use this approach to facilitate communication and to obtain the goal of helping ethnic elders and their caregivers to attain the information and the services that they need. Translated into clinical care, these authors suggest:

LISTEN with an emphasis on understanding what your client is trying to communicate.

EXPRESS the client's concerns in a language appropriate to his or her sociocultural domain.

ACCEPT differences between your world and the client's.

RESTATE your agreed-on suggestions for interventions clearly *and write them down.*

NEVER FORGET the value of a win-win outcome (with each participant in the dialogue feeling that the concerns of each has been heard).

As shown by the demographic projections (Angel and Hogan, 1991), the formal care network will be asked, increasingly, to help ethnic elders and their families. These informal caregivers of ethnic elders will need to work with formal caregiving services as the health of the care recipient declines. The old-old, persons aged 80 and older, are the fastest growing segment of the ethnic elder population (Angel and Hogan, 1991; Manuel, 1988a) and will become an increasing proportion of nursing home residents. Knowledge of the strengths and resources of these ethnic elders and their caregivers will facilitate their interaction with the formal service care network and encourage their seeking needed services.

Finally, when working with the diverse elders of the international community and their families, the importance of family and kinship networks reported among African American, Asian American, and Latino populations residing in the United States remains an important consideration (Baker, 2000; Mollica and Lavelle, 1988; Yamamoto, 1986; Yeo and Gallagher-Thompson, 1996). Cultural and linguistics differences of elders from, for example, the Balkan states, Asia Minor, the Pacific Islands, the Netherlands, Russia, Spain, and South America, need not impede clarification of the specific concerns and needs of these elders and their caregivers. If necessary, working with a competent translator sensitive to the techniques of exploring personal information in the specific culture of the elder will enable clinicians to establish the concerns of the family and to identify the resources that exist within the family and the community. Use of the clinical application of the LEARN model

(Berlin and Fowkes, 1983) will enable clinicians and investigators in the international community to work effectively with their ethnic elders to attain the information they request and to obtain the services that they need.

CONCLUSION

Studies of ethnic elder caregivers have become an increasing focus of research (Aranda, 2001; Connell et al., 2001; Cox, 1995; Cox and Monk, 1996; Fox et al., 1999; Gonzales et al., 1995; Haley et al., 1995, 1996; Henderson et al., 1993; Javenic and Connell, 2001; Kelley, 1994; Lampley-Dallas, 2002; Sterritt and Pokorny, 1998). Compared to other ethnic elders, more literature exists about African American and Latino caregivers whose care recipients have dementia, cancer, cardiac disease, stroke, or who are addressing the issue of nursing home placement (Bullock et al., 2003; Collins et al., 2003; Covinsky et al., 2001; Dilworth, Anderson, and Anderson, 1999; Gallagher-Thompson et al., 2003; Groger, 2002; Hamilton and Sunderlowkski, 2003; Jones et al., 2002; Williams and Dilworth-Anderson, 2002).

Increasing work is appearing to address the Asian American population (Jones et al., 2002) and American Indian caregivers (Jervis and Manson, 2002; John et al., 2001), but few of these studies to date have been population based. Some texts have provided important information concerning these populations (Harper, 1990; Lebowitz et al., 1999; Yeo and Gallagher-Thompson, 1996). Much work remains to be done, particularly in understanding Filipino (McBride and Parreno; 1996), Alaska Native (Aranda, 2001), and Pacific Islander (Yamamoto, 1986) elder care.

ACKNOWLEDGMENT

Special appreciation is expressed to Cathy Moore, M.L.S., medical librarian at the Peninsula Regional Medical Center in Salisbury, Maryland.

REFERENCES

Allen, E. A. 1988. West Indians. In L. Comas-Dias and E. E. H. Griffith (Eds.), *Clinical guidelines in cross-cultural mental health* (pp. 305–33). New York: John Wiley & Sons.

Angel, J. L., and Hogan, D. P. 1991. The demography of minority aging populations. In L. K. Harootyan (Ed.), *Minority elders: Longevity, economics, and health—Building a public policy base* (pp. 1–13). Washington, D.C.: Gerontological Society of America.

Aranda, M. P. 2001. Racial and ethnic factor in dementia care-giving research in the US. *Aging & Mental Health* 5(Suppl. 1): S116–23.

Baker, F. M. 1982. The black elderly: Biopsychosocial perspective within an age cohort and adult development context. *Journal of Geriatric Psychiatry* 15:225–37.

Baker, F. M. 1987. The Afro-American life cycle: Success, failure, and mental health. *Journal of the National Medical Association* 79(6):625–33.

Baker, F. M. 1988. Afro-Americans. In L. Comas-Dias and E. E. H. Griffith (Eds.), *Clinical guidelines in cross-cultural mental health* (pp. 151–81). New York: John Wiley & Sons.

Baker, F. M. 1994. Psychiatric treatment of elder African Americans. *Hospital and Community Psychiatry* 45(1):32–37.

Baker, F. M. 2000. Minority issues. In B. J. Sadock and V. A. Sadock (Eds.), *Comprehensive textbook of psychiatry* (7th ed.) (pp. 3164–74). Baltimore: Lippincott Williams & Wilkins.

Baker, F. M., Lavizzo-Mourey, R., and Jones, B. E. 1993. Acute care of the African American elder. *Journal of Geriatric Psychiatry and Neurology* 6(2):66–71.

Baker, F. M., and Lightfoot, O. B. 1993. Psychiatric care of ethnic elders. In A.C. Gaw (Ed.), *Culture ethnicity and mental illness* (pp. 517–52). Washington, D.C.: American Psychiatric Press.

Berlin, E., and Fowkes, W. 1983. A teaching framework for cross-cultural health care: Application in family practice. *Western Journal of Medicine* 139:934–38.

Boyd-Franklin, N. 2003. Religion and spirituality in African American families. In *Black families in therapy: Understanding the African American experience* (2nd ed.) (pp. 125–43). New York: Guilford Press.

Braithwaite, R. L., and Taylor, S. E. (Eds.). 1992. *Health issues in the black community.* San Francisco: Jossey-Bass.

Bullock, K., Crawford, S. I., and Tennstedt, S. L. 2003. Employment and caregiving: Exploration of African American caregivers. *Social Work* 48(2):150–62.

Collins, W. L., Holt, T. A., Moore, S. E., and Bledsoe, L. K. 2003. Long-distance caregiving: A case study of an African-American family. *American Journal of Alzheimer's Disease and Other Dementias* 18(5):309–16.

Colarusso, C. A., and Nemiroff, R. A. 1987. Clinical implications of adult developmental theory. *American Journal of Psychiatry* 144:1263–70.

Connell, C. M., Shaw, B. A., Holmes, S. B., and Foster, N. L. 2001. Caregivers' attitudes toward their family members' participation in Alzheimer disease research: Implications for recruitment and retention. *Alzheimer Disease and Associated Disorders* 15(3): 137–45.

Coon, D. W., Schulz, R., Ory, M. G. 1999. Innovative intervention approaches with Alzheimer disease caregivers. In D. Biegel and A. Blum (Eds.), *Innovations in practice and service delivery across the lifespan* (pp. 295–325). New York: Oxford University Press.

Covinsky, K. E., Eng, C., Lui, L-Y, Sands, L. P., Sehgal, A. R., Walter, L. C., Wieland, D., Eleazer, G. P., and Yaffe, K. 2001. Reduced employment in caregivers of frail elders: Impact of ethnicity, patient clinical characteristics, and caregiver characteristics. *Journal of Gerontology: Medical Sciences* 56A(11):M707–13.

Cox, C. 1995. Comparing the experiences of black and white caregivers of dementia patients. *Social Work* 40:343–49.

Cox, C., and Monk, A. M. 1990. Minority caregiver or dementia victims: a comparison of black and Hispanic families. *Journal of Applied Gerontology* 9:340–54.

Cox, C., and Monk, A. 1996. Strain among caregivers: Comparing the experiences of African American and Hispanic caregivers of Alzheimer's relatives. *International Journal of Aging and Human Development* 43(2):93–105.

Cuellar, J. B. 1990. Hispanic American aging: Geriatric education curriculum development for selected health professionals—Life expectancy, morbidity, and mortality. In M. S. Harper (Ed.), *Minority aging: Essential curricular content for selected health and allied health professions* (pp. 365–413). Health Resources and Services Administration, Department of Health and Human Services. DHHS Publication No. HRS (P-DV-90-4). Washington, D.C.: Government Printing Office.

Cuellar, N. C. 2002. A comparison of African American and Caucasian American female caregivers of rural, post-stroke, bed-bound older adults. *Journal of Gerontological Nursing* January:36–45.

Dilworth-Anderson, P., and Anderson, N. B. 1999. Dementia care-giving in blacks: A contextual approach to research. In B. Lebowitz, E. Light, and G. Neidereche (Eds.), *Mental and physical health of Alzheimer's caregivers* (pp. 385–409). New York: Springer.

Dilworth-Anderson, P., and Gibson, B. E. 1994. Ethnic minority perspectives in dementia, family caregiving, and interventions. *Generations* 23:40–45.

Elliott, K. S., Di Minno, M., Lam, D., and Tu, A. M. 1996. Working with Chinese families in the context of dementia. In G. Yeo and D. Gallagher-Thompson (Eds.), *Ethnicity and dementia* (pp. 89–100). London: Taylor and Francis Group.

Engle, G. 1980. The clinical application of the biopsychosocial model. *American Journal of Psychiatry* 137:535–44.

Fox, K., Hinton, W. L., and Levkoff, S. 1999. Take up the caregiver's burden: Stories of care for urban African American elders with dementia. *Culture, Medicine, and Psychiatry* 23: 501–29.

Gallagher-Thompson, D., Coon, D. W., Solano, N., Ambler, C., Rabinowitz, Y., and Thompson, L. W. 2003. Change in indices of distress among Latino and Anglo female caregivers of elderly relatives with dementia: Site-specific results from the REACH National Collaborative Study. *Gerontologist* 42:580–91.

Gallagher-Thompson, D., and DeVries, H. M. 1994. Coping with frustration classes: Development and preliminary outcomes with women who care for relatives with dementia. *Gerontologist* 34:548–52.

Gallagher-Thompson, D., Lovett, S., Rose, J., McKibbin, C., Coon, D., Futterman, A., et al. 2000. Impact of psychoeducational interventions on distressed family caregivers. *Journal of Clinical Geropsychology* 6:91–110.

Gallagher-Thompson, D., Solano, N., Coon, D., and Arean, P. 2003. Recruitment and retention of Latino dementia family caregivers in intervention research: Issues to face, lessons to learn. *Gerontologist* 43:45–51.

Gallagher-Thompson, D., and Steffen, A. M. 1994. Comparative effects of cognitive/behavioral and brief psychodynamic psychotherapies for the treatment of depression in family caregivers. *Journal of Counseling and Clinical Psychology* 62:543–49.

Green, J. G., Smith, R., Gardiner, M., and Tinbury, G. C 1982. Measuring behavioral disturbance of elderly demented patients in the community and its effects on relatives: A factor analytic study. *Age and Aging* 11:121–26.

Gonzales, E., Gitlin, L., and Lyons, K. J. 1995. Review of the literature on African American caregivers of individuals with dementia. *Journal of Cultural Diversity* 2(2):40–48.

Gover, K. 2000. Indian entities recognized and eligible to receive services from the United States Bureau of Indian Affairs. *Federal Register* 65:13298–303.

Groger, L. 2002. Coming to terms: African-Americans' complex ways of coping with life in a nursing home. *International Journal of Aging and Human Development* 55(3):183–205.

Haley, W. E., Roth, D. L., Coleton, M. I., Ford, G. R., West, C. A. C., Collins, R. P., and Isobe, T. L. 1996. Appraisal, coping, and social support as mediators of well-being in black and white family caregivers of patients with Alzheimer's Disease. *Journal of Consulting and Clinical Psychology* 64(1):121–29.

Haley, W. E., West, C. A. C., Wadley, V. G., Ford, G. R., White, F. A., Barrett, J. J., Harrell, L. E., and Roth, D. L. 1995. Psychological, social, and health impact of caregiving: A comparison of black and white dementia family caregivers and noncaregivers. *Psychology and Aging* 10(4):540–52.

Hamilton, J. B., and Sandelowski, M. 2003. Living the Golden Rule: Reciprocal exchanges among African Americans with cancer. *Qualitative Health Research* 13(5):656–74.

Harper, M. S. (Ed). 1990. *Minority aging: Essential curricular content for selected health and allied health professions*. Health Resources and Services Administration, Department of Health and Human Services. DHHS Publication No. HRS (P-DV-90-4). Washington, D.C.: Government Printing Office.

Harwood, D. G., Barker, W. W., Cantillon, M., Loewenstein, D. A., Ownby, R., and Duara, R. 1998. Depressive symptoms in first-degree family caregivers of Alzheimer's disease patients: A cross-ethnic comparison. *Alzheimer's Disease and Associated Disorders* 12:340–46.

Henderson, J. N., Gutierrez-Mayka, M., Garcia, J., and Boyd, S. 1993. A model for Alzheimer's disease support group development in African-American and Hispanic populations. *Gerontologist* 33:409–14.

Hennessy, C. H., and John, R. 1995. The interpretation of burden among Pueblo Indian caregivers. *Journal of Aging Studies* 9:215–29.

Hennessy, C. H., and John, R. 1996. American Indian caregivers' perception of burden and needed support services. *Journal of Applied Gerontology* 15:275–93.

Hennessy, C. H., John, R., and Anderson, L. A. 1999. Diabetes education needs of family members caring for American Indian elders. *Diabetes Educator* 25:747–54.

Hinton, L., Haan, M., Geller, S., and Mangas, D. 2003. Neuropsychiatric symptoms in Latino elders with dementia or cognitive impairment without dementia and factors that modify their association with caregiver depression. *Gerontologist* 42:669–77.

Hobus, R. M. 1990. Living in two worlds: A Lakota transcultural nursing experience. *Journal of Transcultural Nursing* 2:33–36.

Janevic, M. R., and Connell, C. M. 2001. Racial, ethnic, and cultural differences in the dementia caregiving experience: Recent findings. *Gerontologist* 41:334–47.

Jervis, L. I., and Manson, S. M. 2002. American Indians / Alaska Natives and dementia. *Alzheimer Disease and Associated Disorders* 16(Suppl. 2):S89–95.

John, R. 1995. *American Indian and Alaska Native elders: An assessment of their current status and provision of services.* Rockville, Md.: U.S. Department of Health and Human Services.

John, R., Hennessy, C. H., Dyeson, T. B., and Garrett, M. 2001. Toward the conceptualization and measurement of caregiver burden among Pueblo Indian family caregivers. *Gerontologist* 41:210–19.

Jones, P. S., Zhang, X. E., Jaceldo-Siegl, K., and Meleis, A. I. 2002. Caregiving between two cultures: An integrative experience. *Journal of Transcultural Nursing* 13(3):202–9.

Kaye, J., and Robinson, K. M. 1994. Spirituality among caregivers. *Image* 26:218–21.

Kelley, J. D. 1994. African American caregivers: Perceptions of the caregiving situation and factors influencing the delay of institutionalization of elders with dementia. *ABNF Journal* July/August:106–9.

Lampley-Dallas, V. T. 2002. Research issues for minority dementia patients and their caregivers: What are the gaps in our knowledge base? *Alzheimer Disease and Associated Disorders* 16(Suppl. 2):S46–49.

Lampley-Dallas, V. T., Mold, J. W., and Flori, D. E. 2001. Perceived needs of African American caregivers of elders with dementia. *Journal of the National Medical Association* 933(2): 47–57.

Lebowitz, B., Light, E., and Neidereche, G. (Eds.). 1999. *Mental and physical health of Alzheimer's caregivers.* New York: Springer.

Lewis, D. I., and Ausberry, M. S. C. 1996. African American families: Management of demented elders. In G. Yeo and D. Gallagher-Thompson (Eds.), *Ethnicity and the dementias* (pp. 167–74). Washington, D.C.: Taylor & Francis.

Manson, S. J. 1995. Mental health status and needs of the American Indian and Alaska Native elderly. In D. K. Padgett (Ed.), *Handbook in ethnicity, aging, and mental health* (pp. 132–47). Westport, Conn.: Greenwood.

Manuel, R. C. 1988. The demography of older blacks in the United States. In J. S. Jackson (Ed.), *The black American elderly: Research on physical and psychosocial health* (pp. 25–48). New York: Springer.

Martinez, C. 1988. Mexican Americans. In L. Comas-Diaz and E. E. H. Griffith (Eds.), *Clinical guidelines in cross-cultural mental heath* (pp. 182–220). New York: John Wiley & Sons.

McBride, M. R., and Parreno, H. 1996. Filipino American families and caregiving. In G. Yeo and D. Gallagher-Thompson (Eds.), *Ethnicity and the dementias* (pp. 123–35). Washington D.C.: Taylor & Francis.

Mintzer, J. E., Rupert, M. P., Loewenstein, D., Gamez, E., Millor, A., Quinteros, R., et al. 1992. Daughter's caregiving for Hispanic and non-Hispanic Alzheimer's patients: Does ethnicity make a difference? *Community Mental Health Journal* 28:293–303.

Mollica, R. F., and Lavelle, J. P. 1988. Southeast Asian refugees. In L. Comas-Diaz and E.E.H. Griffith (Eds.), *Clinical guidelines in cross-cultural mental health* (pp. 262–93). New York: John Wiley & Sons.

Navaie-Waliser, M., Feldman, P. H., Gould, D. A., Levine, C., Kuerbis, A. N., and Donelan, K. 2001. The experiences and challenges of informal caregivers: Common themes and differences among whites, blacks, and Hispanics. *Gerontologist* 41:733–41.

Neugarten, B. L. 1979. Time, age, and the life cycle. *American Journal of Psychiatry* 136:887–94.

Novak, M., and Guest, C. 1989. Application of multidimensional caregiver burden inventory. *Gerontologist* 29:798–803.

Picot, S. J., Debanne, S. M., Manazi, K. H., and Wykle, M. L. 1997. Religiosity and perceived rewards of black and white caregivers. *Gerontologist* 37:89–101.

Pierce, L. L. 2001. Caring and expressions of stability by urban family caregivers of persons with stroke within African American family systems. *Rehabilitation Nursing* 26(3):100–107, 116.

Pinderhughes, E. 1982. Afro-American families and the victim system. In M. McGoldrick, J. K. Pearce, and J. Giordano (Eds.), *Ethnicity and family therapy* (pp. 109–22). New York: Guilford.

Radloff, L. S. 1977. The CES-D scale, a self-report depression scale for research in the general population. *Applied Psychological Measurement* 1:385–401.

Siegel, J. S. 1999. Demographic introduction to racial/Hispanic elderly populations. In Tony P. Miles (Ed.), *Full-color aging: Facts, goals, and recommendations for America's diverse elders* (pp. 1–19). Washington, D.C.: Gerontological Society of America.

Steinmetz, S. R. 1988. Duty bound: Elder abuse and family care. Newbury Park, Calif.: Sage.

Sterritt, P. F., and Pokorny, M. E. 1998. African-American caregiving for a relative with Alzheimer's disease. *Geriatric Nursing* 19(3):127–34.

Strong, C. 1984. Stress and caring for elderly relatives: Interpretations and coping strategies in an American Indian and white sample. *Gerontologist* 24:251–56.

Taylor, R. J., and Chatters, L. M. 1986a. Church-based informal support among elderly blacks. *Gerontologist* 26:637–42.

Taylor, R. J., and Chatters, L. M. 1986b. Patterns of informal support to elderly black adults: The role of family and church members. *Social Work* 31:432–38.

Taylor, R. J., and Chatters, L. M. 1991. Religious life. In J. S. Jackson (Ed.), *Life in black America* (pp. 105–23). Newbury Park: Sage.

Tempo, P. M., and Saito, A. 1996. Techniques of working with Japanese American families. In G. Yeo and D. Gallagher-Thompson (Eds.), *Ethnicity and the dementias* (pp. 109–22). Washington, D.C.: Taylor & Francis.

Teri, L., and McCurry, S. H. 2000. Psychosocial therapies. In C. E. Coffey and J. L. Cummings (Eds.), *Textbook of geriatric neuropsychiatry* (2nd ed.) (pp. 861–90). Washington, D.C.: American Psychiatric Press.

Theis, S. L., Biordi, D. L., Coeling, H., Nalepka, C., and Miller, B. 2003. Spirituality in caregiving and care receiving. *Holistic Nursing Practice* 17(1):458–55.

Torres-Matrullo, C. 1982. Cognitive therapy of depressive disorders in the Puerto Rican female. In R. M. Becorra, M. Karno, and J. I. Escobar (Eds.), *Mental health and Hispanic Americans* (pp. 101–13). New York: Grune & Stratton.

Trimble, J. E. 2000. Social psychological perspective on changing self-identification among American Indians and Alaska Natives. In R. Dana Mahwah (Ed.), *Handbook of cross-cultural and multicultural personality assessment* (pp. 197–222). Mahwah, N.J.: Lawrence Erlbaum Associates.

Valle, R. 1994. Culture-fair behavioral symptoms differential assessment and intervention in dementing illness. *Alzheimer Disease and Associated Disorders* 8(Suppl.):21–45.

Walker, R. D., and LaDue, R. 1986. An integrative approach to American Indian mental health. In C. B. Wilkerson (Ed.), *Ethnic psychiatry* (pp. 143–94). New York: Plenum Medical Book Company.

Wilkinson, C. B. 1986. Introduction. In C. B. Wilkinson (Ed.), *Ethnic psychiatry* (pp. 1–12). New York: Plenum Medical Book Company.

Williams, A. S., Dilworth-Anderson, P., and Goodwin, P. Y. 2003. Caregiver role strain: The contribution of multiple roles and available resources in African-American women. *Aging and Mental Health* 7(2):103–12.

Williams, S. W., and Dilworth-Anderson, P. 2002. Systems of social support in families who care for dependent African American elders. *Gerontologist* 42:224–36.

Yamamoto, J. 1986. Therapy for Asian American and Pacific Islanders. In C. B. Wilkerson (Ed.), *Ethnic psychiatry* (pp. 128–31). New York: Plenum Medical Book Company.

Yeo, G., and Gallagher-Thompson, D. (Eds.). 1996. *Ethnicity and the dementias.* Washington, D.C.: Taylor & Francis.

Zarit, S., Anthony, C., and Boutselis, M. 1987. Interventions with caregivers of dementia patients: Comparison of two approaches. *Psychology and Aging* 2:224–32.

Zarit, S. H., Reever, K. E., and Bach-Peterson, J. 1980. Relatives of the impaired elderly: correlates of feelings of burden. *Gerontologist* 20:649–55.

Zarit, S. H., and Zarit, J. M. 1990. *The memory and behavior problems checklist and the burden interview.* University Park: Pennsylvania State University Gerontology Center.

CHAPTER FOURTEEN

The Ethics of Dementia Caregiving

MICHELE J. KAREL, PH.D.
JENNIFER MOYE, PH.D.

As an individual with dementia gradually loses the capacity for self-care and in-formed decision making, family members are confronted with increased pressure to assist and support that person. Sometimes decisions that need to be made for the individual entail conflict—regarding who should be making a particular decision and whose interests should be considered (e.g., how to spend a family's financial resources). Just how to negotiate these difficult dilemmas—in a compassionate, appropriate, and practical manner—comprises the ethics of dementia caregiving.

In this chapter we review three dimensions of the ethics of dementia caregiving. First, we review the most common ethical dilemmas in dementia caregiving. Second, we provide a framework to guide ethical decision making for dementia care-givers. Finally, we review legal and other practical tools to help families protect the preferences and interests of their loved ones with dementia.

ETHICAL DILEMMAS IN FAMILY CAREGIVING FOR DEMENTIA

A bibliometric review of articles published on the topic of ethics and dementia between 1980 and 2000 found four major themes to account for most (64.6%) of the literature published over that time: decision making, end-of-life issues, treatment, and professional care (Baldwin et al., 2003). However, relatively few of the articles (12%) were related to concerns of family caregivers. While the distribution of eth-ical issues addressed was similar in family versus nonfamily articles, the authors recommend caution that families may or may not share the same concerns as professional caregivers; the same themes may have emerged simply because those were the themes asked about by the researchers.

Several studies or reviews have identified major ethical issues in dementia caregiving, from the perspective of family caregivers and/or persons with dementia. The "Fairhill Guidelines on Ethics of the Care of People with Alzheimer's Disease" resulted from a series of monthly meetings among individuals with mild Alzheimer disease (AD), their family caregivers, and an interdisciplinary group of professionals working in the field (Post and Whitehouse, 1995). Through this discourse, six major areas of ethical concern (and suggestions for managing these dilemmas) were identified: (1) *truth telling and diagnosis,* with consensus that individuals with early-stage dementia should be informed of their diagnosis and be offered educational and supportive services; (2) *driving privileges,* stressing the importance of finding a balance between premature restriction of privileges and minding safety concerns, while trying to include the person with dementia in negotiation; (3) *respecting choice: autonomy, capacity, and competence,* with an emphasis on respecting decisions that the person with AD is still capable of making, thinking of capacities as specific rather than global, and engaging in advance care planning while the person with AD is still able; (4) *dilemmas of behavior control,* including support for safe environments, behavioral interventions, avoidance of physical restraints, and appropriate use of medications; (5) *issues in death and dying,* with an emphasis on advance care planning, understanding the extent to which the person with AD wants the family to follow advance directives or to do what they think is best, and awareness of hospice services; (6) *quality of life and treatment decisions,* involving concern for understanding what makes the person with AD feel happy and focusing on comfort at the end stage of the illness.

Two additional reviews outline similar ethical dilemmas common for family caregivers. As part of a larger survey, family caregivers responded to a general open-ended question about "other concerns," and in this context several common ethical concerns were identified (Pratt, Schmall, and Wright, 1987). These included: the nature of family obligation in caregiving and sharing of responsibilities among family members; conflicts between caregiving and responsibilities to oneself, one's career, or to other family members; financing of health care; balancing concern for the patient's autonomy with paternalism; and understanding the patient's responsibility in planning for long-term care. Another review of the ethics of family caregiving (Barber and Lyness, 2001), written from the perspective of a marriage and family therapist, identified the following six ethical dilemmas, which overlap with the findings of Pratt and colleagues: determining the extent of filial responsibility to a parent with dementia; family equity, or how to divide labor among family members; managing competing commitments between work, family, and caregiving; balancing respect for the care recipient's autonomy and safety in making decisions; knowing what care recipients want and when and how to act on their behalf; and, financing the cost of care.

Finally, a study of everyday ethics for dementia care in nursing homes identified four major domains with ethical implications especially relevant for institutional settings (Powers, 2000): learning the limits of intervention, or how much care to "force" when the resident refuses; finding the balance between protecting safety (e.g., through restraint) and respecting residents' rights to take risks; protecting individual choices and preferred routines while also running an institution efficiently; and defining the community norms and values regarding resources spent on various quality-of-life concerns.

In reviewing this literature, we summarize ethical dilemmas common to family dementia caregiving using three major caregiver questions corresponding to the early, middle, and late stages of the disease process: (1) What is the extent of my obligation as a caregiver? (2) How do I respect the preferences of my loved one as well as protect his or her safety if I feel those preferences are unsafe? (3) Toward the end of life, how do I make the right decisions about my loved one's care?

Becoming a Caregiver: Caregiving Obligations, Motivations, and Competing Interests

Why do family members become caregivers? While many demographic, societal, and psychological factors influence caregiving behavior, most cultures place basic value on the family unit and some degree of mutual family responsibility (Brackman, 1995; Jecker, 1995). Family caregivers are often motivated simply by family mutuality, or the idea that family members should take care of each other. A related motivation is the idea of reciprocity, or that one has an obligation to provide care in return for years of devotion or care provided by the person now ill (as one's spouse, parent, sibling, or other). Certainly not all caregiving is motivated by a sense of obligation, but often as an expression of love and friendship, or as a protective response to another person's vulnerability (Pratt et al., 1987; Selig, Tomlinson, and Hickey, 1991).

While few would argue with these basic motivations for family members to take care of ill relatives, ethical dilemmas arise when such questions as the following are considered: Are there any acceptable limits to caregiving obligation? What care is expected from a child to a parent who was abusive in some manner during childhood? What sacrifices to one's own health or financial interests are reasonable in providing care? (Arras, 1995). What is the appropriate balance between family, community, and governmental responsibility in caring for frail elders? Cultural values and norms play a large part in determining the relative weight given to family care obligations, particularly regarding filial responsibility (Dai and Dimond, 1998; Youn et al., 1999) and the question of whose interests are to be prominent in making decisions about care (Dilworth-Anderson and Gibson, 2002; Yeo and Gallagher-Thompson, 1996). Further, in most cultures women take on disproportionate responsibility for family caregiving, raising the question of whether ethical standards for caregiving differ for men and women (Guberman, Maheu, and Maille, 1992; Martin and Post, 1992).

Individual caregivers are also motivated by a wide range of psychological and emotional needs and responses, which may change throughout the caregiving experience (Guberman et al., 1992; Motenko, 1989). Caregiving can provide significant emotional rewards, such as providing a compassionate response to a vulnerable person, having a meaningful role, and experiencing a sense of altruism. Caregiving can also help to compensate for negative feelings, such as guilt or regret for past behaviors. At the same time, caregiving often creates emotional burdens, including grief over the gradual loss of one's loved one through dementia, anger at the situation, embarrassment over the sick person's behaviors, exhaustion and conflict in balancing multiple roles, and feelings of depression or hopelessness about the future (Mace and Rabins, 1999; Martin and Post, 1992; Meuser and Marwit, 2001; Stoller and Pugliesi, 1989).

Ethical dilemmas can arise when decisions based on a caregiver's emotional needs are not viewed as serving the best interests of the person with dementia. Extreme examples might include: a wife who insists on keeping her husband at home even though she can no longer care for him (e.g., he is malnourished, has had multiple falls and fractures), because she could not tolerate the guilt of placing him in a nursing home; a daughter who chooses not to arrange closer oversight of her father because of longstanding anger at his absence while she was growing up; or, a husband who insists on a feeding tube when most of the family knows his wife would not have wanted such, because of his profound grief and inability to let her die. Sometimes the needs of the person with dementia exceed the physical, emotional, or financial resources of potential family caregivers. Further, some family members have significant medical, psychiatric, or substance abuse problems that interfere with their capacity to provide adequate care even before dementia becomes a problem in the family.

Individual caregivers struggle not only with their own emotional needs but also with the dynamics of a family and social system. The power balance in the family shifts when the family elder gets sick (Qualls, 1999); the shifting of various roles and related decision-making powers can entail significant discomfort or conflict. Depending on their roles in the family and relationship to the ill parent, siblings may differ in their approaches to caregiving involvement and decisions for a parent. Balancing the needs and interests of the person with dementia with the roles, responsibilities, and emotional needs of each of several people in the family system can be daunting, and there is rarely one "right" answer for balancing these various interests (Arras, 1995; Moody, 1992; Pratt et al., 1987). Further, families differ in the extent to which they will accept help from various informal (e.g., friends and neighbors) or formal (e.g., home health aide services, nursing home care) sources. Different family systems, and cultural groups, vary in the types of services and solutions that are consistent with their particular values, norms, and comfort (Dilworth-Anderson, Williams, and Gibson, 2002).

Caregiving in Early to Mid-stage Dementia: Promoting Autonomy versus Protecting Safety

Particularly in early to mid-stage dementia, family members are frequently torn between wanting to respect the self-determination of the person with dementia and wanting to protect that person from harm (Moody, 1992; Post and Whitehouse, 1995). Of note, this same tension may also be felt by families whose relative does not (yet) have a formal diagnosis of dementia but who is undergoing noticeable cognitive changes, or "mild cognitive impairment" (MCI). While MCI remains a controversial diagnostic entity, the following ethical dilemmas for caregivers may be relevant (Peterson, 2004; Winblad et al., 2004). As the disease progresses, the person with dementia may have a more difficult time recognizing or admitting the risks inherent in certain situations. Common issues include whether or not the individual can safely live alone, responsibly manage finances, accurately manage medications, or drive safely. It can be humiliating and demoralizing for the person with dementia to be advised how to manage his or her affairs. With strong motivation to remain independent, the person with dementia may be resistant to offers of help or increased supervision. To what extent the family caregiver(s) should step in and suggest or insist on alternative living arrangements, oversight of the checking account, supervision of medications, or taking away the keys to the car are heart-wrenching decisions.

This dilemma represents a conflict between the ethical principles of autonomy and beneficence. One of the foundations of American culture, and therefore the country's health care, is respect for the individual's self-determination. However, another foundation of health and social services is to protect the best interests and to "do no harm" to the individual. In general, if an individual is believed to have the capacity to make a particular decision—that is, to understand and appreciate the risks and benefits of that decision in accordance with long-standing values— then the principle of autonomy usually prevails; the individual has the right to engage in risky behavior so long as it does not pose danger or unwelcome burden to others.

The person with early-stage dementia may be in a "gray area" of decision-making capacity, so that it is not always clear whether the person truly appreciates the risks taken by, for example, continuing to live alone. Further, people differ greatly in their risk tolerance—how much risk can be tolerated to allow the person with dementia to maintain independence? At some point, when the person is assessed to be incapable and/or the risk too high to tolerate, family caregivers step in to override the wishes of the person with dementia for the sake of his or her well-being or the well-being of others (such as risks of unsafe driving). Further, the preferences of the person with dementia may not be followed if there are conflicting interests among other stakeholders; for example, just because mom decides she wants to move in with her daughter who is already struggling to balance work and child care doesn't mean this is the best plan for everyone.

This dilemma also arises regarding institutional or other formal care of people with dementia. Nursing homes, for example, must balance concerns for their residents' health and safety with the basic rights and preferences of individual "customers." Efficient operation of an institution usually minimizes opportunity for individual preference, such as choice in food and timing of meals. Further, nursing homes historically place greater interest on protecting the safety of residents rather than optimizing their quality of life (Kane, 2001; Powers, 2000). Family caregivers often remain active advocates for their loved ones who reside in nursing homes or who receive other formal services in the community. Thus family caregivers interface with professional care teams in resolving dilemmas such as whether to use restraints to prevent falls, when to use psychotropic medications to control agitated behavior, and whether, for example, to allow the patient to eat the chocolate she has always enjoyed despite dietary concerns.

Another important issue is helping a person with dementia decide whether or not to participate in a research study, or making that decision on behalf of the person with dementia. While beyond the scope of this chapter, the ability of individuals with dementia to offer informed consent for research has become a priority area of investigation. Family caregivers may need to help their loved ones consider the risks and benefits of, for example, participating in a drug treatment trial (Karlawish,

Casarett, Klocinski, and Sankar, 2001; Kim, Cox, and Caine, 2002). A related dilemma for Alzheimer disease caregivers is whether to pursue genetic testing, for the person with dementia (Eaton, 1999) and/or for themselves. Ethical issues regarding genetic testing include the predictive accuracy of the tests, potential psychological distress in caregivers, and the fact that there is no definitive cure (Bassett, Havstad, and Chase, 2004; Coon, Davies, McKibben, and Gallagher-Thompson, 1999).

Caregiving in Late-stage Dementia: Identity of the Person with Dementia and Surrogate Decision Making

An important philosophical question, with clear ethical implications, is how to define the "personhood" of an individual gradually losing capacities through the course of dementia. Over the course of dementia, does a person and his or her basic values and satisfactions in life remain stable, or not? The concept of advance care planning, including the use of advance directives, is predicated on the assumption that a person can predict what he or she might want in some future state of illness. However, what if one's values or attitudes change with life experience (e.g., "I never thought I'd want to live if I went blind, but now that I'm blind, I'm coping and am glad to be alive") or with changing cognitive or emotional capacities (e.g., "My mom always said she'd rather die than be in a nursing home, but she seems so happy there now")? Dilemmas regarding how to interpret advance directives and how to weigh potential differences between a person's "predementia" self versus "dementia" self can be quite difficult indeed.

Medical philosophers and ethicists have written about this issue of the self over the course of dementia. For example, "the someone else problem" (Degrazia, 1999) refers to whether the instructions of an advance directive should apply to an individual distinctly different from the person who originally completed the directive. Similarly, the concept of "precedent autonomy" refers to a previously made decision that may no longer be understood by or applicable to the now incapacitated person (Davis, 2002; Dresser, 1992; Newton, 1999). Further, the person with dementia may be conceived to have a "then self" and a "now self," the latter with potentially changed interests and motivations due to the impact of the illness (Koppelman, 2002).

The ethical challenge for the family caregiver acting as surrogate decision maker is how best to make decisions with respect for the dignity, wishes, and values of someone who has been changing over time. While "substituted judgment" (making the same decision we believe the person would make if that person were still able to) remains the ethical standard for surrogate decision making when possible, the complexity of medical treatment decisions often makes ascertaining exactly what the person would have wanted—and whether that is still what the person would want—quite difficult. It is often impossible to apply prior instructional directives (e.g., "I don't want aggressive medical technologies used to prolong my life if I am dying) to a particular clinical situation (e.g., whether to do GI surgery for bowel impaction in advanced dementia). Many now argue that using a strict substituted judgment standard is not necessarily possible or even preferable (Sullivan, 2002). Models of surrogate decision making increasingly address the importance of building consensus by including what is known about a patient's values with careful consideration of the burdens and benefits of different treatment options (Karlawish, Quill, and Meier, 1999) and by integrating what is known about the prior wishes of the "then self" with the apparent "desires, likes, and dislikes of the now self" (Koppelman, 2002, p. 81).

In fact, evidence suggests that many older adults and families prefer a collaborative, consensus-based decision making process that considers the best interests of the patient and his or her loved ones (High, 1988; Rosenfeld, Wenger, and Kagawa-Singer, 2000). Even if there were a true answer to "what a persons with dementia would have wanted if she could tell us," we know that family members and care providers are not good at predicting what someone would want (Hare, Pratt, and Nelson, 1992; Seckler, Meier, Mulvihill, and Cammer Paris, 1991; Suhl, Simons, Reedy, and Garrick, 1994). When patients are asked whether they want their advance directives followed closely, or for family to do what they feel is best at the time, most say "do what's best at the time" (Puchalski et al., 2000). The majority of family surrogates for persons with dementia say they make decisions based on their understanding of what the patient would have wanted *and* based on what they and family feel is the most reasonable choice for all involved *and* based on what the doctor says is in the patient's best interest (Mezey, Kluger, Maislin, and Mittelman, 1996). Additionally, cultural factors are extremely important in approaches to decision making. Individual autonomy is not the primary value in many cultural groups, and respect for the individual—both before and after incapacity associated with dementia—entails considering decisions from the perspective of the needs of the family and community (Blackhall et al., 1995; Ersek et al., 1998; Hornung et al., 1998).

Certainly, end-of-life decisions are among the most difficult ones faced by family caregivers. Evidence suggests that persons with dementia often do not receive optimal care at the end of life, in part due to the difficulty in predicting the course of illness in advanced dementia and in making decisions regarding nutrition, fluids, and antibiotics. Palliative care for people with dementia, which often entails withholding these seemingly routine treatments, can sometimes leave family members feeling that they are directly "causing" the death of their loved one (Sachs, Shega, and Cox-Hayley, 2004). To make ethical decisions, family caregivers may need improved education about the process of dying and options for palliative care in dementia (Volicer, 2001) and emotional support in coping with guilt and grief so that they can collaborate with care teams in making decisions in the best interest of their loved ones (Forbes, Bern-Klug, and Gessert, 2000; Sachs et al., 2004).

A FRAMEWORK FOR ETHICAL DECISION MAKING

Analysis of ethical decision making entails clarifying the values and goals of relevant stakeholders, identifying the (often conflicting) ethical principles for the particular dilemma at hand and comparing the risks and benefits of alternative solutions (Aulisio et al., 2000; Doolittle and Herrick, 1992). In the realm of dementia caregiving, a critical piece of the dilemma is often who has the capacity and the right to make a particular decision. Major ethical principles that can come into conflict include: autonomy and respect of persons, beneficence (to do good, to promote well-being), nonmaleficence (to avoid causing harm), justice (fair distribution of benefits, risks, and costs), and fidelity or veracity (to be truthful and trustworthy in relationships) (Beauchamp and Childress, 2001; Doolittle and Herrick, 1992). Sorting through difficult caregiving decisions is often best achieved through a process of collaborative communication and consensus.

In the realm of dementia caregiving, we consider five steps for working through ethical dilemmas: (1) Defining the issue and relevant values for the stakeholders; (2) determining the decision-making capacity of the person with dementia; (3) including the person with dementia in the decision-making process to the extent possible; (4) implementing surrogate decision making if necessary and considering alternative solutions; (5) implementing, evaluating, and reevaluating the outcome as needed. Table 14.1 provides suggestions for clinicians who are working with caregivers to negotiate ethical dilemmas, through each of these steps.

The Decision-making Process

Step 1: Defining the issue and relevant stakeholder values. It is important to define exactly what decisions need to be made, how serious or risky the consequences are, and who is affected by the outcomes. What is the impact of the decision on the person with dementia, on his or her family, and on the community at large? Can people agree on the nature of the problem and who has the responsibility to contribute to a solution? What additional information is needed to clarify the problem as well as the range of viable solutions?

TABLE 14.1
*Suggestions for Clinicians in Helping Family Dementia Caregivers
to Negotiate Ethical Dilemmas*

Step for Working Through Ethical Dilemmas in Dementia Caregiving	Suggestions for Clinicians
1. Define the issue and relevant stakeholder values	• Offer a collaborative, problem-solving stance • Communicate that decisions are often complex and rarely have obvious "right" or "wrong" answers • Help caregivers define (1) the problem, (2) which people will be affected by decision outcomes, and (3) which people should contribute to the solution
2. Determine decision-making capacity	• Help caregivers understand that, to the extent the person with dementia is able to understand the risks and benefits of decisions, he or she maintains the right to contribute to the decision-making process • Help caregivers understand that decision-making capacity is not an "all or none" concept, and that their loved ones may maintain certain abilities while needing increased help and support in other areas • Facilitate a referral for evaluation of decision-making capacity (usually to a psychologist, psychiatrist, or geriatric specialist) when there are questions about the patient's capacities related to particular family concerns (e.g., managing finances, independent living, driving)
3. Optimize preferred decision-making participation	• Encourage caregivers to include the person with dementia in making decisions to the extent that he or she wants to participate and is able (i.e., caregivers should avoid "taking over" all decisions while the person with dementia remains able to communicate valid values and preferences) • Model collaborative communication by speaking directly to the person with dementia while the family is present, rather than talking about that person as if he or she were not in the room
4. Implement surrogate decision-making and consider alternative solutions	• Encourage persons with dementia to designate preferred surrogate decision makers (e.g., durable power of attorney for health or finances) while they are still able to do so • Work collaboratively with surrogates to consider the risks and benefits of particular decisions in light of what they know of the patient's values and preferences and in light of reasonable interests of the family • If there appears to be intractable conflict among potential surrogates and/or with the health care team, consult an ethics advisory committee • Regarding end-of-life decisions, use language that avoids making surrogates feel solely responsible for decisions to discontinue life-sustaining therapies; provide information, support, and validation for issues of loss and grief
5. Evaluate outcomes and reconsider decisions over time	• Help caregivers understand that the needs and interests of the person with dementia, and the family, will change over time and that decisions therefore need to be reevaluated over time (e.g., for safety of independent living, driving, medication monitoring) • Plan reevaluation of relevant capacities and family caregiver concerns as part of usual clinical care

For example, how might a family begin to consider whether or not the person with dementia should still be driving? Many complicated questions arise here. For example, an older man with early Alzheimer disease, Joe, feels perfectly capable of driving and sees no other way of getting to his shopping, medical appointments, and social activities. His wife, Catherine, who does not drive, worries about his driving because he has become lost on several occasions. Questions here include whether Joe's ability to drive safely is actually compromised, what level of risk he and his family are willing to tolerate, and what other transportation options exist if he stops driving. For example, their son Robert, who lives locally, works full-time and could help with weekend driving, but he would have to use vacation or sick time from his job to take his parents to weekday appointments. In their suburban location, there are limited options for public transportation. Taxi service would be needed for weekday social activities. At what point is the risk of driving high enough to warrant taking away this man's independence and to incur significant costs of arranging alternative transportation? Does this man's primary doctor have a recommendation? We will return to this example in the final step below.

Step 2: Determining decision-making capacity. The extent to which persons with dementia can be included in making decisions for themselves depends on their decision-making capacity. Early in the illness, the individual should still be able to communicate opinions and preferences and in general will be able to participate in decision making (Moye, Karel, Azar, and Gurrera, 2004). However, as the disease progresses, the individual will have increased difficulty with decision making, owing to problems with remembering important information and weighing the risks and benefits of that information as it applies to his or her situation (Marson, Chatterjee, Ingram, and Harrell, 1996). As such, the individual with dementia becomes dependent on others to make decisions about basic care, residence and, ultimately, life and death medical care (Karlawish et al., 2002).

A person with decisional incapacity is defined as someone who (1) has a clinically diagnosed disease or disorder that results in (2) cognitive or psychiatric impairment that causes (3) specific behavioral or decisional disabilities, to the extent that (4) the individual lacks the ability to meet the most basic requirements for health, safety, or self-care (Moye, 2003). Sometimes the term *competence* (or *competency*) is also used, although technically that is a legal term. Decision-making capacity is not a global, fixed, or "black-and-white" concept, and it may vary according to domain, situation, context, or time. For example, across domains, a person may maintain capacity to make simple medical decisions but not to manage a checkbook. Across situations, a person may be able to manage a checking account but not a complex portfolio of investments. Across contexts, a person may be able to live alone in a small urban apartment with neighbors to help, but not in a large suburban house with limited supports for transportation or supervision. Across time, a person may temporarily lose the capacity to manage his or her medications during an episode of confusion but later regain this capacity (Moye, 2003).

Determination of a person's decision-making capacity is not always obvious, and even experts can reach different opinions on this matter (Marson et al., 1997). In brief, a capacity evaluation should include an evaluation of the individual's diagnosis and the cognitive symptoms of the diagnosis (e.g., memory, judgment, attention, etc). Also, the evaluation should include an assessment of the specific task or decision in question, as close to real life as possible. For example, if the question is financial management capacity, a functional evaluation of the person's ability to manage bills, money, assets, and avoid fraud should be given. If the question is capacity to drive safely, a driving test should be given (Moye, 1999). (For a detailed discussion of ethical issues related to dementia and driving, see Berger and Rosner, 2000). Decisional capacity should not be determined on the basis of a diagnosis alone or a brief cognitive screen. Brief screening scores do not have adequate sensitivity to specific capacity impairments (Kim and Caine, 2002).

The key is to think about the individual with dementia as someone who has capacity for a decision or else has diminished capacity. Only in very late stages does it make sense to think about incapacity. In the diminished capacity range, the caregivers' job is to consider how they can support and assist the individual to make good decisions.

Step 3: Optimizing preferred decision making participation. People differ in the extent to which they play an active role in making important decisions in their lives. While some people value self-determination, other people feel more comfortable having family or others take a more active role in making decisions for them. Certainly, important cultural differences influence the extent to which decisions are made by, and in the best interests of, the individual versus the family or community unit (Yeo and Gallagher-Thompson, 1996). Generational differences exist in which older cohorts have been socialized to defer to physicians' judgments about medical care, while younger cohorts expect to take a more active role in their medical treatment plans. In addition, particular personality styles, belief systems, or interpersonal dynamics influence an individual's desire to take an active role in decision making (e.g., Wallston and Wallston, 1978).

During the early to middle stages of dementia, it is important to optimize the person's ability to participate in decision making if he or she so desires. Several strategies should help to maximize capacity: presenting information in short, structured, organized formats; incorporating illustrations and summaries of information; offering corrective feedback or multiple learning trials (Dunn and Jeste, 2001). Obviously, attending to any problems in hearing or vision and addressing anxiety are also important to respecting the dignity of the individual. However, overly "helping" an individual to make independent decisions is not always the most respectful course of action. Certainly, a person with dementia who says he trusts others to make particular decisions on his behalf can best be respected by understanding whom he trusts to make which types of decisions.

Step 4: Implementing surrogate decision making and considering alternative solutions. When a person with dementia can no longer actively participate in making certain decisions, it is usually family caregivers who assume that responsibility, either formally or informally. Formal legal mechanisms for designating surrogate decision makers include the durable power of attorney for health and/or financial issues, and guardianship; these and other legal tools are discussed further below. Often, these formal designations are not in place, but families still contribute to surrogate decision making about their loved ones' care. Dilemmas can arise around both (1) who the appropriate surrogate decision maker should be and, (2) what decisions should be made.

Often, families agree on a plan of care and the closest "next of kin" (often the spouse or adult child) becomes the primary spokesperson for the person with dementia, for example, in interacting with medical providers, housing directors, or bank officials. In general, the model of a sole surrogate decision maker is not entirely realistic, in that most decisions affect and are negotiated by multiple parties, and even legally designated health care proxies often need and wish to have input and support from others (Lane and Dubler, 1997; Moody, 1992). However, when there is significant conflict within a family, or there is no close kin, it can be difficult to determine the most appropriate surrogate decision maker if the person with dementia did not make such designations ahead of time.

How should conflict among family or other caregivers or providers be negotiated? Guidelines usually respect next of kin in the following order: spouse, adult child, parent, sibling. However, those guidelines do not apply to all families. Sometimes the person who knows the patient best, or who is in best position to make objective decisions, is not the spouse or adult child. Sometimes there is a long-time partner who is not a spouse, either homosexual or heterosexual. Or perhaps there is a close cousin or friend. If adult children are available, it can be difficult to determine which child has final say if there is conflict among the children. In such cases, especially with serious decisions, mediation with an ethics advisory committee or other providers is helpful.

Even when there is a clear surrogate decision maker, it is often difficult for that person—with or without the support of others—to determine what is the "right thing to do" in any particular circumstance. The current standard for surrogate decision making is a "substituted judgment" standard; the surrogate attempts to make a decision as he or she thinks the person with dementia would have made it, using what is known about that person's values, beliefs, and life priorities. However, when surrogates don't have enough information to make a substituted judgment, they are to be guided by a "best interest" standard, that is, to base a decision on what would generally be considered to best serve the interests of the now incompetent person (Dresser, 1992). Determining what is in someone's best interest often entails careful and collaborative weighing of the costs and benefits of alternative solutions, with respect for the dignity of the person with dementia, as well as the health and well-being of the caregivers (Arras, 1995). Competing interests are almost inevitable and are not necessarily "bad"; that is, what is in the patient's best interest is not always in the caregiver's best interest. Caregivers are not ethically required to become physically or mentally ill providing care, nor to spend their entire life savings providing care. Open acknowledgment and respect for competing interests, as well as for the values and obligations motivating dementia caregiving, is critical for reaching ethical care decisions.

Step 5: Evaluating outcomes and reconsidering decisions over time. Many decisions in dementia caregiving are not final ones. Circumstances change over time and decisions need to be reevaluated, especially those regarding the level of supervision needed to protect the person with dementia or the types of medical interventions viewed to be in that person's best interest. For example, decisions about driving safety are certainly among the most difficult faced in early stages of dementia. While many people with mild dementia can still drive safely, all people with progressive dementia ultimately become unable to drive.

In the case example, a family meeting with Joe's doctor led to referral for further neuropsychological testing and a driving evaluation. Recommendations were that Joe could drive locally, preferably with a companion to serve as a memory aide when needed, but that he should avoid longer trips to unfamiliar areas. Their son Robert agreed that he and his sister, who lived an hour's drive away, would take more responsibility for driving their parents to visit other family members in the state. Further, it was made clear by the neuropsychologist and driving evaluator that Joe's ability to drive safely would decline and that he would eventually lose that privilege. It was acknowledged that Joe might not be a reliable judge of his driving safety and that the family would have to monitor this carefully. Joe was not happy with the challenge to his driving ability, but felt included and respected in planning how to proceed. This family will have to evaluate and reevaluate the decision to allow Joe to continue local driving, and it may or may not face a difficult confrontation with Joe when he is no longer safe in operating a vehicle.

TOOLS AND RESOURCES TO AID
ETHICAL DEMENTIA CAREGIVING
The Purpose of Tools

Most of the legal and clinical tools described here were developed to help protect and/or promote the self-determination of people with decisional incapacity, or to protect the interests of a person who may be at risk of neglect, abuse, or exploitation. Several tools are intended for use by competent individuals in planning for potential future incapacity, that is for use in advance care planning. Other tools are legal mechanisms to assure protection of the person or assets of someone who can no longer care for him- or herself.

Tools for Advance Care Planning

Advance directives are legal documents that allow a competent adult to document preferences for future medical decision making in the event of future incapacity to make decisions for oneself. With the durable power of attorney for health care, sometimes known as the health care proxy, an adult designates another person to make surrogate decisions during a time of future incapacity. Usually an alternative surrogate is also named, in case the first one is not available or able to take on the responsibility. The transfer of decision-making authority to the surrogate occurs only when the adult has been determined by the health care provider(s) to be incapable of making decisions. Many individuals with dementia do remain able to designate a health care proxy (Mezey et al., 2000).

Instructional directives, such as the living will, allow an adult to specify particular wishes for types of medical intervention desired or not desired at some point in the future. Living wills often entail endorsement of a general statement such as the following used in the Veterans Health Administration's living will form: "If I should have an incurable or irreversible condition that will cause my death, or am in a state of permanent unconsciousness from which, to a reasonable degree of medical certainty there can be no recovery, it is my desire that my life not be artificially prolonged by administration of 'life-sustaining' procedures. If, at that time, I am unable to participate in decisions regarding my medical treatment, I direct my physician to withhold or withdraw procedures that merely prolong the dying process and are not necessary to my comfort or freedom from pain." Patients can then indicate any additional, particular preferences or other instructions. Sometimes living will documents can be quite specific, with forms available to indicate which of several interventions one would prefer in various states of future health (e.g., coma, dementia) (Emanuel and Emanuel, 1989).

Advance directives, particularly designation of a health care proxy, can be particularly important when the person's preferred decision maker is not the obvious next of kin (e.g., a cousin rather than one's spouse, a lesbian partner rather than one's brother). However, advance directive documents alone have many limitations and are useful only to the extent that they are known to exist and can be accessed at a time of need and, more importantly, provide an opportunity for communication among patients and their families before the time of a crisis (Covinsky et al., 2000; Miles, Koepp, and Weber, 1996; Moody, 1992). Instructional directives alone are often difficult to interpret and apply to particular clinical situations (Hoffman, Zimmerman, and Tompkins, 1996). The following are effective tools used in advance care planning.

1. *Values Histories.* While not legally binding documents, there are increasing numbers of "values history" tools that allow individuals to clarify, document, and communicate the basic values and beliefs they hold that might influence future care decisions (Karel, 2000). For example, individuals can be encouraged to think through their own conceptions of quality of life and consider at what point they might feel life is no longer worth living, to specify religious or cultural beliefs bearing on care decisions, or to indicate the extent to which they wish their own interests and the interests of their family to be considered when care decisions are made. Values history tools include patient workbooks on various aspects of values and medical decision making (Pearlman et al., 1998), interviews intended for providers and/or families to review with patients (Gibson, 1990; Hammes and Rooney, 1998; Karel, Powell, and Cantor, 2004), or forms to accompany advance directive completion (Doukas and McCullough, 1991). Individuals in early-stage dementia can often contribute quite meaningfully to discussions about their values and preferences (Moye et al., 2004).

2. *Advance Proxy Plans.* Some long-term care settings advocate the use of advance proxy planning, in which families and the care team communicate to define the goals of care for the person with dementia, particularly when that person did not leave prior instructional directives (Veterans Health Administration, 2001; Cantor and Pearlman, 2003; Hurley, Bottino, and Volicer, 1994). Certainly, if the patient is still able to participate in defining his or her goals for care, he or she is included in the discussion (Gillick, Berkman, and Cullen, 1999). For example, according to

Gillick et al.'s model, residents and family members are asked to rank three major goals of care—life prolongation, maintenance of physical and cognitive function, and maximization of comfort; the relative rankings of these goals are then translated to define pathways, or levels of care, to guide particular decisions about whether or not to perform diagnostic tests, provide certain treatments, or transfer the patient to a hospital.

3. Durable Power of Attorney. A power of attorney allows a capable adult to give another adult the authority to manage one's property, whereas a durable power of attorney allows another adult to maintain that authority through times of incapacity. A person with early dementia may assign a durable power of attorney to assure that, at the time of future incapacity, assets are managed by a trusted person. Whereas the durable power of attorney is intended to grant authority over the management of financial affairs, the durable power of attorney for health care grants such authority over medical care decisions only.

4. Will (Last Will and Testament). Many adults choose to complete a will that instructs their survivors on how to manage or distribute their estate after their death. Again, individuals with early dementia can protect their own wishes by making a will while they are still capable of doing so.

5. Caregiver's Plans. When the individual with dementia is being helped to plan ahead for future incapacity, the caregiver should also be advised to consider these issues. In addition to protecting their own self-determination in case of future incapacity, caregivers may also wish to make plans in case they are no longer able to provide care for the person with dementia (Mace and Rabins, 1999).

Tools for Protecting the Incompetent Adult

1. Conservatorship. Conservatorship is a legal mechanism established by a court after a hearing that empowers one party to make financial decisions for another (e.g., management of assets, businesses, making contracts, making wills, making gifts). Note that in some states the term *conservatorship* denotes all types of guardianship.

2. Guardianship. Guardianship is a legal mechanism established by a court after a hearing that empowers one party to make financial (see "conservatorship") and/or personal decisions (e.g., regarding a wide range of issues—health care, where to live, where to travel, business arrangements, lawsuits) for another individual. Increasingly, courts are crafting limited guardianships that specifically limit the powers of the guardian in regard to specific decisions. This limiting is in response to evolving understanding that competence is not an all-or-none matter, but that capacities often vary across different domains.

3. Alternatives to Guardianship. As guardianship is a fairly extreme measure used to protect persons unable to make their own decisions, with significant loss of legal rights to the individual, any services or mechanisms that help that individual to function while preserving legal rights to self-determination are important resources. For individuals who are not at risk of serious harm to themselves or others, nor vulnerable to significant exploitation, services to assist with in-home care (e.g., nursing, home health aid, case management, homemaking, provision of meals) or mechanisms to provide decisional assistance (e.g., health care proxy, durable power of attorney, trusts/trustee, representative payee) should be explored before guardianship proceedings.

Processes/Programs for Working through Conflicts

1. Health Care Teams. In the health care setting, interdisciplinary geriatric health care teams are often very helpful resources for helping families consider difficult medical treatment decisions. Depending on the setting (hospital, nursing home, rehabilitation facility, clinic), the health care team may include physicians, nurses, social workers, nutritionists, pharmacists, psychologists, physical therapists, and others. While a particular family member may be the designated surrogate needing to make difficult decisions (e.g., whether or not to pursue tube feeding), the health care team should provide a collaborative and supportive role in helping families to clarify goals for the patient's care, to understand the risks and benefits of various treatment options, and to make recommendations when appropriate. Often, clarification of information can help to resolve conflicts that stem from misunderstandings or unrealistic expectations (Mezey et al., 2002).

2. Ethics Committees. Many health care organizations now have ethics advisory committees that provide consultation to clinical teams, families, or the organization about resolving ethical dilemmas (Aulisio et al., 2000). Most ethics committees comprise health care professionals representing a range of disciplines and views and providing administrative, legal, and consumer perspectives. When there is conflict among a health care team, between the health care team and the patient and/or patient's family, or between various members of the patient's family, the ethics advisory committee can help to clarify questions of decision-making authority, frame issues in terms of conflicting values, and provide a structure to facilitate consensus guided by ethical principles.

3. Adult Protective Services. State offices on aging must include adult protective service functions. Suspicions of abuse or neglect of an elderly individual can be reported and investigated by adult protective services; in fact, most health and social service professionals are required by state law to report suspected elder abuse (physical, emotional, or financial) or neglect. Individuals with dementia are particularly vulnerable to abuse and neglect. When families are not protecting the health, safety, or financial interests of the person, either because of insufficient resources or through frank criminal intent (e.g., stealing money), then it becomes the responsibility of the community—through the powers of the state—to protect that individual. Frequently, families are offered additional supports in helping their loved ones, or if that is not feasible, other arrangements for supervised or institutional care can be made. Detailed information about senior services and links to local program information can be found on the Administration on Aging web site at www.aoa.gov. Further information about elder abuse and neglect can be found on the web site of the National Center on Elder Abuse, www.elderabusecenter.org.

4. *Ombudsman Programs.* In the United States, the Long-Term Care Ombudsman Program, mandated by the Older Americans Act and managed in each of the states, provides a system to "identify, investigate, and work to resolve complaints initiated by, or on behalf of, residents in nursing homes, board- and care-homes, or similar adult care facilities" (Huber et al., 2001, p. 264; Nelson, Huber, and Walter, 1995). Families who are concerned about an older adult's care in any of these institutional settings can bring complaints to the local ombudsman, usually a volunteer who has received training. Information about the Long-Term Care Ombudsman Program can be found on the Administration on Aging web site at www.aoa.gov.

5. *Guardian ad litem.* A guardian ad litem is a person, often an attorney, appointed by the court to represent the best interests of an incapacitated person. Often, the guardian ad litem investigates the circumstances surrounding a request for guardianship and makes recommendations to the court.

6. *Courts.* In most states, guardianship hearings are held in a probate court. In general, courts should be used as the last option for negotiating difficult family ethical conflicts.

CONCLUSION

Family caregivers for persons with dementia face many potential ethical dilemmas, which include defining the extent of their caregiving obligation, balancing concerns for autonomy versus safety of the person with dementia, and making end-of-life care decisions for someone no longer able to communicate his or her preferences. A process of values clarification and collaborative decision making, in which respectful attention to the interests of the person with dementia and those of the family and community, can help family caregivers to determine a range of potential solutions to caregiving dilemmas. By their very nature, ethical dilemmas rarely have one "right answer," and the values of the particular patient, family system, and cultural group will help to define a range of acceptable solutions. Tools to aid advance care planning, involving an ongoing process of communication about goals and preferences for long-term and medical care decisions, can help families to face difficult decisions with greater clarity. When families, or other involved individuals, are not able to make decisions in the best interest of a person with dementia, legal mechanisms exist to help protect that person's health, safety, and financial interests.

REFERENCES

Arras, J. D. 1995. Conflicting interests in long-term care decision making: Acknowledging, dissolving, and resolving conflicts. In L. B. McCullough and N. L. Wilson (Eds.), *Long-term care decisions: Ethical and conceptual dimensions* (pp. 197–217). Baltimore: Johns Hopkins University Press.

Aulisio, M. P., Arnold, R. M., Youngner, S. J., et al. 2000. Health care ethics consultation: Nature, goals, and competencies. *Annals of Internal Medicine* 133:59–69.

Baldwin, C., Hughes, J., Hope, T., Jacoby, R., and Ziebland, S. 2003. Ethics and dementia: Mapping the literature by bibliometric analysis. *International Journal of Geriatric Psychiatry* 18:41–54.

Barber, C. E., and Lyness, K. P. 2001. Ethical issues in family care of older persons with dementia: Implications for family therapists. *Home Health Care Services Quarterly* 20:1–26.

Bassett, S. S., Havstad, S. L., and Chase, G. A. 2004. The role of test accuracy in predicting acceptance of genetic susceptibility testing for Alzheimer's disease. *Genetic Testing* 8:120–26.

Beauchamp, T. L., and Childress, J. F. 2001. *Principles of biomedical ethics* (5th ed.). Oxford: Oxford University Press.

Berger, J. T., and Rosner, F. 2000. Ethical challenges posed by dementia and driving. *Journal of Clinical Ethics* 11:304–8.

Blackhall, L. J., Murphy, S. T., Frank, G., Michel, V., and Azen, S. 1995. Ethnicity and attitudes toward patient autonomy. *Journal of the American Medical Association* 274:820–25.

Brackman, S. V. 1995. Filial responsibility and long-term care decision making. In L. B. McCullough and N. L. Wilson (Eds.), *Long-term care decisions: Ethical and conceptual dimensions* (pp. 181–96). Baltimore: Johns Hopkins University Press.

Cantor, M. D., and Pearlman, R. A. 2003. Advance care planning in long-term care facilities. *Journal of the American Medical Directors Association* 4:101–8.

Coon, D.W., Davies, H., McKibben, C., and Gallagher-Thompson, D. 1999. The psychological impact of genetic testing for Alzheimer disease. *Genetic Testing* 3:121–31.

Covinsky, K. E., Fuller, J. D., Yaffe, K., Johnston, C. B., Hamel, M. B., Lynn, J., Teno, J. M., and Phillips, R. S. 2000. Communication and decision-making in seriously ill patients: Findings of the SUPPORT project. *Journal of the American Geriatrics Society* 48:S187–93.

Dai, Y., and Dimond, M. F. 1998. Filial piety: A cross-cultural comparison and its implications for the well-being of older parents. *Journal of Gerontological Nursing* 24:13–18.

Davis, J. K. 2002. The concept of precedent autonomy. *Bioethics* 16:114–33.

Degrazia, D. 1999. Advance directives, dementia, and "the someone else problem." *Bioethics* 13:373–91.

Dilworth-Anderson, P., and Gibson, B. E. 2002. The cultural influence of values, norms, meanings, and perceptions in understanding dementia in ethnic minorities. *Alzheimer Disease and Associated Disorders* 16:S56–63.

Dilworth-Anderson, P., Williams, I. C., and Gibson, B. E. 2002. Issues of race, ethnicity, and culture in caregiving research: A twenty-year review (1980–2000). *Gerontologist* 42:237–72.

Doolittle, N. O., and Herrick, C. A. 1992. Ethics in aging: A decision-making paradigm. *Educational Gerontology* 18:395–408.

Doukas, D. J., and McCullough, L. B. 1991. The values history: The evaluation of the patient's values and advance directives. *Journal of Family Practice* 32:145–53.

Dresser, R. S. 1992. Autonomy revisited: The limits of anticipatory choice. In R. H. Binstock, S. G. Post, and P. J. Whitehouse (Eds.), *Dementia and aging: Ethics, values, and policy choices* (pp. 71–85). Baltimore: Johns Hopkins University Press.

Dunn, L. B., and Jeste, D. V. 2001. Enhancing informed consent for research and treatment. *Neuropsychopharmacology* 24:595–607.

Eaton, M. L. 1999. Surrogate decision making for genetic testing for Alzheimer disease. *Genetic Testing* 3:93–97.

Emanuel, L. L., and Emanuel, E. J. 1989. The medical directive: A new comprehensive advance care document. *Journal of the American Medical Association* 261:3288–93.

Ersek, M., Kagawa-Singer, M., Barnes, D., Blackhall, L., and Koenig, B. A. 1998. Multicultural considerations in the use of advance directives. *Oncology Nursing Forum* 25:1683–90.

Forbes, S., Bern-Klug, M., and Gessert, C. 2000. End-of-life decision making for nursing home residents with dementia. *Journal of Nursing Scholarship* 32:251–58.

Gibson, J. M. 1990. National values history project. *Generations* 14(suppl.):51–64.

Gillick, M., Berkman, S., and Cullen, L. 1999. A patient-centered approach to advance medical planning in the nursing home. *Journal of the American Geriatrics Society* 47:227–30.

Guberman, N., Maheu, P., and Maille, C. 1992. Women as family caregivers: Why do they care? *Gerontologist* 32:607–17.

Hammes, B. J., and Rooney, B. L. 1998. Death and end-of-life planning in one midwestern community. *Archives of Internal Medicine* 158:383–90.

Hare, J., Pratt, C., and Nelson, C. 1992. Agreement between patients and their self-selected surrogates on difficult medical decisions. *Archives of Internal Medicine* 52:1049–54.

High, D. M. 1988. All in the family: Extended autonomy and expectations in surrogate health care decision-making. *Gerontologist* 28:46–51.

Hoffman, D. E., Zimmerman, S. I., and Tompkins, C. J. 1996. The dangers of directives or the false security of forms. *Journal of Law, Medicine, and Ethics* 24:5–17.

Hornung, C. A., Eleazer, G. P., Strongers, H. S., Wieland, G. D., Eng, C., McCann, R., and Sapir, M. 1998. Ethnicity and decision-makers in a group of frail older people. *Journal of the American Geriatrics Society* 46:280–86.

Huber, R., Borders, K. W., Badrak, K., Netting, F. E., and Nelson, H. W. 2001. National standards for the Long-Term Care Ombudsman Program and a tool to assess compliance: The Huber Badrak Borders scales. *Gerontologist* 41:264–71.

Hurley, A. C., Bottino, R., and Volicer, L. 1994. Nursing role in advance proxy planning for Alzheimer patients. *Caring* 13:72–76.

Jecker, N. S. 1995. What do husbands and wives owe each other in old age? In L. B. McCullough and N. L. Wilson (Eds.), *Long-term care decisions: Ethical and conceptual dimensions* (pp. 155–80). Baltimore: Johns Hopkins University Press.

Kane, R. A. 2001. Long-term care and a good quality of life: Bringing them closer together. *Gerontologist* 41:293–304.

Karel, M. J. 2000. The assessment of values in medical decision making. *Journal of Aging Studies* 14:403–22.

Karel, M. J., Powell, J., and Cantor, M. D. 2004. Using a Values Discussion Guide to facilitate communication in advance care planning. *Patient Education and Counseling* 55:22–31.

Karlawish, J., Casarett, D., Klocinski, J., and Sankar, P. 2001. How do AD patients and their caregivers decide whether to enroll in a clinical trial? *Neurology* 56:789–92.

Karlawish, J. H. T., Casarett, D., Propert, K. J., James, B. D., and Clark, C. M. 2002. Relationship between Alzheimer's disease severity and patient participation in decisions about their medical care. *Journal of Geriatric Psychiatry and Neurology* 15:68–72.

Karlawish, J. H. T., Quill, T., and Meier, D. E. 1999. A consensus-based approach to providing palliative care to patients who lack decision-making capacity. *Annals of Internal Medicine* 130:835–40.

Kim, S. Y. H., and Caine, E. D. 2002. Utility and limits of the mini mental state examination in evaluating consent capacity in Alzheimer's disease. *Psychiatric Services* 53:1322–24.

Kim, S. Y. H., Cox, C., and Caine, E. D. 2002. Impaired decision-making ability in subjects with Alzheimer's disease and willingness to participate in research. *American Journal of Psychiatry* 159:797–802.

Koppelman, E. R. 2002. Dementia and dignity: Towards a new method of surrogate decision making. *Journal of Medicine and Philosophy* 27:65–85.

Lane, A., and Dubler, N. N. 1997. The health care agent: Selected but neglected. *Bioethics Forum* 13:17–21.

Mace, N. L., and Rabins, P. V. 1999. *The 36-hour day: A family guide to caring for persons with Alzheimer disease, related dementing illnesses, and memory loss in later life* (3rd ed.). Baltimore: Johns Hopkins University Press.

Marson, D. C., Chatterjee, A., Ingram, K. K., and Harrell, L. E. 1996. Cognitive predictors of capacity to consent in Alzheimer's disease using three different legal standards. *Neurology* 46:666–72.

Marson, D. C., McInturff, B., Hawkins, L., Bartolucci, A., and Harrell, L. E. 1997. Consistency of physician judgments of capacity to consent in mild Alzheimer's disease. *Journal of the American Geriatrics Society* 45:453–57.

Martin, R. J., and Post, S. G. 1992. Human dignity, dementia, and the moral basis of caregiving. In R. H. Binstock, S. G. Post, and P. J. Whitehouse (Eds.), *Dementia and aging: Ethics, values, and policy choices* (pp. 55–68). Baltimore: Johns Hopkins University Press.

Meuser, T. M., and Marwit, S. J. 2001. A comprehensive, stage-sensitive model of grief in dementia caregiving. *Gerontologist* 41:658–70.

Mezey, M. D., Cassel, C. K., Bottrell, M. M., Hyer, K., Howe, J. L., and Fulmer, T. T. (Eds.). 2002. *Ethical patient care: A case book for geriatric health care teams.* Baltimore: Johns Hopkins University Press.

Mezey, M., Kluger, M., Maislin, G., and Mittelman, M. 1996. Life-sustaining treatment decisions by spouses of patients with Alzheimer's disease. *Journal of the American Geriatrics Society* 44:144–50.

Mezey, M., Teresi, J., Ramsey, G., Mitty, E., and Bobrowitz, T. 2000. Decision-making capacity to execute a health care proxy: Development and testing of guidelines. *Journal of the American Geriatrics Society* 48:179–87.

Miles, S. H., Koepp, R., and Weber, E. P. 1996. Advance end-of-life treatment planning: A research review. *Archives of Internal Medicine* 156:1062–68.

Moody, H. R. 1992. *Ethics in an aging society*. Baltimore: Johns Hopkins University Press.

Motenko, A. K. 1989. The frustrations, gratifications, and well-being of dementia caregivers. *Gerontologist* 29:166–72.

Moye, J. 1999. Assessment of competency and decision making capacity. In P. Lichtenberg (Ed.), *Handbook of geriatric assessment* (pp. 488–528). New York: Wiley.

Moye, J. 2003. Guardianship and conservatorship. In T. Grisso (Ed.), *Evaluating competencies: Forensic assessments and instruments* (2nd ed.) (pp. 309–90). New York: Plenum Pub Corp.

Moye, J., Karel, M. J., Azar, A., and Gurrera, R. 2004. Capacity to consent to treatment: Empirical comparison of three instruments in older adults with and without dementia. *Gerontologist* 44:166–75.

Nelson, H. W., Huber, R., and Walter, K. L. 1995. The relationship between volunteer long-term care ombudsmen and regulatory nursing home actions. *Gerontologist* 35:509–14.

Newton, M. J. 1999. Precedent autonomy: Life-sustaining intervention and the demented patient. *Cambridge Quarterly of Healthcare Ethics* 8:189–99.

Pearlman, R., Starks, H., Cain, K., Rosengreen, D., and Patrick, D. 1998. *Your life, your choices: Planning for future medical decisions: How to prepare a personalized living will* (PB#98159437). Springfield, Va.: U.S. Department of Commerce, National Technical Information Service.

Peterson, R. C. 2004. Mild cognitive impairment as a diagnostic entity. *Journal of Internal Medicine* 256:183–94.

Post, S. G., and Whitehouse, P. J. 1995. Fairhill guidelines on ethics of the care of people with Alzheimer's disease: A clinical summary. *Journal of the American Geriatrics Society* 43:1423–29.

Powers, B. A. 2000. Everyday ethics of dementia care in nursing homes: A definition and taxonomy. *American Journal of Alzheimer's Disease* 15:143–51.

Pratt, C., Schmall, V., and Wright, S. 1987. Ethical concerns of family caregivers to dementia patients. *Gerontologist* 27:632–38.

Puchalski, C. M., Zhong, Z., Jacobs, M. M., Fox, E., Lynn, J., Harrold, J., Galanos, A., Phillips, R. S., Califf, R., and Teno, J. M. 2000. Patients who want their family and physician to make resuscitation decisions for them: Observations from SUPPORT and HELP. *Journal of the American Geriatrics Society* 48:S84–90.

Qualls, S. H. 1999. Realizing power in intergenerational family hierarchies: Family reorganization when older adults decline. In M. Duffy (Ed.), *Handbook of counseling and psychotherapy with older adults* (pp. 228–41). New York: Wiley.

Rosenfeld, K. E., Wenger, N. S., and Kagawa-Singer, M. 2000. End-of-life decision making: A qualitative study of elderly individuals. *Journal of General Internal Medicine* 15:620–25.

Sachs, G. A., Shega, J. W., and Cox-Hayley, D. 2004. Barriers to excellent end-of-life care for patients with dementia. *Journal of General Internal Medicine* 19:1057–63.

Seckler, A. B., Meier, D. E., Mulvihill, M., and Cammer Paris, B. E. 1991. Substituted judgment: How accurate are proxy decisions? *Annals of Internal Medicine* 115:92–98.

Selig, S., Tomlinson, T., and Hickey, T. 1991. Ethical dimensions of intergenerational reciprocity: Implications for practice. *Gerontologist* 31:624–30.

Stoller, E. P., and Pugliesi, K. L. 1989. Other roles of caregivers: Competing responsibilities or supportive resources. *Journal of Gerontology* 44:S231–38.

Suhl, J., Simons, P., Reedy, T., and Garrick, T. 1994. Myth of substituted judgment: Surrogate decision making regarding life support is unreliable. *Archives of Internal Medicine* 154:90–96.

Sullivan, M. D. 2002. The illusion of patient choice in end-of-life decisions. *American Journal of Geriatric Psychiatry* 10:365–72.

Veterans Health Administration, National Ethics Committee. 2001. *Advance proxy planning for residents of long-term care facilities who lack decision-making capacity* (VHA Information Letter IL 10-2001-007). Washington, D.C.: Veterans Health Administration.

Volicer, L. 2001. Management of severe Alzheimer's disease and end-of-life issues. *Clinics in Geriatric Medicine* 17:377–91.

Wallston, K. A., and Wallston, B. S. 1978. Development of the Multidimensional Health Locus of Control (MHLC) scales. *Health Education Monographs* 6:160–70.

Winblad, B., Palmer, K., Kivipelto, M., et al. 2004. Mild cognitive impairment: Beyond controversies, towards a consensus: Report of the International Working Group on Mild Cognitive Impairment. *Journal of Internal Medicine* 256:240–46.

Yeo, G., and Gallagher-Thompson, D. (Eds.). 1996. *Ethnicity and the dementias*. Washington, D.C.: Taylor & Francis.

Youn, G., Knight, B. G., Jeong, H., et al. 1999. Differences in familism values and caregiving outcomes among Korean, Korean American, and white American caregivers. *Psychology and Aging* 14:355–64.

Index

Page numbers followed by *f* indicate figures; page numbers followed by *t* indicate tables.